Forensic Science and Quality Management

Published and Forthcoming Titles in the Forensic Science in Focus Series

Published

The Global Practice of Forensic Science
Douglas H. Ubelaker (Editor)

Forensic Chemistry: Fundamentals and Applications
Jay A. Siegel (Editor)

Forensic Microbiology
David O. Carter, Jeffrey K. Tomberlin, M. Eric Benbow, and Jessica L. Metcalf (Editors)

Forensic Anthropology: Theoretical Framework and Scientific Basis
Clifford Boyd and Donna Boyd (Editors)

The Future of Forensic Science
Daniel A. Martell (Editor)

Forensic Anthropology and the United States Judicial System
Laura C. Fulginiti, Kristen Hartnett-McCann, and Alison Galloway (Editors)

Forensic Science and Humanitarian Action: Interacting with the Dead and the Living
Roberto C. Parra, Sara C. Zapico, and Douglas H. Ubelaker (Editors)

Disaster Victim Identification in the United States in the 21st Century: An Evolving Discipline
John A. Williams and Victor W. Weedn (Editors)

Anthropology of Violent Death: Theoretical Foundations for Forensic Humanitarian Action
Roberto C. Parra and Douglas H. Ubelaker (Editors)

Burnt Human Remains: Recovery, Analysis and Interpretation
Sarah Ellingham, Joe Adserias-Garriga, Sara C. Zapico, and Douglas H. Ubelaker (Editors)

Artificial Intelligence (AI) in Forensic Sciences
Katrin Franke and Zeno Geradts (Editors)

Forensic Science and Quality Management: Addressing the Era of Standardization in Challenging Environments
Roberto C. Parra and Allan G. Alvarez-Godoy (Editors)

Forthcoming

Forensic Skeletal Trauma: Scientific Foundation and Guide to Professional Practice
Donna C. Boyd

Forensic Science and Quality Management

Addressing the Era of Standardization in Challenging Environments

EDITED BY

Roberto C. Parra

The Specialized Forensic Team of the United Nations Joint Human Rights Office (UNJHRO) in the Democratic Republic of the Congo

Allan G. Alvarez-Godoy

International Forensic Consultant, The Hague, Netherlands

AAFS AMERICAN ACADEMY OF FORENSIC SCIENCES

WILEY

Registered Offices
John Wiley & Sons, Inc., 111 River Street, Hoboken, NJ 07030, USA
John Wiley & Sons Ltd, New Era House, 8 Oldlands Way, Bognor Regis, West Sussex, PO22 9NQ, UK

For details of our global editorial offices, customer services, and more information about Wiley products visit us at www.wiley.com.

The manufacturer's authorized representative according to the EU General Product Safety Regulation is Wiley-VCH GmbH, Boschstr. 12, 69469 Weinheim, Germany, e-mail: Product_Safety@wiley.com.

Wiley also publishes its books in a variety of electronic formats and by print-on-demand. Some content that appears in standard print versions of this book may not be available in other formats.

Library of Congress Cataloging-in-Publication Data:
Names: Parra, Roberto C. editor | Alvarez-Godoy, Allan G. editor
Title: Forensic science and quality management : addressing the era of standardization in challenging environments / edited by Roberto C. Parra and Allan G. Alvarez-Godoy.
Description: Hoboken, NJ : Wiley, 2026. | Collection of essays by Pierre Perich and others. | Includes bibliographical references and index.
Identifiers: LCCN 2025047379 (print) | LCCN 2025047380 (ebook) | ISBN 9781394240371 hardback | ISBN 9781394240395 epdf | ISBN 9781394240388 epub
Subjects: LCSH: Forensic sciences–Standards | Human rights
Classification: LCC HV8073 .F58357 2026 (print) | LCC HV8073 (ebook)
LC record available at https://lccn.loc.gov/2025047379
LC ebook record available at https://lccn.loc.gov/2025047380

Cover Design: Wiley
Cover Image: Courtesy of Roberto C. Parra

Set in 10.5/13.5pt Meridien LT Std Roman by Straive, Chennai, India

Contents

About the Editors

Roberto C. Parra

Roberto is a Peruvian anthropologist with over 25 years of experience in forensic science, human rights investigations, and humanitarian action in contexts of mass violence, war crimes, disasters, and migration crises. Since 2002, he has worked in highly complex operational environments across Africa, the Middle East, and Latin America, combining scientific rigor with a deep understanding of social and cultural dynamics in conflict and post-conflict settings. His professional expertise lies in the strategic development, implementation, and oversight of forensic systems and quality management frameworks, focusing on strengthening institutions, ensuring operational integrity, and promoting sustainable forensic practices. Roberto has led the design of forensic strategies, action plans, and organizational structures for high-impact operations, integrating international standards such as ISO/IEC 17025, ISO 9001, ISO 14001, and ISO 45001 into forensic workflows. Roberto has served as a member of the International Committee of the Red Cross (ICRC) Forensic Unit, as a senior advisor to the Peruvian Institute of Legal Medicine and Forensic Sciences, and since 2018 as part of the specialized forensic team of the United Nations Joint Human Rights Office (UNJHRO) in the Democratic Republic of the Congo. His work bridges forensic science, institutional governance, and quality management, contributing to accountability, justice processes, and the defense of human dignity through scientifically robust and ethically grounded forensic operations.

Allan G. Alvarez-Godoy

Allan is a forensic medical practitioner with over 17 years of experience in complex field environments. He presently conducts medico-legal evaluations in investigations of crimes against humanity, converting clinical and forensic results into coherent, substantiated evidence. He previously contributed to United Nations efforts in conflict-affected areas, assisting in investigations into war crimes and significant human rights violations. In Mexico and Central America, he collaborated with the International Committee of the Red Cross on issues pertaining to missing persons, mass-fatality incidents, migration-related fatalities, and urban violence. His experience encompasses the medico-legal recording of torture and ill-treatment, sexual and gender-based violence (SGBV/GBV), and crimes against children (CAC), consistently employing a victim-sensitive, evidence-based methodology. Allan has dedicated his career in promoting forensic methodologies that are both legally robust and practically applicable in the field. He trains investigators, physicians, and legal professionals to apply international standards in resource-limited settings, and he incorporates technology and data platforms to enhance forensic analysis, traceability, and decision-making. His endeavors are driven by a dedication to veracity, responsibility, and human decency.

List of Contributors

Denise Abboud
International Committee of the Red Cross (ICRC), Geneva, Switzerland

Omer O. Adjibode
The Specialized Forensic Team of the United Nations Joint Human Rights Office (UNJHRO) in the Democratic Republic of the Congo

Allan G. Alvarez-Godoy
International Forensic Consultant
The Hague, Netherlands

Eva Bruenisholz
Forensics Command, Australian Federal Police, Canberra, Australia

Daniel Castellanos
University of Antioquia, Medellin
Colombia

Bérarė Doudoulgou
Forensic Physician at the University Hospital Center (CHU) of Bogodogo
Ouagadougou, Burkina Faso

Ruth Garcia-Marroquin
Forensic Science Laboratories
INACIF-Guatemala
Guatemala City, Guatemala

Pierre Guyomarc'h
International Committee of the Red Cross (ICRC)
Geneva, Switzerland

Marleny Huerta-Valdivia
Institute of Legal Medicine and Forensic Sciences of Peru
Lima, Peru

Gian Carlo Iannacone
Institute of Legal Medicine and Forensic Sciences of Peru
Lima, Peru

Sami El Jundi
International Forensic Consultant
Coimbra, Portugal

Ratouissamda Kagambega
Forensic Physician at the University Hospital Center (CHU) of Bogodogo
Ouagadougou, Burkina Faso

José Vicente Pachar Lucio
Institute of Legal Medicine and Forensic Sciences of Panama, Panama

Vincent Mazraani
International consultant with the International Committee of the Red Cross (ICRC)
Geneva, Switzerland

John Mbewu-Bodji
Center of Forensic Medicine and Criminalistics of Kananga
DR Congo

Maria Dolores Morcillo Mendez
International Committee of the Red Cross (ICRC)
Geneva, Switzerland

Roberto C. Parra
The Specialized Forensic Team of the United Nations Joint Human Rights Office (UNJHRO) in the Democratic Republic of the Congo

Pierre Perich
International Forensic Consultant
Marseille, France

Michael Pollanen
Ontario Forensic Pathology Service
Ontario, Canada

Norbert W. Ramde
Forensic Physician at the University Hospital Center (CHU) of Bogodogo
Ouagadougou, Burkina Faso

Claude Roux
Centre for Forensic Science
University of Technology Sydney
Sydney, Australia

Rafael De Abreu E Souza
International Committee of the Red Cross (ICRC)
Geneva, Switzerland

Jane Taylor
International Committee of the Red Cross (ICRC)
Geneva, Switzerland

Daouda Traore
The Specialized Forensic Team of the United Nations Joint Human Rights Office (UNJHRO) in the Democratic Republic of the Congo

Jorge L. Vasquez-Guerrero
Institute of Legal Medicine and Forensic Sciences of Peru
Lima, Peru

Preface

The pursuit of excellence in forensic practice is a noble endeavor, all the more difficult in contexts affected by armed conflict, institutional breakdown, and erosion of the rule of law, like many in today's world, where forensic practitioners face a range of daily challenges to carry out their work, including scarcity of basic resources and dire security constraints.

This is a book that gives a voice to those working, often heroically, in such contexts: to learn from them about their remarkable experiences and lessons learned in carrying out ethically sound, scientifically robust, and reliable forensic case work in the face of apparently insurmountable challenges.

As importantly, we learn from them how existing international standards of forensic best practice, such as the *United Nations Revised Manual on the Effective Prevention and Investigation of Extra-legal, Arbitrary and Summary Executions,* better known as the *Minnesota Protocol on the Investigation of Potentially Unlawful Death,* can guide and assist forensic practitioners confronted with challenges described in this book to ensure that their investigations meet the requirement of international law.

The present book is also an inspiring reminder for all forensic practitioners of the unique value and growing contribution of forensic science for the protection of human rights and human dignity.

Dr. Morris Tidball-Binz
United Nations Special Rapporteur on extrajudicial, summary, or arbitrary executions; Adjunct Clinical Professor in Forensic Medicine, Monash University; Visiting Senior Research Associate, Pozen Center for Human Rights, University of Chicago; Visiting Professor, University of Coimbra and Visiting Professor, University of Milan.

Series Preface

The forensic sciences represent diverse, dynamic fields that seek to utilize the very best techniques available to address legal issues. Fueled by advances in technology, research, and methodology, as well as new case applications, the forensic sciences continue to evolve. Forensic scientists strive to improve their analyses and interpretations of evidence and to remain cognizant of the latest advancements. This series results from a collaborative effort between the American Academy of Forensic Sciences (AAFS) and Wiley to publish a select number of books that relate closely to the activities and objectives of the AAFS. The book series reflects the goals of the AAFS to encourage quality scholarship and publication in the forensic sciences. Proposals for publication in the series are reviewed by a committee established for that purpose by the AAFS and also reviewed by Wiley. The AAFS was founded in 1948 and represents a multidisciplinary professional organization that provides leadership to advance science and its application to the legal system. The 11 sections of the AAFS consist of Criminalistics, Digital and Multimedia Sciences, Engineering Sciences, General, Pathology/Biology, Questioned Documents, Jurisprudence, Anthropology, Toxicology, Odontology, and Psychiatry and Behavioral Science. There are over 7000 members of the AAFS, originating from all 50 states of the United States and many countries beyond. This series reflects global AAFS membership interest in new research, scholarship, and publication in the forensic sciences.

Zeno Geradts
Senior forensic scientist
Netherlands Forensic Institute
of the Ministry of Justice
Netherlands
Series Editor

Acknowledgments

Sincere thanks are extended by the editors and authors to the anonymous reviewers of each of the chapters in this volume, whose critical insights and academic rigor have greatly enhanced the work's quality and soundness.

We are also extremely appreciative of the American Academy of Forensic Sciences (AAFS), whose sponsorship was essential to making this project a reality, and Wiley for their consistent and expert assistance during the publication process.

Introduction

Roberto C. Parra[1] and Allan G. Alvarez-Godoy[2]
[1] *The Specialized Forensic Team of the United Nations Joint Human Rights Office (UNJHRO) in the Democratic Republic of the Congo*
[2] *International Forensic Consultant, The Hague, Netherlands*

Quality Management, a crucial component of contemporary forensic science, has gained a lot more attention since the last few decades of the 20th century, which has resulted in the development of globally accepted, internationally standardized practices (Pereira, 1985, Willis, 2010; Neuteboom et al., 2023; Wilson-Wilde, 2018; Doyle, 2019; Berger, 2025). However, demands for accountability, transparency, reproducibility, replicability, and overall quality assurance of findings have increased alongside this increased visibility and need for forensic science. Despite this, the global forensic science community is currently facing a broader scientific crisis, marked by issues of trust, reproducibility, and credibility. Serious concerns have been raised by high-profile cases of forensic failures, as well as the lack of consistent scientific validation across numerous procedures (Saks and Faiman, 2008; Koehler et al., 2023; Crispino et al., 2021; and many others). Crispino et al. (2021) have eloquently highlighted a explicit paradox in forensic science: on the one hand, the reports of the U.S. National Academy of Sciences (2009) and the *President's Council of Advisors on Science and Technology* (PCAST, 2016) emphasize a structural crisis in forensic science. They highlight a lack of methodological rigor, the fragmentation of the disciplines that comprise it, and the absence of clear and uniform standards. Furthermore, they underscore the weight of experts'[1] cognitive biases, insufficient impartiality, and weaknesses in quality control. All of this has led to flawed and even erroneous reports, with serious consequences such as judicial errors and wrongful convictions (Saks and Faiman, 2008; Koheler et al., 2023). This delicate situation raises the need for profound reform and an epistemological framework that provides greater coherence and legitimacy to forensic practice (Koheler et al., 2023; Crispino et al., 2021).

[1] The use of the term forensic expert can be controversial, so we use this word with caution, although it will be found throughout the text, although we prefer to use it as forensic scientist. Following Luis Fondebrider (2025), he criticizes that the term "expert" is used too freely in forensic science because it is unclear and can cause problems. According to him, people often use it without specifying what training, experience, or certifications actually support that level of expertise, which can cause confusion and lead to an exaggeration of authority. He also states that the label can be used in court or by the media to make people appear to be experts in areas in which they are not very competent. Fondebrider believes that being called an "expert" does not always mean acting with scientific rigor or moral responsibility and that using the term incorrectly hinders the pursuit of justice. See Luis Fondebrider post https://www.linkedin.com/posts/luis-fondebrider-00547b64_experts-ive-never-liked-the-word-expert-activity-7373264334862450689-N1nk/?utm_source=chatgpt.com

On the other hand, social, media, and commercial perceptions offer a completely different picture. Forensic science appears to be an effective and almost infallible field, equipped with cutting-edge technologies and capable of solving complex crimes, including cold cases. It is attributed a central role in the fight against crime, and great expectations are placed on its future thanks to artificial intelligence. The paradox lies in the fact that, while its scientific soundness is questioned in the courts, in the public sphere it is exalted as an almost magical and effective science (Crispino et al., 2021).

To ensure the validity, reliability, and relevance of forensic science in the modern world, a profound reform has been demanded (Koehler et al., 2023). A reinvention that prioritizes methodical research, exhaustive method validation, and transparency of the process is suggested as a way to reverse this situation. Establishing unequivocal standards, fostering a culture of critical evaluation, and supporting continuous development are necessary for this change. Furthermore, the importance of reproducible results and an interdisciplinary approach that combines scientific knowledge with judicial needs is emphasized. Adopting these measures would allow forensic science to respond more successfully to new methodological and technological challenges while improving its real reputation with the public and the legal system (Koheler et al., 2023; Roux et al., 2022; Ross et al., 2025). In parallel with this context of innovation and transformative development, forensic science is also moving toward technical standardization (Ballentyne and Wilson-Wilde, 2020; Wilson-Wilde, 2018; Berger, 2025). Increasing capacity ("more"), improving quality ("better"), shortening execution times ("faster"), reducing costs ("cheaper"), and strengthening the integration of all stages of the workflow ("easier and safer") seem to be the path to modern globalizing forensic science. A true machine, ideally automated, to produce results at low cost, in mass, and with technically standardized precision and constant validation between internationally constructed networks.

An international regulatory framework has been established in the field of forensic science to ensure traceability, quality, and transparency in all procedures. Under such a framework, every step, from the identification and collection of evidence to the presentation of findings in court, would be based on internationally accepted technical standards (Berger, 2025; Wilson-Wilde, 2018; Doyle, 2019). It is argued that these efforts would reduce arbitrary practices, while strengthening the reliability of findings, improving institutional credibility, and facilitating the acceptance of evidence in judicial contexts. In this situation, international standards would be considered necessary to integrate best practices in forensic management, promote continuous improvement, and harmonize procedures. These objectives would be supported by a comprehensive set of ISO standards (ISO 21043-1, ISO 21043-2, ISO 21043-3, ISO 21043-4, ISO 21043-5, ISO/IEC 14001:2015, ISO/IEC 15189:2012, ISO/IEC 17020:2012, ISO/IEC 17025:2017, ISO/IEC 9001:2015) governing terminology, evidence collection, analysis, interpretation, and reporting. Guidelines could also be implemented for quality control, environmental sustainability, inspection agency operations, and laboratory competency. Together, this regulatory framework would provide a crucial system that would strengthen confidence in forensic science as a vital field for the efficient functioning of the legal system. All of this is developed and designed from a Global North perspective, which also involves rigorous accreditation and audit procedures (Neuteboom et al., 2023; Neuteboom and Ross, 2024; Ross and Neuteboom, 2020).

The benefits of this advancement include promoting international comparability of results and strengthening institutional confidence in administrative management. However, a fundamental challenge with its rapid growth and the growing anxiety about the global standardization and automation of processes and procedures is how to ensure that these standards also consider the diversity of environments and needs, especially in situations where conditions are far from ideal, as is clearly the case in the Global South?

This is where the idea of challenging environments comes into play. These settings, which are usually found in the Global South, are distinguished by institutional instability, resource scarcity, structural limitations, enduring inequality, and frequently violent or humanitarian crisis situations. The transfer of models created for forensic environments in the Global North may not work in these challenging environments and may often even ignore the operational and social realities that impact the effectiveness of forensic science. Forensic science that pursues an industrial model, with an emphasis on technical advancement, improvement, and automation as ends in themselves, does not always capture the complexity of these heterogeneous and challenging environments nor does it ensure that forensic science achieves its primary objective: contributing to justice, and the fight against impunity.

The goal of this volume is not to fully address every facet of this discussion. Instead, it aims to create an environment that supports critical but constructive evaluation of how standardization can advance forensic science while maintaining awareness of the variety of contexts in which it works. The chapters collected here caution that accreditation alone does not provide a 100% guarantee of quality, far from casting doubt on its value. In fact, it can lead to false impressions or "mirages" that create a false sense of security among justice officials, the general public, and even the forensic community if institutional strengthening is not continued.

The authors, who have extensive experience working in demanding environments, illustrate this tension throughout the work with case studies, comparative analyses, and theoretical reflections. Examples of how quality is attained by not only meeting standards but also incorporating them into an ethical, adaptable, and contextually relevant operating framework are provided, ranging from the investigation of new tools like artificial intelligence to the contextualized adaptation of international instruments like the Minnesota Protocol. Forensic quality necessitates both technical and scientific rigor, but more importantly, ethical and social sensitivity, as evidenced by cases like deaths in custody in the African region of Burkina Faso, the forensic humanitarian efforts of the International Committee of the Red Cross worldwide, or the forensic documentation of sexual violence in armed conflicts.

Similar to this, the national experiences of Guatemala, Peru, and Panama show that accreditation procedures can spur development if they are supported by plans to bolster administrative, technical, and human resources, as well as political, logistical, and most importantly, financial will. In the absence of this assistance, there is still a chance that accreditation will turn into a stand-alone goal that is more closely related to getting official recognition than to actually improving practices. The "accreditation mirage" concept, which is used in the final chapter to summarize these lessons, serves as a reminder that genuine quality necessitates institutional resilience, social relevance, and scientific integrity rather than just documentary compliance. To put it simply, standards are useful instruments, but they cannot take the place of expert judgment, contextual knowledge, or the ethical commitment necessary for forensic work. This book's ultimate goal is to promote thoughtful consideration, acknowledging both the advantages of accreditation and standardization and their drawbacks when used in isolation from the unique circumstances of each setting. By situating regulatory frameworks within a larger ecosystem of quality that blends technical rigor, contextual sensitivity, and a dedication to upholding justice, the intention is not to erode but to strengthen trust in them.

Therefore, the pages that follow are an invitation to a thoughtful and productive discussion. Through a variety of perspectives and experiences, we suggest a shift toward a forensic quality model that recognizes that, in a diverse world, formal homogeneity will never take the place of sound, modified, and socially responsible scientific responses while maintaining international standards.

Building authentic forensic quality in demanding environments necessitates a more comprehensive approach than conventional control and certification systems (Ross and Neuteboom, 2020; Neuteboom and Ross, 2024). Forensic science must be viewed as a discipline that operates at the nexus of empirical research, the service of justice, and interaction with diverse communities (Roux et al., 2023; Ross et al., 2025). Measuring excellence solely by adhering to documentation requirements or standardizing procedures is insufficient (Ross and Neuteboom, 2020; Neuteboom and Ross, 2024). In this way, quality needs to be viewed as a dynamic equilibrium between contextual relevance, institutional capacity, and scientific integrity. Applying proven techniques rigorously is a requirement of scientific integrity, but so is being willing to review, modify, or even replace them in response to operational needs or empirical data. Institutional capacity includes governance frameworks that promote openness, responsibility, and technical independence in addition to the availability of resources and skilled labor. According to contextual relevance, forensic procedures must address the social, cultural, political, and economic realities of the setting in which they are used (Ross et al., 2025). This means avoiding foreign solutions that, while perfect in theory, turn out to be ineffectual or even detrimental in practice.

According to this vision, international standards must be adaptable instruments that can be incorporated into various forensic environments without compromising their scientific basis (Roux et al., 2022). This suggests a cultural change in how organizations view quality as well as how auditors, certifiers, and regulatory agencies evaluate performance. As long as methodological rigor and result traceability are upheld, excellence can and should be expressed in a variety of ways. This is not about loosening the requirements (Neuteboom and Ross, 2024). Accreditation models that value not only formal compliance but also the capacity to innovate and adjust to challenging situations are made possible by this approach, which views quality assessment as a dynamic process that is always changing.

Similarly, developing authentic forensic quality necessitates a consistent dedication to professional development and continuing training (Ross et al., 2025). Investing in people is just as important as investing in infrastructure or technology in demanding settings where employee turnover, work overload, and resource scarcity are prevalent. Forensic quality is upheld by everyone's ability to grow, adapt, and learn rather than by decree or certification (Ross et al., 2025; Wayermann et al., 2023; Roux et al., 2022; Willis 2010; among many others). This necessitates developing an organizational culture that encourages interdisciplinary cooperation, values empirical data, and stimulates critical thinking (Crispino et al., 2021).

In the end, pursuing an inclusive and contextualized forensic quality model will help the public's trust in forensic science as a foundation of justice in addition to benefiting organizations and industry professionals. The best assurance that forensic quality won't be a mirage but rather a tangible, sustainable reality that is genuinely focused on the service of truth and justice is provided by an approach that integrates international standards with local adaptations, rewards both technical coherence and social relevance (Ross et al., 2025), and puts people, professionals and communities, at the center of the process.

References

Ballantyne, K.N. and Wilson-Wilde, L. (2020) Assessing the reliability and validity of forensic science An industry perspective. *Australian Journal of Forensic Sciences*. Advance online publication. https://doi.org/10.1080/00450618.2019.1711182.

Berger, C.E.H. (2025) Finally a really forensic worldwide standard: ISO 21043 Forensic sciences, Part 4, Interpretation. *Forensic Science International: Synergy*, **10**, 100589. https://doi.org/10.1016/j.fsisyn.2025.100589.

Crispino, F., Weyermann, C., Delémont, O., Roux, C., and Ribaux, O. (2021) Towards another paradigm for forensic science? *Wiley Interdisciplinary Reviews: Forensic Science*, **e1441**. https://doi.org/10.1002/wfs2.1441.

Doyle, S. (2019) *Quality Management in Forensic Science*. Academic Press (Elsevier). https://doi.org/10.1016/C2015-0-04588-9.

ISO 21043-1. (n.d.) Forensic sciences–Part 1: Vocabulary. https://www.iso.org/standard/87128.html.

ISO 21043-2. (n.d.) Forensic Sciences–Part 2: Recognition, recording, collection, transport and storage of items. https://www.iso.org/standard/88665.html.

ISO 21043-3. (n.d.) Forensic sciences–Part 3: Analysis. https://www.iso.org/standard/72040.html.

ISO 21043-4. (n.d.) Forensic sciences–Part 4: Interpretation. https://www.iso.org/standard/72039.html.

ISO 21043-5. (n.d.) Forensic sciences–Part 5: Reporting. https://www.iso.org/standard/73896.html.

ISO/IEC 14001:2015. (n.d.) Environmental management systems–Requirements with guidance for use. https://www.iso.org/obp/ui/#iso:std:iso:14001:ed- 3:v1:en.

ISO/IEC 15189:2012. (n.d.) Medical laboratories–Requirements for quality and competence. https://www.iso.org/standard/56115.html.

ISO/IEC 17020:2012. (n.d.) Conformity Assessment–Requirements for the Operation of Various Types of Bodies Performing Inspection. https://www.iso.org/standard/52994.html.

ISO/IEC 17025:2017. (n.d.) General Requirements for the Competence of Testing and Calibration Laboratories. https://www.iso.org/standard/66912.html.

ISO/IEC 9001:2015. (n.d.) Quality management systems–Requirements. https://www.iso.org/iso-9001-quality-management.html.

Koehler, J.J., Mnookin, J.L., and Saks, M.J. (2023) The scientific reinvention of forensic science. *Proceedings of the National Academy of Sciences*, **120**(41), e2301840120. https://doi.org/10.1073/pnas.2301840120.

Margot, P. (2011) Commentary on the need for a research culture in the forensic sciences. *UCLA Law Review*, **58**, 795–801.

National Research Council (2009). *Strengthening Forensic Science in the United States: A Path Forward*. Washington, DC: The National Academies Press.

Neuteboom, W. and Ross, A. (2024) Shall the twain ever meet? *Australian Journal of Forensic Sciences*. Advance online publication. https://doi.org/10.1080/00450618.2024.2363823.

Neuteboom, W., Ross, A., Bugeja, L., Willis, S., Roux, C., and Lothridge, K. (2023) Quality management in forensic science: A closer inspection. *Forensic Science International*, **111779**. https://doi.org/10.1016/j.forsciint.2023.111779.

PCAST, President's Council of Advisors on Science and Technology (2016). *Forensic Science in Criminal Courts: Ensuring Scientific Validity of Feature-Comparison Methods* (Report to the President). Executive Office of the President. https://obamawhitehouse.archives.gov/sites/default/files/microsites/ostp/PCAST/pcast_forensic_science_report_final.pdf?utm_source=chatgpt.com.

Pereira, M. (1985) Quality assurance in forensic science. *Forensic Science International*, **28**, 1–6. https://doi.org/10.1016/0379-0738(85)90159-8.

Ross, A., Lennard, C., and Roux, C. (2025) Forensic science: Where to from here? *Forensic Science International*, **366**, 112285. https://doi.org/10.1016/j.forsciint.2024.112285.

Ross, A. and Neuteboom, W. (2020) ISO-accreditation–Is that all there is for forensic science? *Australian Journal of Forensic Sciences*. Advance online publication. https://doi.org/10.1080/00450618.2020.1819414.

Roux, C., Crispino, F., Ribaux, O., Walsh, S.J., and Margot, P. (2022) The Sydney Declaration: The principles of forensic science. *Forensic Science International: Synergy*, **4**, 100216. https://doi.org/10.1016/j.fsisyn.2022.100216.

Saks, M.J. and Faigman, D.L. (2008) Failed forensics: How forensic science lost its way and how it might yet find it. *Annual Review of Law and Social Science*, **4**, 149–173.

Weyermann, C., Willis, S., Margot, P., and Roux, C. (2023) Towards more relevance in forensic science research and development. *Forensic Science International,* **348**, 111592. https://doi.org/10.1016/j.forsciint.2023.111592.

Willis, S. (2010) Power, process, people–A presentation on quality and competence in forensic science delivered at EAFS2009. *Science & Justice,* **50**(1), 23–25. https://doi.org/10.1016/j.scijus.2009.11.079.

Wilson-Wilde, L. (2018) The international development of forensic science standards—A review. *Forensic Science International.* Advance online publication. https://doi.org/10.1016/j.forsciint.2018.04.009.

CHAPTER 1

Forensic Quality Management and Era of Standardization: Where the Rubber Meets the Road in Challenging Environments

Roberto C. Parra[1,*], Eva Bruenisholz[2], and Claude Roux[3]

[1]*The Specialized Forensic Team of the United Nations Joint Human Rights Office (UNJHRO) in the Democratic Republic of the Congo*

[2]*Forensics Command, Australian Federal Police, Canberra, Australia*

[3]*Centre for Forensic Science, University of Technology Sydney, Sydney, Australia*

1.1 Introduction

The journey of quality management in forensic science stretches from its medieval roots in European guild systems to its current status as a prominent global normative framework (Ross and Neuteboom, 2020a). This chapter aims to examine how standardization and quality assurance (QA) have shaped forensic science, particularly when confronted with operational realities marked by complexity, resource limitations, and institutional instability. Recognizing that it is ludicrous to envisage forensic science without QA, this chapter broadens the debate by asking: Can the logical framework and application tools developed in industrial settings genuinely serve the purposes of and complex demands from forensic science, or do they risk constraining the field's scientific autonomy and interpretive flexibility? The relevance of this question is accentuated in complex and high-risk operational contexts. A foundational framework for its resolution is derived from the Sydney Declaration (SD) (Roux et al., 2022), which is further elaborated in this chapter.

1.1.1 Historical Development and the Rise of Standardization

Throughout history, the idea of quality has changed significantly. Quality was first associated with artisanal excellence in medieval guilds, where standards

*The views expressed herein are those authors and do not necessarily reflect the views of the United Nations.

Forensic Science and Quality Management: Addressing the Era of Standardization in Challenging Environments, First Edition. Edited by Roberto C. Parra and Allan G. Alvarez-Godoy.

were determined by each artisan's level of skill (Juran, 1995). However, as industrial capitalism grew, quality became institutionalized. Inspection systems were created during the Industrial Revolution (1760–1840) to keep an eye out for product flaws because mass production required consistency. Quality as a managerial and technical concept originated from this (Juran, 1995; Garvin, 1988).

The Industrial Revolution ushered in a factory-based logic centered on efficiency, scale, and quality control via end-point inspection. In the early 20th century, Frederick W. Taylor (1911) developed scientific management, or Taylorism, which was key to future developments. To increase productivity and efficiency, Taylor promoted the standardization of work tasks, the study of motion and time, and stringent control over work procedures. Taylorism prioritized conformity over creativity and succeeded in rationalizing industrial production, but it also treated workers like mere cogs in a machine. Under Taylorism, the terms "quality" and "uniformity," and "control" came to mean attributes that could be quantified, managed, and enhanced. Organizations' approaches to quality in the ensuing decades would be significantly impacted by this mechanistic viewpoint. This approach measured quality after production rather than addressing root causes of error. The subsequent advent of statistical quality control in the 1920s represented a shift toward prevention, advocating that quality should be embedded within each step of the process.

The influential "quality gurus" of the 20th century, such as Walter Shewhart, W. Edwards Deming, Joseph Juran, and Kaoru Ishikawa, established principles like cause-and-effect analysis, control charts, quality circles, and continuous improvement cycles (e.g., the PDCA cycle: plan-do-check-act or Deming Cycle). Deming (1986) questioned the Taylorist rigidity (Juran, 1995). This signaled the shift from quality control to quality culture, a paradigm where quality is a result of institutional commitment, values, and behaviors as well as processes (Juran, 1995; Garvin, 1988). A quality culture is more than just following rules; it is a shared philosophy where everyone in the company takes ownership of enhancing performance. It places more emphasis on learning than blame, teamwork over hierarchy, and reflexivity over routine (Garvin, 1988). People's thoughts, decisions, and relationships with the goal of their work are all influenced by quality. It also acknowledges the importance of judgment, context, and ethical discernment, as not all values can be expressed in metrics.

While developed for manufacturing, these concepts gradually found their way into fields like forensic science (Ross and Neuteboom, 2020a,b; Hazard et al., 2014). In this field, this cultural view of quality is especially pertinent (Hazard, 2014; Margot, 2011). Industry standards like ISO/IEC 17025 had a significant impact on forensic laboratories' adoption of quality management systems in the late 20th century (Ross and Neuteboom, 2020a). These systems, which reflected the Taylorist legacy of control and uniformity, placed a strong emphasis on personnel qualifications, equipment calibration, traceability, and procedural documentation. However, drawbacks emerged when these models were applied within forensic contexts.

According to Hazard et al. (2014: 1772), "The forensic science community struggles today with the comprehensive quality approach because it failed to develop its own approach, instead mistakenly copying the work from the manufacturing sector." This claim draws attention to a structural shortcoming in forensic science: the lack of a high-quality model derived from its unique features. Forensic science is concerned with the detection, recognition, examination, and interpretation of traces – vestiges of past events that are often imperfect, incomplete, and not reproducibly or statistically generated, as they arise from uncontrolled and usually unpredictable circumstances (Weyermann and Roux, 2021). Further, forensic procedures require expert interpretation, disciplinary diversity, and adaptation to particular judicial contexts. For these reasons, the adoption of normative models, while offering some control mechanisms, is insufficient to guarantee their dependability and applicability (Olson and Ramsay, 2025). While forensic practice necessitates methodological flexibility and a rigorous scientific approach that transcends procedural formalism (Mousseau et al., 2025), the industrial model is predicated on repetition and the standardization of production processes that are ill-fitted to the nature of forensic science.

The novel ISO 21043 standard seeks to provide forensic science with an international framework tailored to its specific needs (Berger, 2025; Morrison et al., 2025). ISO 21043 aims to capture the complexities of forensic processes, from evidence collection to interpretation and reporting. While ISO/IEC 17025 has long been a more general reference point, but one that would work in tandem with the new ISO standard. Berger (2025) identifies Part 4, focusing on interpretation, as a fundamental contribution. It includes a structured decision tree and standardized vocabulary that aim for greater clarity and consistency. However, the pursuit of uniformity can also unintentionally generate rigidity, hampering the necessary adaptability in jurisdictions characterized by diverse and contradictory legal traditions, resources, and institutional practices, as is particularly the case in the Global South. On the other hand, from a forensic data science perspective, Morrison et al. (2025) offer a more critical review. They value the focus on empirical validation and the likelihood-ratio framework as ways to ensure clarity and robustness of processes. However, they point out conceptual flaws, such as unclear definitions of key terms, and assert that ISO 21043 is not intended as an accreditation standard. This limits its immediate practical impact, making it more of a goal than a rule.

The views of Berger (2025) and Morrison et al. (2025) clarify the dual essence of ISO 21043: it would serve, on the one hand, as a tool for possible harmonization and, on the other hand, as a reminder of the persistent problems of global inequality. If we fail to recognize the differences in resources and experience between the Global North and the Global South, the idea of true international uniformity could remain a utopian ideal rather than becoming operationally functional. In any case, the epistemological essence, semiotic scope, and rigor remain a deficiency that must be resolved.

In the context of forensic science, these industrial practices were adopted to foster institutional trust, deliver consistent outcomes, and enable external audits. Over time, a logic of "structural control," including protocols, accreditations, validations, and document traceability, began to replace reliance on individual expert competence. This transition, presented as necessary for public trust and traceability (Wilson-Wilde, 2018; Ballantyne and Wilson-Wilde, 2020), redefined forensic work as a series of validated, auditable, and measurable steps, akin to a production chain spanning from crime scene to court report.

However, there has been ongoing discussion in the field about this "era of standardization." On the one hand, supporters contend that industrial manufacturing-based quality systems are necessary to uphold the validity and consistency of practice. Others caution that rigorous adherence to these frameworks may jeopardize scientific autonomy and diminish the importance of expert judgment, particularly in complex or unique cases that are challenging to adapt to standard operating procedures (Hazard, 2014; Crispino et al., 2022; Mousseau et al., 2025). This raises a crucial query: To what extent do these systems fit the purposes of forensic science?

1.1.2 Refocusing on Quality: From Checklist Culture to Scientific Judgment

In forensic science, discussions about quality are often limited to management tools, accreditation, and protocols. Despite their necessity, these mechanisms risk losing their meaning if separated from the conceptual foundations that support them. True quality must be based on solid foundations of logical reflection, semiotics, and epistemology (Roux et al., 2022; Crispino, 2024; Illes et al., 2020; Cole, 2013; Margot, 2011).

From an epistemological perspective, forensic science must clarify the types of knowledge it generates, as well as its limits and scope. It is important to critically examine the concepts of certainty, probability, and plausibility rather than taking them for granted. In the absence of this, quality control could guarantee uniformity of the process, ignoring the true reliability of the findings. Forensic science reveals deficiencies in reasoning and case-specific research, primarily attributable to training that emphasizes specialization and repetitive methodologies (Cole, 2013; Illes et al., 2020). To tackle this issue, active learning strategies are suggested, incorporating problems, projects, and real-world experiences that enhance critical thinking and teamwork (Illes et al., 2020). At the same time, its practice takes place in a unique epistemic culture that is shaped by data that cannot be repeated, institutional rules, and the pressure of courts, all of which affect how forensic knowledge is produced and validated (Cole, 2013). The semiotic aspect is equally significant (Crispino, 2024; Crispino et al., 2022; Roux et al., 2022). According to Crispino (2024), forensic science must be reimagined from its foundations, as a trace is not merely a tangible object; it is a sign that requires recognition and interpretation to uncover its meaning. Although Bayesian statistics and regulatory reforms help, they are unable to completely eradicate bias or the intricacy of judicial reasoning (Dror, 2025). Bayesian statistics offers a useful prescriptive framework for logically organizing evidence, but its applicability is constrained by the interpretative intricacies of judicial processes. Peirce's semiotics[1] enhances this quantitative methodology by incorporating the examination of meanings and contexts into the evaluation of the probative value of forensic evidence (Crispino, 2024: Roux et al., 2022). This semiotic proposal emphasizes that all inferences are interpretive, with various meanings being assigned by laypeople, judges, and scientists. Therefore, without incorporating the human element, technical quality alone is inadequate. The strength of forensic science lies in its ability to articulate findings within their context, following a coherent and logical argumentative framework that clearly demonstrates their value (Crispino, 2024; Roux et al., 2022). Forensic traces, consisting of specific signs such as fingerprints, genetic profiles, bone fractures, and injuries in general, for example, "do not speak for themselves," but rather must be deciphered. Interpretive frameworks influenced by context and conventions give them probative value. Evaluating the reliability of forensic interpretations requires understanding this semiotic mediation (Crispino, 2024). Finally, logic serves as the basis for the reasoning that connects hypotheses to evidence. Clear and compelling argumentative structures are just as important to quality as technical precision (Roux et al., 2022).

The notion of quality in forensic science has always attracted scrutiny. As early as the 1980s, during a presentation to a meeting of the International Association of Forensic Sciences (IAFS) in Oxford, UK in 1984, Margaret Pereira (1985) questioned whether implementing quality management was affordable. Her own response continues to resonate to this day: "The real question is whether we can afford not to" (Neuteboom et al., 2023). This early viewpoint signaled a significant turning point by highlighting that quality is a necessity for credible and valid forensic findings, not a luxury. Ross and Neuteboom (2020a) frame the evolution of forensic quality management as a deliberate, adaptive process rather than a passive adoption of outside standards. They describe it as an "odyssey" requiring robust organizational commitment, a culture of continuous improvement, and sufficient resources, operational and financial.

The increasing focus on compliance in professional and scientific fields could unintentionally turn quality into just a matter of following the rules. Formal systems and standardized procedures are essential for maintaining

[1] The value of Peirce semiotics lies in the necessary and sufficient triadic decomposition of signs, in which the perception of the sign (representation or ground) results in another signification (the object) via a necessary Interpretant, which can be a function, a resultant, a thought, or a judgment (Crispino, 2024).

accountability and consistency; however, they may unintentionally restrict professional activities to bureaucratic efficiency at the expense of substantive excellence. In these situations, critical thinking, creativity, and epistemological reflection are pushed to the side, which makes it hard for professionals to question their assumptions, deal with complex uncertainties, or adapt to new problems. Relying too much on checklists can also give you a false sense of security, hiding deeper weaknesses that only expertise, experience, and scientific reasoning can reveal. Forensic science requires more than just following the rules. It requires the ability to understand scientific principles, the ability to look at traces that may or may not become evidence later in a bigger picture, and the courage to admit when one does not know something. So, it is important to build a strong scientific culture. This involves not only enhancing technical skills but also fostering critical reflection, promoting continuous learning, and implementing rigorous assessments to evaluate the depth of knowledge. QA should find a middle ground between keeping procedural safeguards in place and giving experts the freedom to use their professional judgment in ways that make their fields more reliable and trustworthy.

1.1.3 Balancing Standardization and Professional Autonomy

According to Willis (2010), the true quality of forensic science is determined by the practitioner's judgment, training, cognitive ability, and adaptability. Excessive focus on compliance and documentation can stifle discourse about the evidential significance, boundaries of expertise, and the abductive reasoning central to forensic interpretation. This is especially problematic in challenging environments, such as conflict zones or humanitarian crises, where adaptability, contextual awareness, and epistemic sensitivity are indispensable. In such settings, quality must be a reflexive, logical practice, not simply a certificate of compliance.

Neuteboom and Ross (2024) notably distinguish between "adopters" (often institutional managers, seeking comfort in standards and procedures) and "skeptics" (typically forensic scientists, valuing flexibility and critical thought). They argue this divide need not be irreconcilable; quality systems should cultivate environments for open scientific discourse, not close them off. This tension, between rigid, document-driven approaches and dynamic, adaptive practice, lies at the heart of contemporary forensic science.

1.1.4 The Epistemic Gap and the Need for Scientific Culture

Forensic science is defined as "a case-based research-oriented, science-based endeavor to study traces" (Roux et al., 2022: 2). The value of a trace is determined not only by procedural conformity but also by its epistemic meaning within a logical explanatory narrative (Hazard, 2014). Interpreting traces requires cognitive abilities, critical thinking, reasoning, logic, and hypothesis formation (Kelty et al., 2011, 2017, 2023, 2024), rarely addressed in current quality systems (Neuteboom et al., 2023). Even though ISO/IEC 17025 stipulates competence requirements (clause 6.2), assessments often focus on practical and technical skills, leaving cognitive and interpretive competencies under-evaluated. This gap exposes a preference for documentary compliance over well-informed scientific judgment (Neuteboom et al., 2023). In this situation, certain changes have been made to meet the needs of forensic laboratories. ANAB[2] AR 3125:2023 is one example[3]. It adds forensic-oriented requirements to ISO/IEC 17025, covering topics like ethics, safety, environmental conditions, and staff education. ILAC G-19:06/2022[4] also encourages a modular approach to the forensic process, from gathering evidence to interpreting it. It shows how to use ISO/IEC 17025 and ISO/IEC 17020 in forensic situations. The ISO 21043 series also covers the whole forensic science process (Morrison et al., 2025; Berger, 2025), from terminology (Part 1) to recognition, recording, transport, and storage (Part 2), analysis (Part 3), interpretation (Part 4), and reporting (Part 5) (Morrison et al., 2025). This makes each step of forensic practice stronger (Berger, 2025). The critique by Neuteboom et al. (2023) remains entirely valid, notwithstanding recent adaptations. Forensic practice remains at risk of prioritizing checklists and administrative procedures over the development and application of cognitive and interpretive expertise. This reinforces the need for accreditation systems to encourage more critical thinking.

Standardization, moreover, has sometimes prioritized process over purpose, sidelining the forensic discipline's core aims: reconstructing, preventing, and understanding criminal phenomena (and others harmful to society) (Roux et al., 2021). This dissociation between means and ends has resulted in an instrumental and fragmented vision that privileges formal compliance over substantive understanding. As Margot (2011) argues, what is needed is not just a culture of quality, but a culture of forensic science itself, built on research, critical training, and philosophical reflection.

1.1.5 From Administrative Compliance to Critical Forensic Science

The true value of quality in forensic science does not reside in codified norms, but in integrating those norms with scientific reasoning and context-specific practice. Willis (2010) warns that accreditation can create a false sense of infallibility; technical compliance does not guarantee correct results (Olson and Ramsay, 2025). The most recent and telling illustration of this point is the problems experienced by the Queensland DNA laboratory in Australia.

[2] See https://webstore.ansi.org/?source=blog&_gl=1*1dztitn*_gcl_au*MTExNDM0NjE2MS4xNzU2ODE3MTE4

[3] See https://blog.ansi.org/anab/what-is-ar-3125/?utm_source=chatgpt.com

[4] See https://ilac.org/latest_ilac_news/revised-ilac-g19-document-published/?utm_source=chatgpt.com

Despite significant work undertaken by management to address the problems, many reports (Sofronoff, 2022; Bennett, 2023; Walvisch et al., 2024; Budowle, 2025; Wright et al., 2025) confirmed that accreditation does not suffice to guarantee quality (Olson and Ramsay, 2025).

Technical reform alone will not work unless there is a significant change in culture as well. Therefore, while professionalization has emphasized certification and accreditation, the field must now seek a deeper transformation: the cultivation of a robust and reflective scientific culture. Forensic practice inherently relies on expert interpretation (Hazard, 2014; Crispino et al., 2022). Quality goes beyond just avoiding mistakes; it includes inference, context, and coherence, and it requires both epistemological and administrative evaluation. It also includes relevance, purpose, continuous improvement, and long-term impact that goes beyond just following the rules. This means recognizing the diversity of forensic work, from state-of-the-art laboratories to resource-limited field sites, and promoting principles that guide practice beyond mere procedure. It is important to emphasize that basic scientific foundations like those described in Roux et al. (2022) do not go against QA; instead, they work together. Fundamental principles establish the conceptual and ethical framework for sound scientific practice, guaranteeing that research is valid, transparent, and pertinent. QA is a way to set those principles into action and strengthen them through standards, controls, and procedures.

1.1.6 Chapter Roadmap

These theoretical and practical tensions, between standardization and scientific judgment, compliance and critical reflection, and process and purpose, are present in all forensic contexts. However, they become significantly magnified in operational settings marked by structural violence[5], institutional and financial instability, or fragmented regulatory landscapes. In such challenging environments, the risks of over-reliance on procedural norms, the under-development of expertise, or the neglect of context-specific judgment can have profound consequences not only for scientific credibility but for justice and humanitarian outcomes. It is precisely here that the scientific foundation assumes special importance.

Recognizing these challenges, the remainder of this chapter critically examines the potential and limits of forensic quality management, focusing particularly on how these systems function (or fail) under the pressure of real-life, high-stakes contexts. A key argument is that broader foundational frameworks, such as the SD, can play a fundamentally complementary role in maintaining quality when conventional mechanisms are insufficient. Importantly, the SD is not

[5] Structural violence is a form of violence that is not seen but is caused by social, economic, and political inequalities that are built into institutions. It restricts opportunities, rights, and access to essential resources, causing suffering and exclusion without direct aggression. It shows up as poverty, racism, discrimination, and inequality in the system (Galtung, 1969; Farmer, 2004).

intended to replace traditional quality frameworks, but rather to provide a comprehensive strategic foundation for forensic science that remains valid in all environments, both standard and nonstandard. By rooting practice in its core principles, it enables reliability, effectiveness, and scientific integrity where conventional quality control frameworks may fail. It thus ensures that forensic science remains agile, transparent, and relevant in a rapidly changing world.

By exploring how forensic scientists address the intersection of ever-evolving standards, resource constraints, and complex cases, the chapter seeks to illuminate both the paths forward and the pitfalls to avoid. In doing so, it advocates for a model of forensic science that is not only procedurally rigorous but also resilient, reflective, and sensitive to the diverse real complexities in which it is practiced, especially based on rigorous scientific foundations.

1.2 Quality Management in Forensic Science: From Tradition to Transformation

1.2.1 Purposes and Institutional Justification

The primary justification for forensic quality management has historically been the need to strengthen public and judicial confidence in forensic science. Lentini's (2009) "*Forensic Quality Triangle*" is a common way to show that forensic science is of high quality. It includes three important parts: certification, accreditation, and standardization. These components function interdependently to enhance the reliability of forensic evidence and to maintain public and judicial confidence in its application.

Certification is all about how good someone is at doing something. It requires more than mere education or experience; practitioners must empirically validate their proficiency in the accurate and consistent application of established methodologies. Ballantyne and Wilson-Wilde (2020) contend that competence can solely be demonstrated through blind proficiency testing conducted in conditions that replicate actual casework. Certification, then, makes professionals responsible, enhances clarity, and gives the courts confidence that expert testimony is based on proven skill.

Accreditation, on the other hand, is about how well an institution can do its job. It means that independent groups officially recognize that laboratories follow international standards like ISO/IEC 17025 or the new ISO/IEC 21043 and have strong quality management systems. According to Wilson-Wilde (2018), accreditation proves that laboratories not only have the technical skills they need but also have processes that are consistent, can be audited, and are focused on continuous improvement. This dimension is directly related to institutional QA systems, which use documentation, peer review, and internal audits to lower the chances of mistakes, contamination, or bias in the forensic process.

Standardization is the base that gives us the common set of methods and procedures. International efforts, like those led by ISO/TC272, set standards that everyone agrees on that set the minimum standards for collecting, analyzing, interpreting, and reporting evidence. Lentini (2009) emphasized that without recognized standards, both certification and accreditation lose effectiveness, as there would be no clear criteria for defining and evaluating good practice. These three pillars, along with strong institutional QA systems, make sure that forensic science gives results that are valid, reliable, and can be compared across countries. They also protect the validity of forensic evidence in court decisions and boost public trust in forensic institutions.

In legal contexts, where expert evidence can decisively influence decisions that affect fundamental rights, ensuring the reliability and transparency of forensic findings is an ethical, scientific, and legal imperative. From this perspective, quality systems aim to minimize errors, document decision-making, reduce operator variability, and establish formal mechanisms for continuous improvement (Neuteboom et al., 2023). However, beyond its technical-operational function, forensic quality has acquired symbolic and strategic value within institutions. In many countries, especially those with weakened, transitional, or reforming judicial systems, the implementation of quality systems has been interpreted as a sign of modernization, professionalization, and transparency. Within this framework, accreditation operates not only as a tool for external validation but also as an instrument of institutional governance, allowing laboratories to align with international standards, position themselves within globalized networks, and access funding and international cooperation.

In this sense, quality in forensic science should not be understood solely as a set of standardized procedures, but as an institutional practice aimed at ensuring the epistemic integrity of forensic knowledge, its legal utility, and its social relevance. That is, the ultimate purpose of forensic quality management is not only to optimize processes but mainly to build legitimacy and public trust before the public, the judicial system, and the scientific community.

The implementation of quality systems thus constitutes a form of epistemic governance that harmonizes multiple dimensions: technical, legal, organizational, and ethical.

It is a scaffolding that contributes to stabilize forensic practices, mitigate the risk of errors or biases, and promote a more rigorous dialogue between science and law. At the same time, as various critical voices have pointed out (Roux et al., 2022; Crispino and Roux, 2017; Crispino et al., 2022; Ross and Neuteboom 2020a,b; Neuteboom and Ross, 2024; Willis, 2010, among other), it also represents a regulatory mechanism that, when applied rigidly or without context, can constrain scientific autonomy and critical thinking.

For this reason, understanding the purposes and institutional justification of forensic quality requires a critical perspective that is historically informed and epistemologically aware. To progress toward quality models that not only adhere to standards but also genuinely elevate the epistemic, ethical, social, and humanitarian values, as well as their diversity in the contexts where forensic science is applied, it is essential to recognize its multifaceted nature and various contexts. Understanding and solidifying basic principles is just as important, since these are the ideas and methods that make forensic practices trustworthy and valid. Without a clear understanding of these principles, any model of quality could end up being just about following the rules instead of encouraging ongoing improvement and strengthening the role of forensic science in society as a whole.

1.2.2 Toward a Forensic Scientific Culture

Addressing the current tensions in forensic quality management requires more than revising technical standards; it calls for the cultivation of a true forensic scientific culture (Kirk, 1963; Margot, 2011; Hazard, 2014). This entails educating and training professionals who are not only proficient in following protocols but who can integrate quality principles with critical thinking, interpretive reasoning, and epistemic sensitivity (Kelty et al., 2011, 2017, 2023, 2024). Quality should not be reduced to the mechanical application of procedures; rather, it must be understood as a deliberative and reasoned practice, where forensic inference is not merely documented but thoroughly justified.

The interpretation of traces in forensic science requires professional judgment, use of appropriate inference (in particular abductive reasoning and analogy), and adaptation to specific contexts (Weyermann and Roux, 2021). These aspects, which are highly dependent on the practitioner and the environment, are difficult to codify into universal procedures and often fall outside the scope of quality systems. As a result, quality runs the risk of being equated with procedural conformity rather than the validity of inference. This view can lead to an "illusion of reliability" based more on documentary compliance than on the actual epistemic value of the forensic inference (Weyermann and Roux, 2021; Crispino et al., 2022; Roux et al., 2022).

The implementation of standards or the use of structural controls as stand-ins for scientific proficiency is insufficient to characterize a culture of quality in forensic science. A genuine forensic science culture is built upon practitioners with rigorous scientific training, grounded in strong university education, and deeply engaged with the unique challenges and questions specific to the field (Margot, 2011; Bruenisholz et al., 2024). Many laboratories were founded in institutional structures where hierarchy took precedence over the critical advancement of knowledge. This led to disjointed forensic practices, undertrained staff, and a tendency to function as mere producers of results, particularly in the field of DNA (Margot, 2011). Because every case is a real investigative challenge, a culture of forensic science excellence requires not only a strong scientific basis but also the analytical and reflective ability to detect, examine, and evaluate traces in complicated contexts. This procedure acknowledges forensic science as a distinctive field that includes the responsible communication of its findings, critical interpretation, and acceptance of uncertainty (Roux et al., 2022; Hazard, 2014; Ballantyne et al., 2024).

In forensic reasoning, Hazard (2014) asserts that relevance is not an inherent characteristic of a trace; instead, it arises from the relationship between the trace and the case context, facilitated by inferences and interpretive methodologies. In this context, a trace possesses no intrinsic value; its significance emerges only when the trace is acknowledged, chosen, and interpreted by the scientist, who employs their training, experience, intuition, and contextual understanding to ascribe meaning to it. Relevance is understood as a dynamic and relational construct that surpasses the material attributes of the trace, situating it within a particular explanatory and operational context.

Different ways of reasoning are used to build relevance. The trace is linked to reasonable hypotheses that try to explain why the trace is present in the situation being looked into by using abductive, inductive, or deductive reasoning. This cognitive process enables the conversion of the trace into a clue, which serves as a sign with explanatory significance within the narrative of events (Crispino, 2024; Weyermann and Roux, 2021; Crispino et al., 2022). So, relevance does not just depend on the trace itself; it also depends on how well the scientist can fit it into a useful and rational story about the investigation (Weyermann and Roux, 2021; Crispino et al., 2022).

Hazard (2014) also emphasizes that relevance is always relative, contextual, and temporal. There is no single rule that can objectively and definitively say which trace is important; its importance depends on the situation, the organization, and the person. In this context, two dimensions can be identified: factual relevance, which pertains to the acknowledged connection between the trace and the case, and appropriate relevance, which assesses whether the resources expended in gathering and analyzing the trace are warranted by the anticipated informational advantages. The significance of the trace is established through an interpretive and contextual process that embodies forensic culture alongside the scientist's expertise and experience. Bitzer et al. (2015) assert that the evaluation of traces in forensic settings has conventionally depended on what they term external indicators. These are standardized and generalizable criteria, like how often a certain trace occurs statistically, how reliable the analytical methods are, how well it matches records or databases, or how well it can be used in court. These indicators give an objective frame of reference, but they are mostly not connected to the specific situation of the investigation. The authors, on the other hand, talk about the idea of the utility of the clue, which moves the focus from these outside factors to the investigation's internal logic. From this standpoint, the utility of a trace is not solely contingent upon its rarity or technical precision, but rather on its efficacy in facilitating the resolution of the particular case, whether by diminishing uncertainty, reinforcing or undermining hypotheses, or recalibrating the investigative approach. Bitzer et al.'s (2015) proposal seeks to transcend the static perspective of external indicators by contextualizing the evaluation of the trace within the dynamic interplay between the informational potential of the clue and the cognitive requirements intrinsic to the investigative process. The authors also suggest the idea of "expected utility" as a way to figure out which traces are most important before doing the analysis. In this way, conscious and efficient selection is encouraged, redundancies are avoided, and the contribution of forensic science is maximized.

Crispino (2024) underscores that these deficiencies cannot be rectified solely through protocols, accreditations, or technical enhancements, as the fundamental issue resides in the essence of the trace and in the assignment of meaning within decision-making frameworks. His proposal to advance forensic semiotics through the integration of Peirce's framework opens a novel and largely unexplored trajectory in the field. In this context, the concept of the interpretant elucidates the human contribution to the construction of meaning in forensic findings, highlighting its biases, limitations, and possibilities. In the current era of artificial intelligence in forensic science (see Chapter 2), it is essential to distinguish the contributions of these technologies, effective in data management and pattern recognition, from the reflective reasoning of the human brain. Crispino (2024) underscores that interpretive judgment, grounded in semiotic logic, will remain indispensable: only the human intellect can ascribe meaning to signs within their judicial and social contexts. We should not forget this aspect today when trying to build trust in a system that is increasingly using automation and artificial intelligence.

This approach emphasizes the value of instructional strategies that develop interpretive skills, moving beyond purely technical instruction to promote reflective practice and genuine scientific literacy. Ultimately, building a forensic scientific culture means fostering a professional ethos centered on inference, transparency, and epistemic responsibility. In such a culture, quality is not an external imposition but the natural outcome of scientifically engaged and critically aware practitioners.

1.3 The Standardization Era: The Forensic Shift and Industrial Ideals

One of the most significant, and contentious, changes in the field's recent development is the consolidation of standardization as the predominant paradigm in forensic science. This movement, which was initially motivated by the justifiable need to increase public and judicial confidence in forensic results, progressively embraced the concepts, metaphors, and working logic of industrial production. Key manufacturing concepts like consistency, efficiency, control, and repeatability were incorporated into the institutional jargon of forensic quality management. Accreditation became a strategic and symbolic objective as laboratories were reorganized around technical documentation, procedural compliance, and performance metrics.

These modifications had unexpected epistemological repercussions even though they brought about much-needed accountability and error-reduction mechanisms. Originally intended to be a field based on contextual reasoning based on the examination of isolated incidents, forensic science started to lose sight of its original purpose. Procedural completeness was frequently given precedence over the deeper significance of scientific reasoning due to the emphasis on process control and conformance. Because of this, there is less room for professional judgment that includes using inference with contextual sensitivity.

Furthermore, the industrial paradigm frequently prioritizes quantifiable results over qualitative findings. This reinforces a concept of quality that runs the risk of becoming synonymous with bureaucratic correctness rather than scientific robustness by creating a tension between what can be measured and what cannot. This change affects how forensic work is perceived, practiced, and valued in addition to how it is managed, as many commentators have pointed out (Neuteboom and Ross, 2024; Willis, 2010). According to Neuteboom and Ross (2024), this adoption has been so intense that in many institutional settings a "compliance culture" has taken root, one that replaces scientific deliberation with documentary adherence. In their analysis of the divide between "adopters" (managers, auditors, technicians) and "skeptics" (forensic scientists, researchers), the authors describe a system in which compliance trumps critical thinking, and where the effectiveness of procedures is assessed more by their auditability than by their epistemic relevance. A narrow and technocratic view of forensic practice is implied when forensic science quality is reduced to rigorous adherence to accreditation systems and standardized procedures. The forensic professional, who is in charge of producing and interpreting knowledge, is reduced to a supporting role in this framework, while the emphasis is placed on external auditors and evaluators, who ultimately end up having undue control over the process (Willis, 2010).

Form over substance, documentary conformance over scientific reasoning and the expert's critical autonomy are all weakened by this logic. As a result, forensic procedures may be formally sound but may be shallow in their interpretation and insensitive to context. As the foundation of forensic quality, competency, which is defined as both technical knowledge and the ability to reason, communicate, and make sense of complex situations, needs to be strengthened immediately. This is done through rigorous scientific training and a professional judgment ethic.

1.3.1 Mean vs. Purpose

A type of operational fragmentation has been facilitated by the extensive use of standardization in forensic science, whereby the trace examination and interpretation are separated into distinct technical tasks. The expert's integrated responsibility over the overall narrative is weakened by this compartmentalization, which also tends to impede holistic reasoning. The growing gap between means and purpose is highlighted by Roux et al. (2021), who note that standardization tends to prioritize the how over the why, which frequently weakens the contextual meaning of findings.

Therefore, forensic work runs the risk of becoming less of a scientifically significant investigation and more of a procedural compliance exercise. Instead of evaluating professionals' critical interpretation, epistemic reflexivity, or judicial reasoning skills, this "bureaucratization" of forensic knowledge has fostered a culture where professionals are primarily judged on their ability to complete forms, adhere to established workflows, and pass audits. According to Neuteboom et al. (2023), technical conformance is given disproportionate weight in current quality management frameworks, which rarely evaluate cognitive or interpretive competence. According to their global survey, formal competence standards did not consistently identify, evaluate, or track critical thinking, logical reasoning, hypothesis formulation, and judgment, all of which are critical cognitive skills. Rather, quality systems continue to be primarily concerned with procedural results.

This change has significant ramifications. The development of propositions at the heart of forensic science cannot be replaced by standard operating procedures (SOPs), even though they may guarantee consistency in quantifiable steps. According to Roux et al. (2021), forensic science may lose its investigative and inferential character if quality is confused with compliance, which would undermine its capacity to make a significant societal contribution beyond the presentation of evidence in Court. Further, Neuteboom et al. (2023) underscore a critical concern in forensic science: the pronounced disparity between the focus on technical competencies and the insufficient emphasis on cognitive competencies. The former are typically well-defined and consistently evaluated through standardized protocols, whereas the latter are inadequately defined and infrequently subjected to formal evaluation mechanisms. This imbalance is an issue because forensic practice involves more than just using tools; it also includes critical thinking, logical reasoning, making informed decisions, and coming up with hypotheses in situations where there is a lot of uncertainty. The absence of systematic recognition and evaluation of these skills poses the risk of cultivating professionals who possess technical proficiency yet remain inadequately equipped to navigate the interpretative complexities intrinsic to the field. Consequently, Neuteboom et al. (2023) emphasize the necessity for quality management frameworks that explicitly incorporate cognitive competencies as a fundamental aspect of forensic practice.

In the end, an overemphasis on procedural fidelity runs the risk of transforming forensic science into a system of "quality on paper," where real scientific robustness is replaced by the appearance of rigor. Quality frameworks must reintegrate cognitive competence, interpretive reasoning, and the ability to deal with uncertainty in order to restore purpose. These are qualities that cannot be pre-programmed and must be developed through education, mentoring, and a change in institutional culture.

1.3.2 The Forensic Quality Paradox

Modern forensic science faces a structural paradox brought about by the era of standardization: the more standardized practice grows, the more likely it is to stifle its critical, interpretive, and inferential elements. In addition to being theoretical, this paradox shows up in the day-to-day work of forensic specialists, who must balance the need to follow established protocols with the need to draw conclusions that are supported by science in situations that are frequently complicated and uncertain. According to Willis (2010), the shift from science to process has left less room for scientific contemplation, creating a perilous false sense of technical certainty that does not always equate to improved outcomes.

The forensic professional is often reduced to an executor of protocols rather than an active interpreter of evidence, which creates a sort of epistemic alienation (Willis, 2022). Current quality systems, as Crispino et al. (2022) caution, have a tendency to assess the proper application of the procedure rather than the applicability of the reasoning, which can validate results that are technically correct but scientifically dubious. Compliance, not comprehension, is being measured. The fundamental cause of the forensic quality paradox is this discrepancy between operational validation and epistemological validity. Moreover, the paradox is made more apparent in situations where the ideal laboratory that the standards model differs greatly from the actual working conditions, as happens in Latin America (e.g., see Chapters 7–10). Additionally, the stress of keeping records, following rules, and conquering these obstacles is frequently a tiresome conundrum in real life. According to Willis (2010), quality that is only concerned with processes can fall short in situations where experience, ethical awareness, and contextual judgment are more important than strict adherence to a process. It is true that forensic quality cannot be boiled down to a technical assurance. It must be viewed as an ethical and epistemological practice that involves taking accountability for the interpretation of the evidence, the reasoning behind conclusions, and the communication of uncertainties. Hazard (2014) notes that the ability of forensic reasoning to produce sound, explicit, and verifiable inferences, rather than the process followed, is what gives it legitimacy. Although helpful, the quality system should critically support scientific discussion rather than take its place.

Therefore, the paradox is not that quality is a barrier in and of itself, but rather that its careless and decontextualized application may actually erode the very thing it was meant to enhance: public confidence in forensic science (Zhang and Lu, 2025). Gaining this trust requires more than just accreditation and certification credentials; it also requires methodological openness, sound judgment, and the capacity to adjust to actual difficulties. Rebalancing the axis between means and ends is the answer. Standards are means, not ends in and of themselves. If we lose this distinction, we may start to value things that are easier to measure more highly than those that are important (Roux et al., 2021).

1.4 Quality in Challenging Environments: Where the Rubber Meets the Road

In complex, demanding, and challenging forensic situations, such as those that occur during armed conflicts, mass violence, large-scale disasters, or serious human rights violations, the quality systems that are often recommended internationally present significant strategic, operational, and ethical problems. Operationally, insecurity, lack of resources, and time constraints make it difficult to strictly adhere to standardized protocols, which could even slow down urgent responses. Strategically, the presence of numerous actors and interests requires a level of flexibility and adaptability that inflexible frameworks often fail to consistently provide. The mechanical application of procedures can conflict with ethical principles such as valuing victims and being sensitive to different cultures. Also, worrying about strictly following standardized systems and protocols can make people forget about the epistemological core of forensic work for a number of reasons. First, strict adherence to procedures may prioritize compliance over critical reflection, turning complex reasoning into routine mechanical tasks. Second, protocols are often made to make sure that things are done consistently and that people are held accountable, but they have difficulty to capture the nuances that give meaning to traces in an investigation. Third, when practitioners concentrate excessively on evading procedural errors, they may overlook the interpretative and inferential aspects that genuinely produce knowledge. As a result, forensic science may be diminished to mere technical proficiency instead of its epistemic. For these reasons, we need a more flexible and context-sensitive quality management system. It must balance technical rigor with ethical imperatives and remain true to the primary goal of forensic science.

The rigid application of standards designed for controlled laboratory environments can prove unsuitable or even counterproductive in these settings. As evidenced in forensic investigations conducted in the Democratic Republic of the Congo, quality management must adapt to environments marked by chronic uncertainty, insecurity, and deep technical and logistical constraints, without compromising the integrity of the evidence or the safety and dignity of victims (Komar et al., 2021). Currently, using and maintaining one of these standardized international mechanisms in this scenario is very difficult, if not impossible. The 2002 Bali bombing and the MH17 crash investigation serve as prime examples of how forensic science must adapt when conventional ISO-compliant and validation-based procedures are no longer fully applicable

(AFP 2022, 2024,). Since the crash of MH17 took place in an area of active conflict, approved protocols like chain-of-custody controls, verified collection techniques, and ISO 17025 laboratory conditions could not be implemented right away (Ranson, 2015). Under strict limitations, forensic teams were forced to rely on triage principles, scientific integrity, and adaptable interagency coordination. Similar to the Bali bombing, which featured a scene of widespread casualties and fragmented infrastructure, the scope and urgency of victim identification exceeded the stringent deadlines and documentation required by traditional quality systems.

Such conditions highlight the need to rethink the concept of quality through a more flexible, contextual, and purpose-driven lens. Rather than imposing externally developed standards that often are disconnected from challenging environments, it becomes imperative to construct situated quality models that prioritize methodological coherence, transparency in reasoning, and epistemic awareness. These frameworks should aim not only guarantee the technical credibility of forensic results but also to ethically engage with the lived realities of affected populations and the professionals working under extreme conditions. This includes acknowledging that many forensic processes in these environments require creative adaptation, expert judgment, and moral discernment that cannot be fully captured by prescriptive procedures.

Such an approach does not imply abandoning the core principles of quality, such as reliability, traceability, or continuous improvement, but rather reconfiguring them to advance forensic science as a human endeavor, centered on traces, responsive to context, and grounded in inference. Quality, in this sense, must transcend mere procedural compliance to become an enabler of meaningful investigation, scientific integrity, and posthumous dignity. It should be understood as a dynamic and adaptive framework that reinforces the legitimacy of forensic work not only in the eyes of judicial systems, but also among victims' families, local communities, and the community at large.

Ultimately, reimagining quality in this way opens the door to a more resilient and ethically grounded forensic practice, one capable of operating effectively in the face of structural inequalities, institutional fragility, and profound humanitarian challenges. In these complex scenarios, quality should be a means of supporting justice, and human rights, not an obstacle to them.

Accredited forensic laboratories and their quality management systems often appear robust, but this often ignores or distorts the reality of forensic work, generating a popular myth among judicial authorities: if you are not accredited, your results lack scientific quality. In Africa and Latin America, where there is a high demand for forensic services, many efforts have been made and important experiences have been gained that go against the idea that only accredited laboratories can produce scientifically valid results. These areas, which are often limited by a lack of resources and red tape, have shown that it is possible to create strict standards and make a real difference in justice systems even when they are not formally accredited. This shows that scientific quality doesn't just depend on an accreditation seal; it also depends on how dedicated professionals are, how innovative they are, and how well they can meet society's urgent needs (see Chapters 7–). Unfortunately, certification and accreditation are not necessarily or always present, but that does not mean their quality is diminished. The chaotic, unstable, and resource-limited conditions found in real-life settings, particularly those affected by armed conflict, institutional fragility, or systemic violence, rarely resemble the controlled and regulated environment of the laboratory, or expected in standards.

Forensic professionals in many areas are forced to operate with little equipment, under duress from authorities, communities, or security threats, and with limited access to logistical support and training. Without modification, following procedures that are simple to execute in an ISO-accredited laboratory become nearly impossible. For instance, in situations where refrigeration is unavailable, electricity is unstable, or legal protections are inadequate, it can be extremely challenging to maintain chain of custody, ensure sample integrity, or complete standardized documentation.

Furthermore, the applicability, viability, and even morality of forensic interventions may be compromised by strict adherence to international standards without contextual calibration. In these situations, forensic quality needs to be redefined as adaptive competence – the ability to uphold scientific integrity while adapting to changing and resource-constrained circumstances, rather than procedural perfection. In addition to technical proficiency, this calls for cultural awareness, fortitude, and moral discernment. A constructive way forward would be to recognize these constraints openly and to promote flexible, context-sensitive mechanisms that can complement or substitute for full ISO-style procedures when resources are scarce. Rather than dismissing the work of laboratories or professionals who cannot meet every formal requirement, justice systems could encourage the adoption of minimum quality standards, simplified documentation models, and locally adapted practices that still protect the integrity of evidence. International organizations and regional networks might also play a role by providing technical guidance, training, and peer support aimed at strengthening reliability without imposing unattainable benchmarks. Such approaches would allow forensic professionals to operate responsibly in adverse environments while preserving the credibility of their work, demonstrating that scientific rigor is possible even outside ideal laboratory conditions.

For these situations, the SD (Roux et al., 2022) could provide a broader strategic perspective that would allow forensic practitioners to uphold scientific integrity while adapting to operational constraints. Indeed, the SD recommends strategic application of forensic principles, such as openness, critical thinking, and flexibility, guaranteeing that scientific integrity can be maintained even in the absence of completely controlled settings (Olckers and Ben Khelil, 2024).

1.4.1 Brief Overview of the Sydney Declaration

Forensic science has been under the microscope for decades and in more recent time deemed "in crisis" (Roux et al., 2015, 2021; Koheler et al., 2023). If the NRC (2009) and PCAST (2016) reports are probably still fresh in mind, Paul L. Kirk was already pointing out in 1963 that in forensic science "progress has been technical rather than fundamental, practical rather than theoretical, transient rather than permanent" (Kirk, 1963: 235). As highlighted by Roux et al. (2015, 2021, 2022), the crisis may be attributed to an absence of a unified vision and a commonly held understanding of forensic science, coupled with the imperative to reorient the discipline from methodological means toward its foundational purpose. Therefore, in 2022, after decades of questioning, and in a context of growing technological fragmentation within the scientific discourse on forensic science, an informal collective of eminent forensic scientists (academics and practitioners) leveraged the organization of 2023 International Academy of Forensic Science (IAFS) conference in Sydney, Australia, to initiate a critical and holistic reflection on forensic science directions and core principles as a discipline in its own right (Roux et al., 2022; Crispino et al., 2022). The Sydney Declaration was born[6].

The SD constitutes a significant rethinking of forensic science as a practice based on basic epistemic principles (Roux et al., 2022; Olckers and Ben Khelil, 2024; Ribaux et al., 2024; Buzzini, 2024). The SD, which puts the trace at the epistemological center and places it above technology or legal disciplines, has been praised as a daring attempt to rethink forensic science from the ground up. It has had a good initial impact, as evidenced by its promotion in a variety of fora across the globe, its translation into many different languages, and its utility being demonstrated in event reconstruction (Miranda et al., 2023), forensic science development, and operations, for example. The large number of citations in peer-reviewed literature further showed how helpful the SD is to place various forensic practices within a common framework, particularly in interdisciplinary and reflexive contexts (Ribaux et al., 2024). However, this promising initial support should be contrasted against some commonly reported challenges like the perceived ambiguity around the SD's purpose, the use of complex academic language, and uncertainty about its relationship to existing QA frameworks. This conversation within the forensic science community and its stakeholders is ongoing and necessary to bridge the gap between theory and practice. Ultimately, the SD's legitimacy will be determined by its capacity to unite a forensic community that is able to withstand the system's centrifugal forces and validate forensic science as a separate, important, and socially relevant discipline (Ribaux et al., 2024).

[6] An audiovisual resource specially prepared can also be freely viewed at the following link: https://www.youtube.com/watch?v=AaZwQkEpyKE&t=5s

The SD aims to establish a "shared understanding and acceptance of the essence of forensic science, its purpose, and fundamental principles. It provides a definition of forensic science and seven fundamental principles that emphasize the pivotal role of the trace as a vestige, or remnant of an investigated activity." The principles address critical features of forensic science, "such as context, time asymmetry, the continuum of uncertainties, broad scientific knowledge, ethics, critical thinking, and logical reasoning" (Roux et al. 2022: 1).

The SD defines forensic sciences as: "a case-based (or multi-case-based) research-oriented, science-based endeavor to study traces, the remnants of past activities (such as an individual's presence and actions), through their detection, recognition, recovery, examination, and interpretation to understand anomalous events of public interest (e.g., crimes, security incidents)" (Roux et al., 2022: 2). It also comprises of seven principles, articulating "the nature and ground of this discipline:

1. Activity and presence produce traces that are fundamental vectors of information.
2. Scene investigation is a scientific and diagnostic endeavor requiring scientific expertise.
3. Forensic science is case-based and reliant on scientific knowledge, investigative methodology and logical reasoning.
4. Forensic science is an assessment of findings in context due to time asymmetry.
5. Forensic science deals with a continuum of uncertainties.
6. Forensic science has multidimensional purposes and contributions.
7. Forensic science findings acquire meaning in context." (Roux et al., 2022: 2)

The SD offers a foundational reconceptualization of forensic science, shifting the focus from procedural compliance and technical outputs to the essence of what forensic science is and does. Through its definition, the Declaration recenters the discipline around its core epistemology: understanding past events through traces. This definition moves beyond the constraints of laboratory-bound or accreditation-driven models. It acknowledges that forensic science is inherently investigative, interdisciplinary, and dynamic, an approach that resonates particularly well in complex, uncertain, and resource-limited contexts. It recognizes that forensic work is not just about producing laboratory reports but about generating meaningful, contextually situated knowledge that can inform decisions in justice, security, and humanitarian domains. The seven fundamental principles further solidify this framework by grounding forensic science in its scientific and contextual nature The SD embodies the semiotic essence of forensic science (Crispino, 2024).

One common criticism of the SD is that it does not seem to accurately reflect the quality standards and procedures used in accredited forensic laboratories.

This comes from the fact that the SD does not explicitly refer to methods or quality management practices. But this omission should not be seen as opposition. The Declaration does not compete with or replace accreditation frameworks; instead, it sets out general rules that work well with them. It is important to make this difference clear so that there are no misunderstandings and to show that the Declaration and accreditation have different but important roles in forensic science. This impression stems from the fact that the SD does not directly address standardized methods or quality management systems such as those found in ISO frameworks. However, this lack of action should not be interpreted as opposition. Rather, it demonstrates the purpose of the Declaration: to establish universal and transversal principles to guide forensic practice in all operating systems. In this context, quality is not limited to compliance with control standards; it also includes ensuring that results are truly fit for purpose. ISO systems provide the technical basis for control and assurance, but the SD offers the big picture that unites these changes but in a different dimension, a foundational dimension. The SD was meant to stay neutral about organizational structures and accreditation systems from the start. It is not meant to replace them, but to complement them by ensuring that all technical standards are grounded in enduring, fundamental principles.

1.4.2 The Sydney Declaration as an Overarching Strategic Quality Framework for Challenging Environments

As shown above, traditional QA frameworks like ISO/IEC 17025 in forensic science are meant to protect scientific integrity, technical competence, and consistency in settings with a lot of resources. These frameworks make sure that everything can be traced and that people are held accountable by setting strict rules for how things should be done and how they should be documented. But forensic work can't stop just because these kinds of systems are not available or are not practical. In this way, the SD offers a flexible, scientifically sound, and principle-based framework that not only works with current QA systems but can also be used as a guiding framework when formal accreditation is not possible. Even when traditional standards exist, the SD provides the foundational epistemological framework upon which these systems are built. The SD does not compete with ISO-based approaches; instead, it strengthens their legitimacy and fills important gaps in high-pressure, resource-limited, or ethically sensitive environments. This allows forensic science to move forward with integrity and flexibility. The Declaration helps forensic practitioners maintain scientific integrity while adapting to the realities of high-pressure, time-sensitive, or resource-limited settings (Olckers and Ben Khelil, 2024).

For example, within the African context, the SD presents a valuable opportunity to serve as a guiding framework that acknowledges the continent's unique structural complexities, institutional limitations, and sociopolitical diversity.

Its implementation goes beyond a mere statement of principles, offering practical guidance and relevance to the diverse forensic landscapes found across Africa (Olckers and Ben Khelil, 2024; Nkonyane, 2025).

This approach emphasizes the value of expert reasoning and contextual analysis as pillars of sound practice, rather than focusing on tools or infrastructure. Rather than prescribing rigid processes or techniques, the SD offers a set of foundational principles that guide forensic practice when standard operating procedures or validated methods are inaccessible, inapplicable, or underdeveloped. Rooted in the core scientific and philosophical foundations of forensic science, it enables practitioners to produce meaningful and defensible results in dynamic and uncertain contexts. The Declaration provides a strategic anchor for practice by emphasizing the "why" and "how" of forensic science, tracing human activity through scientific inquiry, while allowing flexibility at the operational and tactical levels to adjust methods, tools, and reporting strategies based on the context.

Key contributions of the SD in challenging environments include, but are not limited to:

1. Bridging the gap between rigid QA expectations and on-the-ground realities
2. Enabling transparent practice when conventional validation or accreditation pathways are unavailable
3. Maintaining scientific integrity without reliance on infrastructure-heavy models
4. Supporting adaptability in high-pressure, politically complex, or resource-constrained settings
5. Legitimizing innovation and responsive thinking in the face of novel challenges

In such environments, the Declaration enhances key aspects of forensic science, including reliability, effectiveness, relevance, flexibility, adaptability, and innovation, supporting the long-term resilience, and credibility of the discipline.

1.4.2.1 Enhancing Reliability Through Scientific Grounding

One of the core contributions of the SD lies in its ability to maintain scientific reliability even when traditional indicators of quality – such as accreditation, full validation, or formal SOPs – cannot be met. The Declaration emphasizes:

The trace as the central vector of information (Principle 1), focusing practitioners on the evidential link between presence, activity, and material remnants.

The use of a diagnostic during scene investigation (Principle 2), reinforcing the need for scientific rigor from the outset, including documentation, observation, and hypothesis testing.

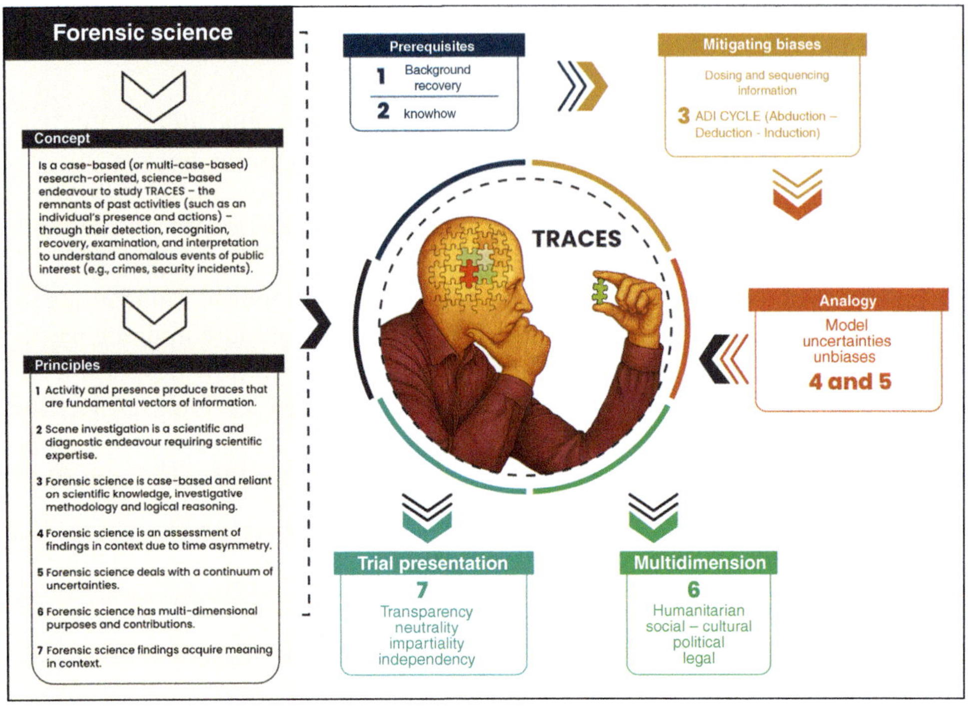

Figure 1.1 A conceptual summary and the theoretical framework that supports the epistemological and operationalizable orientation of the SD (Roux et al., 2022).

The need for contextual interpretation (Principles 4 and 7), ensuring that findings are not assessed in isolation but within the case narrative and investigative goals (Figure 1.1).

By grounding forensic science in the trace and the logic of interpretation, rather than solely in procedural conformity, the Declaration allows for transparent, reproducible reasoning even when technical repeatability is compromised. It encourages evidence-based justification of methods and decisions, reinforcing the trustworthiness of findings under challenging conditions.

1.4.2.2 Ensuring Relevance

In complex or resource-constrained environments, the relevance of forensic science should not be measured solely by its alignment with court-admissibility standards or formal QA frameworks. These settings, such as humanitarian operations, post-conflict investigations, or disaster response, often demand forensic contributions that extend beyond traditional legal proceedings. In such contexts, relevance is defined by the ability to provide timely, meaningful, and contextually appropriate information that supports broader goals, including intelligence, justice, fact-finding, human rights protection, public safety, or reconciliation.

The SD directly addresses this expanded notion of relevance. By recognizing the multidimensional contributions of forensic science (Principle 6), the Declaration broadens the scope of what is considered valuable work – moving beyond court-admissibility alone. It legitimizes forensic work that is strategically aligned with diverse objectives – even when traditional validation pathways or legal infrastructures are absent. This reframing enables practitioners to demonstrate value through impact rather than mere procedural compliance.

1.4.2.3 Supporting Effectiveness and Relevance in Diverse Contexts

The Declaration recognizes that forensic science is fundamentally case-based (Principle 3) and that its primary function is to support understanding of anomalous or criminal events through the study of traces. In doing so, it supports fit-for-purpose practices that respond to the specific demands, timelines, and contextual constraints of each case. This increases the likelihood that forensic outputs are meaningful and actionable within investigative, judicial, or humanitarian settings. In challenging environments, this means:

- Prioritizing relevance of results over rigid process conformity.
- Enabling triage-based approaches where full procedural adherence is not feasible but core scientific principles are still followed.
- Supporting multidisciplinary and cross-jurisdictional collaboration through a shared philosophical framework.

1.4.2.4 Enabling Flexibility and Adaptability

Modern forensic practice increasingly requires agility in the face of rapidly evolving operational conditions. And when standard QA models, designed for static environments, fail to accommodate the complexities of forensic engagements in challenging environments, the Declaration fosters a culture of adaptability and flexibility in the face of uncertainty into its foundational thinking (Principle 5) that is both scientifically grounded and ethically responsible through:

- Reflective practice in the presence of incomplete data
- Innovation in the use of methods and tools to study traces
- Iterative interpretation as more information becomes available

This makes the Declaration inherently responsive to change, whether technological, environmental, or geopolitical, allowing practitioners to adapt in real time, provided they remain grounded in the core principles of trace-based inquiry and contextual understanding.

1.4.2.5 Encourage Innovation While Maintaining Integrity

The SD recognizes that it is not always feasible to follow every QA step to the letter. In these situations, forensic professionals can still uphold forensic integrity by:

- Focusing on critical steps that preserve the chain of custody and the accuracy of results, even when some procedural elements might be simplified or altered.
- Ensuring transparent documentation of any deviations from standard practices, explaining the reasons behind these changes, and the efforts made to maintain scientific accuracy despite the limitations.
- Implementing "compensatory" quality control techniques that are suitable for the specific environment, such as creating additional safeguards or cross-checks, when full QA procedures cannot be followed.

Further, by encouraging foundational thinking, the Declaration creates space for methodological innovation, including new forms of data integration, interdisciplinary collaboration, and use of emerging technologies. Forensic science is not static; it evolves in response to new challenges and emerging technologies. The Declaration facilitates creative problem-solving in situations where established methods do not yet exist or cannot be applied as intended. In this way, the SD functions not only as a fallback when QA systems fail, but as a strategic compass for the future of forensic science, ensuring that the discipline remains scientifically robust, ethically grounded, and contextually responsive even as environments, technologies, and societal expectations continue to evolve. The SD positions forensic science as a discipline with multidimensional purposes and contributions (Principle 6). This view supports innovation not just in technologies or techniques, but in how forensic science aligns with justice, public interest, and human rights. By stepping beyond the constraints of narrow compliance models, the Declaration allows for:

- The development of context-sensitive methodologies,
- The inclusion of non-traditional actors and disciplines in forensic inquiry,
- The advancement of ethical, transparent, and socially responsible science.

Building on the foundational discussion of the African context, recent analyses by Olckers and Ben Khelil (2024) illustrate how the Declaration's principles are being translated into tangible action. For example, its adoption by key scientific bodies has initiated cross-sector dialogues, enhanced institutional recognition, and promoted ethical standards tailored to local realities. These developments not only strengthen the credibility of forensic work within Africa but also provide valuable models for adaptation in other regions facing similar challenges as well as enable African practitioners to align their work with universal scientific and ethical standards, while promoting institutional recognition and appreciation for their efforts (Smith and Horne, 2024).

Furthermore, their proposal highlights how the Declaration can act as a catalyst for transforming fragmented forensic ecosystems into coherent and functional frameworks. The SD has been formally adopted as a founding reference by the African Academy of Forensic Sciences (AFSA), which also encourages its translation and dissemination as a pedagogical and policy tool (Olckers and Ben Khelil, 2024). The authors note that its implementation not only guides practitioners in their daily work but also guides policymakers, academics, journalists, and judicial actors in understanding the boundaries and scope of forensic science. As a result, the Declaration not only redefines what forensic science is but also helps create a common language to defend its place in African legal systems (Olckers and Ben Khelil, 2024; Smith and Horne, 2024). In this sense, the Declaration is not only considered a scientific document but also a transformative platform that enables the imagination of a mature, autonomous, and socially and legally grounded African science.

Forensic services face various obstacles in many African countries, such as insufficient funding and training, and institutional deficiencies, including conceptualization. By ignoring local conditions and material constraints, regulatory models imported from more developed regions are often inapplicable. In recognition of such limitations, the International Forensic Strategic Alliance (IFSA) has developed minimum requirements guidelines to provide a foundational standard for forensic practice in resource-limited settings, offering a practical reference point where local protocols are absent or underdeveloped (IFSA, 2024). The absence of laboratories, training centers, and specialized agencies creates a structural dependence on international cooperation, whose solutions do not always address the specificities of the environment, and even if they do, they cannot be sustainable over time.

Alternatively, the Declaration emphasizes that forensic quality depends on the practitioner's ability to apply sound logical reasoning, maintain methodological transparency, and ensure argumentative traceability, and not solely on formal compliance with procedures or available technology. This allows reliable scientific conclusions to be drawn even in environments with inadequate infrastructure. Based on this reasoning, quality becomes a crucial principle guiding expert judgment in the face of ambiguity (Roux et al., 2022). This declaration's call to create a forensic science grounded in the reality of the challenging environment, with its own identity, based on universal values such as impartiality, traceability, and rigor, but adapted to local circumstances, is one of its most revolutionary and noteworthy features. The goal is to create morally sound and practical frameworks for action that address the problems and realities of the country, not to replicate the systems of other countries.

This approach defends scientific integrity and strengthens the ethical commitment to the truth in environments where forensic specialists are subject to institutional pressures or training limitations, even where they do not exist and are still developing. However, this perspective contrasts with the real situation in countries like the Democratic Republic of Congo, where there is virtually no organized forensic infrastructure, and capacity building for specialized human resources is still in its infancy. While international assistance has been crucial, thanks to the Office of the United Nations High Commissioner for Human Rights (OHCHR), through its UNJHRO office in the DRC and its forensic team, it focuses on contexts of violence and the fight against impunity. Its work combines specialized technical assistance, forensic operations, and strengthening access to justice. It also highlights how difficult it is to develop lasting capacities at the national level. A real challenge that is being faced.

In Latin America, the Middle East, and Asia, where forensic practice encounters equally complex and difficult circumstances, experiences akin to those Olckers and Ben Khelil (2024) detailed in the African context can also be seen (Bouzin et al., 2021, 2023; Howes et al., 2024). Forensic science is not always developed in well-equipped laboratories or under unified regulatory frameworks in these contexts, which are characterized by structural inequality, institutional limitations, chronic violence, or political instability. Conversely, forensic specialists must work in unstable, humanitarian, or disjointed justice systems, which emphasizes the applicability of the strategy put forth in the Declaration. As in the African region, the SD provides methodological and ethical guidance in these areas that goes beyond available resources and focuses on the fundamental goals of the discipline, including intellectual honesty in the face of uncertainty, scientific rigor, inferential clarity, and dedication to evidence. As a result, the reflections of Olckers and Ben Khelil (2024) and Roux et al. (2022) take on a universal dimension by reminding us that the principles of forensic science, not its instruments, constitute its true foundation. Consequently, the Declaration serves as a common platform for forensic scientists operating in complex environments globally and who share a steadfast dedication to justice, truth, and human dignity, despite its technical challenges.

1.4.3 Forensic Science in Practice: Intersecting the Mechanisms of Compliance with Epistemic Logic

The SD and conventional QA systems should not be perceived as contradictory or antagonistic criteria, as they operate in different dimensions. QA focuses on control, standardization, and verification. The SD, on the other hand, focuses on fundamentals, establishing the essential epistemological rules for forensic practice. It is also important to remember that the SD is the foundation upon which QA systems can be built or modified. When traditional models are unavailable or difficult to implement, the SD serves as a basis and guide for redesigning relevant frameworks in the operational environment. The SD seeks to rebalance these perspectives, reminding us that the true power of forensic science lies not in repeating steps, but in producing reliable, well-founded, and contextualized interpretations. According to this view, experience and technical tools are subordinated to the logical and persuasive skills of the expert, who assigns meaning to traces with transparency, while adapting to the unique context of each case.

The contemporary debate on quality management in forensic science highlights a tension between external manifestations of quality and its profound scientific content. Standardization through accreditation systems such as ISO 17025 was designed to generate confidence in processes, but has often led to a culture of regulatory compliance in which adherence to procedures is prioritized over the exercise of expert judgment (Neuteboom et al., 2023). This centralization of control can displace the interpretive authority of the scientist, replacing it with the apparent security offered by certificates and external audits (Ross and Neuteboom 2020a). As a result, the critical thinking and flexibility needed to address complex cases risk being overshadowed by the rigidity of protocols and general standards. As Neuteboom and Ross (2024) point out, this tension manifests itself in the gap between managers, who are adopters of standards, and professionals, who are skeptical and demand space for scientific thought, which poses the challenge of balancing transparency and flexibility so as not to sacrifice scientific essence for the sake of bureaucracy.

This phenomenon has been observed to reflect a general trend in the institutional management of forensic science, where respect for scientific thought is subordinated to compliance with procedures. This operational logic, supported by auditing and oversight procedures, reduces the importance of forensic work to the mere existence of official records, without necessarily assessing the quality of the logic that underpins them.

The adoption of mass production models in forensic science has led to this shift being interpreted as a component of an "industrial culture." However, forensic science is not a factory system. Judgment, interpretation, and situated knowledge are essential to its essence. Evidence presented in Court or to other stakeholders consist of deciphered data influenced by its context, the recovery environment, and the inferential chain that allows for the reconstruction of historical events.

Forensic quality management necessitates the equilibrium of normativity and scientific rationality, guaranteeing that formal compliance does not supplant critical reflection while promoting resilient, adaptable processes genuinely aimed at enhancing knowledge. The aim is to ensure that established procedures support, rather than limit, the interpretive abilities of forensic scientists. Practitioners should be equipped not only with operational skills but also with a solid foundation in logic, epistemology, and metacognitive strategies, especially when confronted with evidence that is ambiguous, incomplete, or open to multiple interpretations (Bruenisholz et al., 2024; Neuteboom et al., 2023).

Forensic practice relies heavily on the practitioner's ability to draw reliable inference from scarce and often incomplete or compromised data and resources in critical environments. This is especially the case in African or Latin American contexts, where fully equipped forensic laboratories and robust institutional protocols are generally lacking. In this case, forensic epistemology does not conflict with the absence of standards; rather, it is exemplified by the ability to act with responsibility, rigor, and judgment, even in uncertain situations (Roux et al., 2022).

Modern forensic science should not be viewed as a rigid dichotomy between a mechanistic model, which emphasizes auditability and compliance with formal regulations, and an introspective approach based on fundamentals, on essence. The SD argues that quality in forensic work transcends mere procedural standards and must be based on deeper principles: appropriate logical reasoning and interpretation of findings in context, and utmost commitment to ethics and transparency. Effective control and verification mechanisms are necessary to guarantee that information remains traceable and that processes are transparent and accessible to all. However, these alone do not guarantee the epistemic soundness of conclusions. The Declaration's call for introspection is not intended to supplant these tools; rather, it seeks to incorporate them into a comprehensive framework that views quality as a multidimensional construct encompassing technical rigor, interpretive soundness, and ethical responsibility. The real challenge for forensic science, therefore, is to integrate both levels so that formal procedures can contribute to a reflective, critical, and socially useful practice. In this second horizon, forensic science is emerging as a scientifically rigorous and human-centered discipline, capable of navigating uncertainty, an evolution supported by the SD.

1.5 Conclusion: How Should the Road Actually Appear?

Forensic science is increasingly recognizing the limitations of simplistic models that equate quality with rigid adherence to industrial quality management protocols, signaling a shift toward more nuanced and purpose-driven approaches. Such models could take away the discipline's epistemological depth and turn it into a bureaucratic exercise in following the rules. In this context, the Sydney Declaration (SD) stands out as a key turning point. Its significance does not reside in offering technical recommendations, but in delineating an epistemological and semiotic framework that reinstates forensic science to its scientific core. Crispino (2024) posits that the SD embodies the semiotic assertion of forensic science, acknowledging that the forensic trace is not a mere residue but a sign whose significance must be deciphered through a logical and transparent process aimed at a variety of purposes associated with secure societies.

This acknowledgment represents what could be referred to as Dimension A, the fundamental foundation of the discipline. Dimension A encompasses both ontology, the trace as sign, and axiology, the duty to produce valid, comprehensible, and transparent knowledge. It lays down rules that go beyond technical protocols, such as recognizing the inherent uncertainty of the trace (e.g. being generated by a unique context and compromised or incomplete) and inference (e.g. abduction where an observation may be due to more than on possible cause), clearly explaining reasoning, and making sure that results are shared in a way that non-experts can understand. Dimension A protects the epistemic integrity of forensic practice and stops it from becoming just a procedural or administrative task.

Dimension B, the control logics, is built on this foundation. It includes the methodological and normative frameworks that are meant to put the principles of the SD into action. ISO 21043 is the first international standard that is only for forensic science. ISO 21043 talks about the whole forensic process, from finding items (Part 2), to analyzing them (Part 3), interpreting them (Part 4), and writing reports (Part 5). It also sets up a common vocabulary (Part 1). Part 4: Interpretation is especially important within this framework. Morrison et al. (2025) and Berger (2025) say that it sets up a structured way for experts to think about things, separating investigative interpretation, which tries to come up with hypotheses or explanations, from evaluative interpretation, which looks at competing ideas within the likelihood-ratio framework. The standard says that all data and assumptions must be clearly documented, methods must be validated, and limitations must be clearly stated. This promotes both accountability and consistency across jurisdictions.

Dimension B also includes more general standards that are widely used in forensic practice. For example, ISO/IEC 17025 sets general requirements for the competence of testing and calibration laboratories, and ISO/IEC 17020 sets rules for conformity assessment for inspection bodies, including those that investigate crime scenes. These standards are not only for forensic use, but they are still very important for QA, accreditation, and getting forensic laboratories recognized around the world. In addition to ISO 21043, they make up a set of rules that help forensic science be more comparable, reproducible, and credible.

The relationship between Dimension A and Dimension B is neither linear nor uniform. Instead, it can be viewed as a quantum multiverse where both exist, although not always in the same way. Dimension A is foundational and has its own theoretical nature that can be operationalized on its own, while Dimension B depends on both explicit and implicit conditions. Although the two work well together and would help forensic professionals understand and act much better professionally, this is not often the case, at least in challenging environments. In environments with ample resources, characterized by accredited laboratories, skilled personnel, and reliable infrastructures, Dimension B can be comprehensively executed, integrating ISO 21043 with ISO/IEC 17025 and ISO/IEC 17020 to create stringent QA systems. In such cases, the interplay between foundational epistemic principles (Dimension A) and operational normative frameworks (Dimension B) yields a forensic practice that is both scientifically robust and socially legitimate.

However, in difficult situations where resources are scarce, institutions are weak, or the judicial system is overloaded, Dimension B cannot always be fully put into action. International accreditation schemes often involve significant costs and time commitments, particularly for activities such as periodic audits, technical validations, and proficiency testing. Local resources may not be able to handle all of this. Imposing these frameworks universally may lead to unintended consequences, such as the exclusion of laboratories unable to comply, or the promotion of superficial adherence that creates an illusion of compliance without genuinely enhancing scientific quality.

In these situations, Dimension A's implementation becomes critical. Even without complete quality control systems, the epistemological and semiotic principles of the SD can direct forensic practice in scientifically valid manners. Recognizing the trace as a sign, utilizing clear logical reasoning, and articulating uncertainty offer basic assurances of quality that can be implemented without expensive accreditation programs. In this sense, the ultimate objective is not to do away with regulations, but to return forensic practice to its original scientific meaning, ensuring that forensic science is more than a ritual of compliance and remains an autonomous epistemic endeavor.

This observation has direct implications for numerous regions in Latin America, Africa, and Asia, where forensic systems function amid structural instability. In these kinds of situations, Dimension A is the most important place to start. It enables forensic scientists to formulate clear and logical conclusions, even when operating with limited resources. As economic and institutional conditions improve, elements of Dimension B, such as ISO 21043, ISO/IEC 17025, ISO/IEC 17020, and related frameworks, can be progressively implemented, reinforcing the foundational principles already established.

In conclusion, the SD (Dimension A) and international standards like ISO 21043, ISO/IEC 17025, and ISO/IEC 17020 (Dimension B) are not mutually exclusive options; they are two parts of the same considerations that must work together. The first delineates the epistemological and semiotic underpinnings of forensic science, whereas the second sets the methodological framework for its implementation. In contexts abundant in resources, both dimensions can be fully actualized, resulting in a sophisticated and cohesive forensic practice. In contexts with limited resources, Dimension A must be the most important part, making sure that forensic science stays scientifically and socially valid while also making it possible for Dimension B to be added gradually.

When viewed through this dual lens, forensic science can be seen as a transformative field that maintains its independence, rigor, and social relevance while broadening its scope in response to new challenges. Developing a strong forensic culture, based on thorough education, institutional dedication, and constant innovation, will not only ensure its reliability but also enable the forensic field to appropriately meet standards, improve justice systems, and proactively address the evolving requirements of global society in diverse environments, starting with the most challenging.

References

AFP (2022) Operation Alliance: 2002 Bali Bombings. https://www.afp.gov.au/news-centre/podcasts/operation-alliance-2002-bali-bombings (accessed December 3, 2025).

AFP (2024) Search among the sunflowers. https://www.afp.gov.au/news-centre/podcasts/mh17-10-year-anniversary (accessed December 2025).

Ballantyne, K.N. and Wilson Wilde, L. (2020) Assessing the reliability and validity of forensic science – An industry perspective. *Australian Journal of Forensic Sciences*, **52**(3), 275–281. https://doi.org/10.1080/00450618.2019.1704058.

Ballantyne, K.N., Summersby, S., Pearson, J.R., Nicol, K., Pirie, E., Quinn, C., *et al.* (2024) A transparent approach: Openness in forensic science reporting. *Forensic Science International*, **8**, 100474. https://doi.org/10.1016/j.fsisyn.2024.100474.

Bennett A. (2023) Final report: Commission of inquiry to examine DNA project 13 concerns. Queensland. https://www.dnaproject13inquiry.qld.gov.au/assets/DNA%20Project%2013%20Report.pdf (open in a new window) (accessed December 3, 2025).

Berger, C.E.H. (2025) Finally a really forensic worldwide standard: ISO 21043 Forensic sciences, Part 4, Interpretation. *Forensic Science International: Synergy*, **10**, 100589. https://doi.org/10.1016/j.fsisyn.2025.100589.

Bitzer, S., Albertini, N., Lock, E., Ribaux, O., and Delémont, O. (2015) Utility of the clue — From assessing the investigative contribution of forensic science to supporting the decision to use traces. *Science & Justice*, **55**(6), 509–513. https://doi.org/10.1016/j.scijus.2015.05.005.

Bouzin, J.T., Sauzier, G., and Lewis, S.W. (2021) Forensic science in Seychelles: An example of a micro-jurisdiction forensic delivery system. *Forensic Science International: Synergy*, **3**, 100139. https://10.1016/j.fsisyn.2021.100139.

Bouzin, J.T., Lópes, T., Heavey, A.L., Parrish, J., Sauzier, G., and Lewis, S.W. (2023) Mind the gap: The challenges of sustainable forensic science service provision. *Forensic Science International: Synergy*, **6**, 100318. https://doi.org/10.1016/j.fsisyn.2023.100318.

Bruenisholz, E., Bunford, J., Jones, K., Knott, F., Lam, A., Tahtouh, M., *et al.* (2024) Operational relevance of the Sydney Declaration: The example of the Australian Federal Police (AFP) Forensics Command. *Forensic Science International*, **359**, 112035. https://doi.org/10.1016/j.forsciint.2024.112035.

Budowle, B. (2025) Independent review of operational matters at forensic science Queensland and recommendations for foundational reform – based on specified terms of reference. https://www.parliament.qld.gov.au/Work-of-the-Assembly/Tabled-Papers/docs/5825t0891/5825t891.pdf (accessed December 3, 2025).

Buzzini, P. (2024) Kirk's 'Ontogeny of Criminalistics' revisited under the lens of the Sydney Declaration. *Forensic Science International*, **359**, 112023.

Cole, S.A. (2013) Forensic culture as epistemic culture: The sociology of forensic science. *Studies in History and Philosophy of Biological and Biomedical Sciences*, **44**(1), 36–46.

Crispino, F. (2024) Towards a forensic semiotics. *Forensic Science International*, **357**, 111968. https://doi.org/10.1016/j.forsciint.2024.111968.

Crispino, F. and Roux, C. (2017) Forensic-led regulation strategies: Are they fit for security problem-solving purposes? In: *The Routledge International Handbook of Forensic Intelligence and Criminology* (eds. Q. Rossy *et al.*). Routledge, Abingdon, Oxon, UK, pp. 65–76.

Crispino, F., Weyermann, C., Delémont, O., Roux, C., and Ribaux, O. (2022) Towards another paradigm for forensic science? *Wiley Interdisciplinary Reviews: Forensic Science*, **4**(3), e1441.

Deming, W.E. (1986) *Out of the Crisis*. MIT Center for Advanced Engineering Study. (500 pp.)

Dror, I.E. (2025) Biased and biasing: The hidden bias cascade and bias snowball effects. *Behavioral Sciences*, **15**(4), 490.

Farmer, P. (2004) *An anthropology of structural violence. Current Anthropology*, **45**(3), 305–325.

Galtung, J. (1969) *Violence, peace, and peace research. Journal of Peace Research*, **6**(3), 167–191.

Garvin, D.A. (1988) *Managing Quality: The Strategic and Competitive Edge*. The Free Press.

Hazard, Đ. (2014) La pertinence en science forensique : une (en)quête épistémologique et empirique. Thesis, University of Lausanne. 281pp.

Hazard, Đ., Stauffer, E., and Margot, P. (2014) Forensic science and the paradigm of quality. In: *Encyclopedia of Criminology and Criminal Justice* (eds. G. Bruinsma and D. Weisburd). Springer, New York, NY. https://doi.org/10.1007/978-1-4614-5690-2_141.

Howes, L.M., Julian, R., Wilson, R., and dos Santos, M.C. (2024) Forensic science capacity development: A case study of Timor-Leste. *Forensic Science International: Synergy*, **9**, 100553. https://doi.org/10.1016/j.fsisyn.2024.100553.

Illes, M., Wilson, P., and Bruce, C. (2020) Forensic epistemology: A need for research and pedagogy. *Forensic Science International: Synergy*, **2**, 51–59.

International Forensic Strategic Alliance (IFSA). (2024). Minimum Requirements Documents. https://www.ifsa-forensics.org/minimum-requirements-documents/ (accessed December 3, 2025).

Juran, J.M. (1995) *A History of Managing for Quality: The Evolution, Trends, and Future Directions of Managing for Quality*. McGraw-Hill.

Kelty, S.F., Julian, R., and Robertson, J. (2011) Professionalism in crime scene examination: The seven key attributes of top crime scene examiners. *Forensic Science Policy & Management: An International Journal*, **2**(4), 175–186. https://doi.org/10.1080/19409044.2012.693572.

Kelty, S.F., Robertson, J., and Julian, R. (2017) Beyond technical training to professionalism in crime scene examination: Enhancing cognitive, leadership, and social abilities in career development programs. *Forensic Science Policy & Management: An International Journal*, **8**(3–4), 65–78.

Kelty, S.F., Ribaux, O., and Robertson, J. (2023) Identifying the critical skillset of top crime scene examiners: Why this matters and why agencies should develop top performers. *WIREs Forensic Science*, **5**, 5.

Kelty, S.F., Joshua, P.R., and Robertson, J. (2024) Building on the critical skills framework of top crime scene examiners to recruit high-caliber crime scene investigation candidates. *WIREs Forensic Science*, **6**(5), e1519. https://doi.org/10.1002/wfs2.1519.

Kirk, P.L. (1963) The ontogeny of criminalistics. *Journal of Criminal Law and Criminology*, **54**, 235–238. https://scholarlycommons.law.northwestern.edu/cgi/viewcontent.cgi?article=5166&context=jclc.

Koehler, J.J., Mnookin, J.L., and Saks, M.J. (2023) The scientific reinvention of forensic science. *Northwestern University Law Review*, **117**(3), 743–788. https://doi.org/10.2139/ssrn.4475282.

Komar, D., El Jundi, S., Parra, R.C., and Perich, P. (2021) A comparison of the international protocols for the forensic assessment of conflict-related sexual violence victims. *Journal of Forensic Sciences.*, **66**(4), 1520–1523.

Lentini, J.J. (2009) Forensic science standards: Where they come from and how they are used. *Forensic Science Policy and Management: An International Journal*, **1**(1), 10–16.

Margot, P. (2011) Commentary on the need for a research culture in the forensic sciences. *UCLA Law Review*, **58**(3), 795–801.

Miranda, M.D., Buzzini, P., De Forest, P.R., and Willis, S. (2023) An exercise in scientific problem solving: Illustrating the utility of the principles of the Sydney declaration. *Journal of Forensic Sciences*, **68**(5), 1835–1842.

Morrison, G.S., Eliott, S., Guiness, J., Sonden, L., and Syndercombe Court, D. (2025) A guide to ISO 21043 Forensic Sciences from the perspective of the forensic-data-science paradigm. *Science & Justice*, **65**(5), 101304. https://doi.org/10.1016/j.scijus.2025.101304.

Mousseau, V., Morelato, M., and Roux, C. (2025) The quest for regulating crime scene investigation in forensic science: Can we learn about discretion and standardization from other fields? *Wires*, **7**(2). https://doi.org/10.1002/wfs2.70010.

NRC, National Research Council (2009) *Strengthening Forensic Science in the United States: A Path Forward*. National Academies Press.

Neuteboom, W. and Ross, A. (2024) Shall the twain ever meet? *Australian Journal of Forensic Sciences*. https://doi.org/10.1080/00450618.2024.2363823.

Neuteboom, W., Ross, A., Bugeja, L., Willis, S., Roux, C., and Lothridge, K. (2023) Quality management in forensic science: A closer inspection. *Forensic Science International*, **111779**. https://doi.org/10.1016/j.forsciint.2023.111779.

Nkonyane, N., 2025. The Sidney Declaration: Revisiting the Essence of Forensic Science https://www.linkedin.com/posts/nokuthula-nkonyane-45892115b_forensicscience-sidneydeclaration-collaboration-activity-7299819806021632000-UY3T (accessed December 3, 2025).

Olckers, A. and Ben Khelil, M. (2024) The Sydney declaration – An unique opportunity for Africa. *Forensic Science International*, **357**, 111969. https://doi.org/10.1016/j.forsciint.2024.111969.

Olson, A. and Ramsay, C. (2025) Errors in toxicology testing and the need for full discovery. *Forensic Science International: Synergy*, **11**, 100629. https://doi.org/10.1016/j.fsisyn.2025.100629.

Periera, P. (1985) Quality assurance in forensic science. *Forensic Science International*, **28**(1), 1–6. https://doi.org/10.1016/0379-0738(85)90159-8.

PCAST, President's Council of Advisors on Science and Technology. (2016) Forensic science in criminal courts: Ensuring scientific validity of feature-comparison methods. Executive Office of the President.

Ranson, D. (2015) The loss of Malaysia airlines flight MH17: A forensic and humanitarian task. *Journal of Law and Medicine*, **22**(4), 745–750. PMID: 26349375.

Ribaux, O., Lopes, F.K., and Weyermann, C. (2024) Signs of how the Sydney Declaration article is received in the forensic science literature. *Forensic Science International*, **360**, 112066. https://doi.org/10.1016/j.forsciint.2024.112066.

Ross, A. and Neuteboom, W. (2020a) ISO-accreditation – Is that all there is for forensic science? *Australian Journal of Forensic Sciences.* https://doi.org/10.1080/00450618.2020.1819414.

Ross, A. and Neuteboom, W. (2020b) Implementation of quality management from a historical perspective: The forensic science odyssey. *Australian Journal of Forensic Sciences.* https://doi.org/10.1080/00450618.2019.1704058.

Roux, C., Talbot-Wright, B., Robertson, J., Crispino, F., and Ribaux, O. (2015) The end of the (forensic science) world as we know it? The example of trace evidence. *Philosophical Transactions of the Royal Society B: Biological Sciences,* **370**(1674), 20140260. https://doi.org/10.1098/rstb.2014.0260.

Roux, C., Willis, S., and Weyermann, C. (2021) Shifting forensic science focus from means to purpose: A path forward for the discipline? *Science & Justice,* **61**, 678–686. https://doi.org/10.1016/j.scijus.2021.08.005.

Roux, C., Bucht, R., Crispino, F., De Forest, P., Lennard, C., Margot, P., *et al.* (2022) The Sydney Declaration – Revisiting the essence of forensic science through its fundamental principles. *Forensic Science International,* **332**, 111182. https://doi.org/10.1016/j.forsciint.2022.111182.

Smith, J.H. and Horne, J.S. (2024) Quality management system in forensic science: An African perspective. *Forensic Science International: Synergy,* **8**, 100476. https://doi.org/10.1016/j.fsisyn.2024.100476.

Sofronoff W. (2022) Final report: commission of inquiry into forensic DNA testing in Queensland. Queensland. https://www.health.qld.gov.au/__data/assets/pdf_file/0036/1196685/final-report-coi-dna-testing-qld-dec-2022.pdf (open in a new window).

Taylor, F.W. (1911) *The Principles of Scientific Management.* Harper & Brothers.

Walvisch, J., Kogios, R., and Davey, A. (2024) Forensic science in the justice system: Learnings from the Queensland DNA inquiry. *Australian Journal of Forensic Sciences,* **57**(4), 418–425. https://doi.org/10.1080/00450618.2024.2363816.

Weyermann, C. and Roux, C. (2021) A different perspective on the forensic science crisis. *Forensic Science International,* **323**, 110779. https://doi.org/10.1016/j.forsciint.2021.110779.

Willis, S. (2010) *Power, Process, People: A Critical Look at ISO Accreditation and What it Means for the Forensic Science Community.* National Institute of Forensic Science.

Willis, S. (2022) The professionalisation of forensic science. *WIREs Forensic Science,* **5**(1), e1478. Advance online publication. https://doi.org/10.1002/wfs2.1478.

Wilson-Wilde, L. (2018) The international development of forensic science standards – A review. *Forensic Science International,* **288**(1), 9.

Wright, K., Wilson L., and Sears, A (2025) *Review of Blackburn DNA Analysis.* https://www.parliament.qld.gov.au/Work-of-the-Assembly/Tabled-Papers/docs/5825T0889/5825t889.pdf. (accessed December 3, 2025).

Zhang, A.L. and Lu, H. (2025) When scientists share their struggles: How scientists' self-presentation on social media influences public perceptions, support for science, and information-seeking intentions. *Science Communication.* https://doi.org/10.1177/10755470251322902.

CHAPTER 2

Artificial Intelligence in Forensic Science: An Important Opportunity for Challenging Environments

Roberto C. Parra[1,*], Gian Carlo Iannacone[2], and Allan G. Alvarez-Godoy[3]
[1] *The Specialized Forensic Team of the United Nations Joint Human Rights Office (UNJHRO) in the Democratic Republic of the Congo*
[2] *Institute of Legal Medicine and Forensic Sciences of Peru, Lima, Peru*
[3] *International Forensic Consultant, The Hague, Netherlands*

2.1 Introduction

Artificial intelligence (AI) has changed many fields of science and, among them, forensic science (Geradts and Franke, 2023). It is at the forefront of recent advancements in evidence-based disciplines due to its ability to process large datasets, precisely identify patterns, and automate analytical procedures (Stacey et al., 2025). AI represents a fundamental shift in the way forensic science functions, moving away from manual, expert-dependent methodologies and toward systems powered by intelligent algorithms that can learn, adapt, and even predict complex forensic phenomena (Stacey et al., 2025). This is far from just a fad and it is here to stay.

Practically speaking, AI improves forensic procedures by making workflows more standardized, repeatable, and effective (Geradts and Franke, 2023; Stacey et al., 2025; RTI, 2025; DOJ, 2025). The interdisciplinary reference work "*Artificial Intelligence (AI) in Forensic Sciences*," edited by Zeno Geradts and Katrin Franke, critically analyzes the application of AI in modern forensic practice. From a scholarly and scientific standpoint, the book incorporates theoretical and practical contributions from biometric and genetic pattern analysis to image, audio, and video processing. It is pertinent because it examines ethical, privacy, and standardization concerns in addition to the validity, explainability, and

*The views expressed herein are those authors and do not necessarily reflect the views of the United Nations.

Forensic Science and Quality Management: Addressing the Era of Standardization in Challenging Environments, First Edition. Edited by Roberto C. Parra and Allan G. Alvarez-Godoy.

dependability of algorithms in legal settings. As a result, the book is an essential tool for scholars, forensic specialists, and attorneys who want to comprehend the advantages and disadvantages of AI in the creation and assessment of forensic evidence.

The integration of AI into forensic science signifies a paradigm shift in both administrative management and forensic investigation processing (DOJ, 2025; RTI, 2025; Stacey et al., 2025). An academic forum to methodically examine the opportunities and risks of this technology was provided by the recent symposium titled "Harnessing AI for Forensics,"[1] which was organized by RTI International[2] with assistance from the National Institute of Standards and Technology (NIST)[3] and the Johns Hopkins University Data Science and AI Institute.[4] The symposium was held in August 2025 at the Johns Hopkins University Bloomberg Center (RTI, 2025).[5] Three important application dimensions were found as a result of this event.

The first strategic use of AI is *"resource allocation."* Staffing, equipment, and response time are major limitations for forensic laboratories. AI systems can estimate case length and complexity through predictive analysis of historical data, allowing for more effective resource allocation and empirical support for budget management. In addition to increasing output, this optimization promotes accountability and transparency in the legal system. The second important contribution is the *"prioritization of cases and evidence."* Machine learning algorithms are able to predict which evidence is most promising and automatically categorize cases based on their urgency. By reducing the backlog of less complicated cases and speeding up response times for high-priority crimes, this capability improves equity in access to justice.

Finally, by combining various evidence sources (chemical, fingerprint, and biological) into a single analytical framework, AI promotes more *"cohesive intelligence."* By identifying patterns, correlations, and possible connections between investigations, this integration helps forensic analysts produce more comprehensive and solid knowledge. But in order to keep systems trustworthy, auditable, and free from prejudices that might jeopardize justice, the symposium underlined the necessity of rigorous human oversight.

The symposium highlights that AI should be viewed as a methodological supplement that strengthens the pursuit of justice and truth by augmenting human capabilities in forensic science, rather than as a replacement. This is especially helpful in nations with underdeveloped institutional quality frameworks, where variations in forensic procedures may compromise the validity of results. In countries where quality standards for forensic science processes have not yet been incorporated, as is the case with ISO standards, AI can be applied as a tool

[1] See https://forensicrti.org/harnessing-ai-forensics/
[2] See https://www.rti.org
[3] See https://www.nist.gov
[4] See https://ai.jhu.edu
[5] See https://washingtondc.jhu.edu/news/ai-in-forensics/

to standardize these processes and thus generate more reliable analysis results (Ketsekioulafis et al. 2024). AI technologies provide tools that mimic human decision-making, but they are more reliable and resistant to cognitive bias. In this situation, automation serves as a tool to promote methodological transparency and analytical rigor, two essential components of forensic reliability, rather than just a quick fix.

The ability of AI to replace mechanistic tasks, those repetitive, operationally predictable processes that are frequently subject to strict quality control requirements, is one of its main advantages. These are usually highlighted in regulatory or administrative frameworks that require formal compliance, sometimes without giving enough thought to the analysis's scientific justification. AI can act as a support system in these situations, guaranteeing procedural component standardization, traceability, and error reduction. This frees up human experts to concentrate on what really requires intellectual work: the interpretative and reflexive aspects of forensic practice, where theoretical foundation, judgment, and context are crucial. Therefore, expertise is not replaced by AI; rather, it is shielded from being weakened by excessive bureaucracy.

This development of forensic applications with AI is also compatible with the principles of the Sydney Declaration, which demands that forensic science continue to be sound scientifically, sensitive to context, and relevant to society. This is made possible by AI, which promotes both ethical application and technical accuracy. It supports expert opinions' objectivity and defensibility, both of which are critical in legal proceedings (Barash et al., 2024). When appropriately developed and validated, automated tools help guarantee that forensic findings are repeatable and understandable to nonexpert audiences, including communities and courts, while also minimizing human error.

In this regard, AI and nanotechnology advancements can greatly support two crucial forensic analysis components taken into account in the Sydney Declaration: (1) creating a sufficient crime scene analysis method to gather the most traces and (2) encouraging more objectivity in the processing of traces by employing automated detection and classification techniques. The application of AI in forensics would then be pertinent since it enables automation for increased accuracy and precision, which lowers bias and analysis errors. Additionally, it makes it possible to prepare expert reports, promote multidisciplinary work in real time, and interpret results objectively. This makes it easier to put the Sydney Declaration's recommendations into practice.

However, forensic science must proceed cautiously when integrating AI. The objective is to rethink forensic problem-solving using a new paradigm of intelligent systems, not to digitally duplicate conventional techniques. It also necessitates understanding the moral, legal, and normative ramifications, especially with regard to accountability, equity, and transparency (Stacey et al., 2025). AI has the potential to make forensic science a more dependable, flexible, and scientifically based field, but only if it is integrated carefully and responsibly.

This chapter examines how AI is revolutionizing forensic science, emphasizing how it can streamline procedures, reduce bias, and enhance the general caliber of analysis. AI is positioned as a supplemental tool to assist forensic practitioners rather than to replace human expertise, particularly in repetitive or highly regulated tasks where accuracy and consistency are crucial. AI ensures that forensic practice stays rigorous, scientifically based, and responsive to the intricacies of real-life cases by taking over these mechanistic tasks, freeing up experts to concentrate more on the interpretive and contextual elements of their work.

However, AI plays a strategic role that goes beyond its technical one, providing forensic institutions with chances to improve their scientific integrity and accountability culture. AI has the potential to improve the effectiveness and breadth of forensic investigation by combining various types of evidence and identifying patterns in intricate datasets. It is crucial to remember that our goal is obviously not even a comprehensive analysis of the vast field that this topic of AI encompasses, as new ideas and discussions are produced daily and even the most fantastical ideas can come true. Instead, this chapter seeks to draw attention to new opportunities and critically examine them in order to promote a continuing discussion about how AI can responsibly direct the course of forensic science going forward, especially in difficult situations.

2.2 Impact of Artificial Intelligence on Forensic Sciences Within the Framework of the Principles of the Sydney Declaration

In Chapter 1 of this book, it has been described how the Sydney Declaration can be a valuable opportunity for operationalization in challenging environments. The Sydney Declaration establishes the basic principles for maintaining scientific integrity in forensic practice. In this context, AI has gained relevance over the years and will play a fundamental role in the development of forensic science through its application throughout the stages of forensic processes. The use of AI can optimize data interpretation and decision-making based on verifiable information, making it a key tool for various applications in forensic science, as described below.

2.2.1 Evidence Identification with AI and Nanotechnology

The strategic triad of nanotechnology, AI, and human reasoning is redefining the operational and epistemological underpinnings of modern forensic science (Chango et al., 2024). With nanotechnology expanding the scope of what can be detected, AI improving the ability to analyze and automate, and human reasoning contributing meaning, critical judgment, and ethical responsibility to the interpretive process, each of these elements offers a complementary and essential dimension to address the complexity of contemporary forensic scenarios (Chango et al., 2024).

By creating vast amounts of high-resolution data, nanotechnology in this integrated model makes it possible to access even the smallest traces of evidence via sensors, markers, or sophisticated visualization systems. Then, using trained algorithms, AI acts as an intelligent filter, processing this data, identifying trends, categorizing anomalies, or putting forth initial theories. The results are validated, contrasted, and interpreted by the human expert, who combines their theoretical training, contextual knowledge, and legal sensitivity to create a cohesive, socially relevant, and legally sound scientific narrative.

This equilibrium is essential to prevent an unwarranted dependence on automated systems, particularly when the outcomes have significant legal ramifications. AI can lessen prejudices and systematic mistakes, but it cannot take the place of a human's capacity to assess risks, identify exceptions, or evaluate data in situations that are emotionally, historically, or culturally complex. Additionally, ethical oversight is made possible by human reasoning, which guarantees that technological choices adhere to frameworks of justice, equity, and transparency.

In summary, intelligent articulation between reflexive (human judgment), algorithmic (AI), and micro (nanotechnology) is where the true potential of this convergence lies, not in substitution. Without sacrificing the ethical and epistemic commitment that characterizes the expert's role in the pursuit of truth, this synergy fortifies a more accurate, flexible, and trustworthy forensic practice (Kosta et al. 2024; Chango et al., 2024).

2.2.2 Automation and Robotization in Forensic Analysis

Automation has significantly transformed the collection and analysis of evidence in forensic science, reducing the margin of error and improving the reliability of results. Robots with AI can handle evidence with greater precision than humans, eliminating errors caused by poor handling that lead to contamination and/or degradation from sample collection to processing (Kowalski et al., 2014). Furthermore, these robotic systems are equipped with advanced sensors capable of detecting biological and chemical traces at crime scenes, providing more efficient collection and avoiding external interference. In forensic laboratories, automation has allowed these robots to autonomously classify evidence, ensuring that each sample is processed according to standardized protocols without manual intervention. Another important advantage of using AI robots in forensic analysis is their ability to perform repetitive tasks with high accuracy, speeding up response times in criminal investigations. In some countries, robots have been integrated into forensic units to perform fingerprint scanning and sample collection for DNA analysis without human contact, increasing the objectivity of the processes, reducing the likelihood of human-caused errors (Tiwari 2024).

Determining biases and errors in research: AI plays a critical role in improving the precision and accuracy of forensic investigations by reducing errors and biases that could compromise the validity of analyses (Yang et al., 2024). Using advanced machine learning algorithms, AI can evaluate large volumes of data and identify patterns, such as in examinations of ballistic evidence, fingerprints, DNA analysis, and other forensic evidence. Through a comprehensive analysis, AI can detect inconsistencies in testimony, human errors in the interpretation of evidence, and cognitive biases that can influence the criminal investigation process (Kosta et al., 2024).

Despite their education and experience, forensic specialists are vulnerable to unconscious influences that can skew their judgment, according to a number of cognitive science studies (Dror, 2020, 2023, 2025; Dror et al., 2017). These automatic cognitive biases influence perception, memory, and decision-making, particularly when unrelated contextual information is presented (Dror and Kukucka, 2021; Parra et al., 2024). Methodological models that control the sequence and style of information delivery to the expert (Linear Sequential Unmasking–Expanded, LSU-E) have been put forth in an effort to reduce this risk (Dror and Kukucka, 2021). These models prioritize an initial evaluation that is solely based on empirical evidence before providing any further contextual information. By reducing bias and noise in decision-making, this approach aims to free interpretation from assumptions shaped by outside expectations and instead base it on reliable scientific standards, even in the forensic investigation of complex cases of serious human rights violations (Parra et al., 2024).

In this situation, AI can be very helpful in providing these reasoning models with structural support. Initial analyses can be carried out in a standardized, objective, and repeatable way thanks to systems built to work with decontextualized data, which keeps contaminating information from influencing the primary interpretation. AI is also capable of automatically controlling the order in which information is exposed, creating protocols that maximize relevance and the best time to introduce particular case elements. This technical ability improves the forensic process' traceability and transparency while also boosting analyst consistency. A more error-resistant forensic practice that can incorporate contextual understanding without compromising the analysis's epistemic integrity is created by articulating reflective human reasoning with objective algorithmic analysis flows.

2.2.3 Association of Traces with Context and Time

The ability to associate traces with their temporal, spatial, and causal context is one of the ways AI is significantly changing the reconstruction of forensic scenarios. Shenoy et al. (2023) point out that AI enables forensic analysts to connect pieces of evidence to the exact moment they were created, allowing for more precise chronological reconstructions. Algorithms that combine data from various sources and accurately reconstruct causal sequences are used to accomplish this (Shenoy et al., 2023). Additionally, Piraianu et al. (2023) stress that by embedding various forms of evidence, including DNA, biological remains, fingerprints, and activity patterns, into a logical contextual framework within the crime scene, AI systems can recognize relationships among them because of their capacity to process large-scale datasets. The ability of forensic specialists to comprehend how various traces interact and converge in a single criminal event is greatly improved by this cross-domain integration (Cărcăle, 2025). Furthermore, sophisticated AI algorithms can reliably determine the age of biological and non-biological materials, including chemical residues, textile fibers, and bloodstains. When evaluating the forensic significance of such traces, it is critical to ascertain whether they were created during the pertinent criminal event or at a different time (Cărcăle, 2025). According to Cărcăle (2025), AI also makes it easier to reconstruct event timelines by examining digital sources like call logs, signals from mobile devices, social media activity, and geolocation information. This feature speeds up the creation of testable hypotheses while lowering the possibility of human error in the manual interpretation of data.

Further illustrating AI's usefulness in scene reconstruction and evidence interpretation, a more comprehensive analysis of the technology's effects in forensic science also emphasizes its use in postmortem interval estimation, forensic identification, and pattern recognition in injuries or human remains (Piraianu et al., 2023).

Collectively, these capabilities demonstrate that AI is a powerful analytical assistant in the creation of forensic reports, not just a supporting tool. AI improves reconstruction accuracy and lessens the influence of bias or erroneous assumptions by linking traces to their exact temporal and contextual parameters. This is especially important in complicated cases with a lot of evidence, as human analysis might be too sluggish or prone to mistakes.

The end result is a potent synergy, objective, automated reconstruction systems enhanced by interpretative, critical forensic reasoning, when AI-driven modeling and skilled human validation are combined. The result is a forensic practice that is more scientifically based, context-sensitive, and trustworthy.

2.2.4 Interpretation of Results and Generation of Forensic Reports

The interpretation of forensic results and the creation of expert reports are being increasingly transformed by AI, which is enabling a move toward automated, statistically supported conclusions that improve objectivity and decrease subjectivity. According to Ramchandra et al. (2024), AI-driven systems can generate preliminary forensic reports using machine learning and robust statistical modeling, relieving experts of some of the work so they can concentrate on validating and critically assessing the final outputs. This reorientation streamlines routine interpretive tasks while maintaining the forensic expert's crucial role in maintaining scientific and legal integrity.

AI systems automatically interpret evidence, including digital artifacts, biometrics, and chemical profiles, using probabilistic models and comparisons with extensive, carefully curated forensic databases. This improves accuracy and consistency across cases. Credibility is increased and interpretation variability is reduced when individual evidentiary findings can be cross-referenced against repository-level norms. Farber (2025) also emphasizes how AI-generated expert reports can combine information from various forensic fields, including digital, biological, chemical, and anatomical, and are backed by sophisticated analytical frameworks. However, the final narrative must still be validated by a multidisciplinary human panel. Particularly in complicated cases with a wealth of evidence, this hybrid approach reduces the risk of bias and speeds up case resolutions.

The use of generative AI agents and Large Language Models (LLMs) to aid in report writing has also been explored recently. For example, it has been suggested that frameworks using AutoGen AI agents (such as LLAMA and StarCoder) convert natural language commands into forensic actions, significantly lowering the amount of manual labor. Such systems raise questions about hallucinations and legal admissibility, despite their potential, which emphasizes the significance of strict validation procedures and professional supervision (Wickramasekara et al., 2025; Wickramasekara and Scanlon, 2024).

Farber (2025) explores the use of AI tools, ChatGPT-4, Claude, and Gemini, in forensic image analysis to create personalized AI models for forensic work. After the AI systems independently examined thirty crime scene photos, ten forensic experts evaluated the reports. The results show how helpful AI can be as an additional tool, particularly for rapid screening that supports expert analysis without replacing it. Despite their high accuracy in observations, the tools struggled to identify evidence, and their performance differed depending on the type of crime: they performed better in arson investigations (7.1) than in homicide cases (7.8). The findings show both AI's shortcomings and its potential to increase expert productivity, especially when managing complex evidence or large caseloads. Most importantly, the study calls for legal and ethical frameworks to guide the application of AI in criminal justice, with implications for forensic training, future tool development, and investigative techniques. The AI achieved high observation accuracy and significantly reduced analysis time, from an average of 42 minutes per image to less than two minutes (Farber, 2025), despite the fact that human evaluators performed marginally better overall. These findings demonstrate that, rather than taking the place of expert judgment, interpretative automation can be a useful tool for decision support.

Validation, standardization, and traceability are critical to the accuracy of AI-generated interpretations. To ensure that automated conclusions remain reliable and legally defensible, Solanke and Biasiotti (2022) stress the necessity of standardized evaluation of AI models in digital forensics, including ongoing monitoring, redundancy mechanisms, and expert-in-the-loop oversight (Farber,

2025; Solanke and Biasiotti, 2022). According to Sanna et al. (2024), it is imperative to evaluate the resilience of AI systems in authentic research settings and draw attention to their vulnerability to hostile inputs, which may jeopardize their dependability and security. This research underscores the importance of developing robust AI security measures and defense mechanisms to address these vulnerabilities.

The body of research backs up a number of significant benefits of AI-enhanced forensic reporting, including:

- *Increased efficiency:* without compromising consistency, automated drafting and preliminary interpretation significantly cut down on time-to-report.
- *Increased objectivity:* probabilistic modeling and evidence-based analyses lessen the need for arbitrary human judgment.
- *Multisource integration:* AI is able to compile and display disparate data in a logical manner, including digital logs, chemical assays, and DNA profiles.
- *Accountability and traceability:* all of the AI's statistical judgments and deductions can be recorded and examined.
- However, *there are restrictions on these capabilities:* AI systems need to be open, explicable, and vulnerable to ethic and legal scrutiny. To ensure procedural fairness and evidentiary reliability, forensic AI tools must adhere to strict standards of transparency, accuracy, and explainability, according to the DOJ report on AI in criminal justice (DOJ, 2024). When combined, AI does not replace the role of forensic experts; rather, it reorganizes it by giving machines repetitive, mechanical, or statistical interpretive tasks, leaving human experts in charge of contextual interpretation, legal framing, and final validation. Without sacrificing epistemic integrity, this division of labor improves overall efficiency and report robustness. In conclusion, well-designed AI systems can decrease subjectivity and bias, speed up the processing of complex cases, and produce high-quality forensic reports based on automated and statistical analysis. As a result, skilled practitioners become assessors and verifiers of narratives produced by machines, creating a mutually beneficial human-AI collaboration that enhances forensic reporting's precision and legitimacy.
- *Multidisciplinary work:* AI fosters collaborative and integrated work in forensic analysis, enabling forensic experts from various fields to work more efficiently. Along with technological advancements, communication between forensic scientists and professionals in criminal investigation, such as criminologists and judicial experts, will be strengthened, improving the accuracy and credibility of forensic reports (Tynan, 2024).

AI facilitates the integration of forensic data by connecting multiple sources of information into a centralized platform, ensuring that forensic experts have real-time access to relevant data. Additionally, language processing models enable forensic reports to be translated into more accessible terms for judges and lawyers, minimizing misinterpretations. Its collaborative analysis capabilities also allow investigators in different locations to work simultaneously on forensic analysis, which is crucial for international cases requiring inter-institutional cooperation, as well as complex cases that demand expertise from forensic professionals in other regions of the world (Eurojust, 2024).

In this communication context, AI has been integrated to enhance forensic training through simulations and machine learning tools, providing professionals in training with realistic scenarios without compromising real casework (Parmar, 2023). Finally, its application in standardizing multidisciplinary work reduces discrepancies in result interpretation, ensuring consistency in forensic analyses and the quality of forensic reports.

2.3 Critical Points to Consider in the Implementation of Forensic AI

The implementation of AI applications in the forensic field requires the use of models, which are applied according to the nature of the samples to be analyzed. Among the most commonly used models are neural networks (Prince, 2023) or LLMs (Xiao and Zhu, 2025):

2.3.1 Neural Networks

They are the basis of modern AI and are inspired by the functioning of the human brain. These networks are made up of several interconnected layers: an input layer, where data is entered (such as DNA profiles); one or more hidden layers, where information is processed; and an output layer, which provides the result, such as the prediction of some physical trait. During the training process, the network adjusts the "weights" of its connections to learn to identify patterns, for example, by linking genetic variations to phenotypic characteristics (Sehrawat et al., 2023). In other applications, a neural network can sort through mixtures of DNA obtained at a crime scene.

2.3.2 Large Language Models (LLMs)

LLMs, such as ChatGPT, are large-scale neural networks trained on huge volumes of text to understand and generate human language. For example, although they do not predict traits from DNA, they are extremely useful in the management and analysis of information. They can review textual evidence, analyze previous reports, and find patterns in records of previous investigations, or even detect inconsistencies in witnesses from written testimony. Likewise, if required, models in different applications can be integrated. For example, the AutoGen framework allows for the construction of AI systems composed of multiple collaborative agents (Fatima et al., 2025). It functions like an orchestra conductor, allowing different models (agents) to interact to solve complex tasks as:

- *Agent 1 (Phenotyping):* Analyzes DNA and generates a robot portrait.
- *Agent 2 (Fingerprint):* Searches a database for matches.
- *Agent 3 (Data Analysis):* Tracks the suspect's digital history.
- *Agent 4 (Report):* Synthesizes all the information in a final report for the investigator.

This system makes it possible for the different AIs to work synergistically, overcoming the limitations of a single model and facilitating the resolution of complex cases.

Another factor to be considered for the success of the developed AI system in relation to ensures the validity and reliability of an AI model in forensics, its training must adhere to rigorous principles. The goal is for AI to learn to identify patterns in data to make accurate predictions in the face of new information. Here are the essential principles:

2.3.3 Data Quality and Representativeness

To train robust AI models in forensics, it is essential to have data that is accurate and correctly labeled. In criminalistics, for example, extensive databases are used where each DNA sample with its respective nucleotide variations is linked to confirmed physical traits, such as the color of eyes, hair, or skin of thousands of people (Kayser et al., 2023). These data allow AI to establish reliable relationships between genetics and phenotype. The validation dataset is then used to test the model with unknown cases, evaluating its performance and simulating its effectiveness in real-world scenarios.

2.3.4 Cross-validation

This technique is key to ensuring that the model not only works well with the data it was trained on but is robust and generalizable. It consists of dividing the data into several partitions and performing multiple cycles of training and validation, alternating the sets used (Di Maggio et al., 2025). Thus, bias toward a specific population group is prevented and confidence in the model is increased in the face of any genetic profile, regardless of its origin.

2.3.5 Overfitting

Overfitting occurs when the AI "memorizes" the training data, rather than learning the underlying logic. This can lead to deceptively accurate results with known data, but fail with new samples. To avoid this, it is essential to use more quality data, apply cross-validation, employ regularization techniques, and establish criteria to stop training in time. Thus, the model will be accurate and reliable in cases never before analyzed (Cawley and Talbot, 2010).

2.3.6 Explainability (XAI)

In the legal environment, explainability is indispensable. It's not enough to claim that the software predicted that the suspect had blue eyes. The expert must be able to explain on the basis of which genetic markers this conclusion was reached. Complex AI models, such as neural networks, are often "black boxes" that are difficult to interpret, so the development of explainable and transparent tools is a requirement for the acceptance of evidence in court (Hassija et al., 2024).

2.4 Improving Quality Standards in Countries Without ISO Certification

Forensic analysis's caliber and dependability are crucial to guaranteeing that justice is administered correctly. Forensic services in certain nations have not yet adopted ISO quality standards, and their lack of ISO certification can raise suspicions among the justice administration, who believe that forensic science without accreditation and certification is more prone to mistakes in exam interpretation, thereby compromising the validity of the findings. As argued in Chapter 1 of this book, this is not necessarily the case and needs to be substantially demystified. However, as a form of balance and interrelation with proposed innovations such as the Sydney Declaration, AI can complement these approaches and can be a relevant factor in the standardization of forensic processes by providing automation, auditing, and quality control tools. In other words, AI would take care of the tasks that most interest administrators in justice systems.

The implementation of AI to standardize forensic processes, especially in resource-limited countries, can help establish uniform forensic protocols at low cost by automating evidence analysis and detecting procedural flaws, resulting in the appropriate use of resources. Advanced algorithms can compare samples with databases, ensuring that analyses meet international standards, which also generates savings in validation processes. However, despite its benefits, the implementation of AI in forensic science faces challenges such as the lack of technological infrastructure, essential for its use, and resistance to change on the part of forensic professionals and those involved in these processes. However, investment in forensic training and technology can significantly transform these negative aspects of its implementation and strengthen quality.

Based on fundamental ideas like the significance of the trace, the value of critical thinking, contextual interpretation of the evidence, and the acceptance of the inherent uncertainty in retrospective investigations, the Sydney Declaration has suggested a critical rethinking of the field in this regard. Concurrently, the emergence of AI offers fresh chances to uphold these values, especially in unfavorable settings where conventional quality frameworks are ineffective.

AI, which is defined as technology that can process large amounts of data autonomously, not only improves forensic investigators' analytical skills but also changes the way traces are found, analyzed, and assessed. For example, intelligent systems can find patterns, create inferential models, and suggest hypotheses that a human expert might miss in time in situations where access to laboratories is restricted or the amount of time between the incident and the forensic intervention jeopardizes the integrity of the trace. AI serves as an extension of scientific reasoning, providing a sophisticated approach to the Sydney Declaration's emphasis on the principle of temporal asymmetry and the acknowledgment of uncertainty, rather than taking the place of human labor.

Furthermore, AI encourages the contextual assessment of traces, which is crucial for a field that relies on situated reconstructions rather than universal truths. AI algorithms can produce dynamic event maps that show relationships, trajectories, and causal sequences by processing multiple sources – digital, physical, and testimonial – at the same time. As supported by the semiotic turn in modern forensic science, this ability strengthens the concept of contextual retrodiction, going beyond the conventional idea of "evidence" as discrete data and encouraging its interpretation as a sign.

However, there are systemic barriers to the broad use of AI. The ethical regulatory frameworks and technological infrastructure necessary for successful implementation are absent in many low-resource or structurally violent nations. This calls for a reconsideration of capacity-building and technology transfer strategies to make sure that intelligent systems contribute to the reversal of epistemic asymmetries rather than their reproduction. In this sense, the Sydney Declaration provides a normative compass: AI must be viewed as a tool that complements, never replaces, the practitioner's inferential reasoning, and must be used critically, ethically, and contextually.

Then, at this point the question arises: is it possible to implement forensic AI in countries with fewer resources? and the central answer is related to if the AI makes forensic analysis cheaper or more expensive, then the AI has the potential to reduce analysis costs in the long term, although it requires a significant initial investment, which represents the main barrier to entry.

The high initial costs of AI implementation are related to:

- *Technical infrastructure:* Powerful servers (often with specialized GPUs) and secure storage systems for large volumes of genetic data and digital evidence are indispensable.
- *Software licensing:* Commercial tools such as Parabon Snapshot® can involve high licensing or analytics costs.

- *Human capital:* A multidisciplinary team (experts in AI, data science and forensics) is needed, whose training and recruitment requires a considerable investment.
- However, *long-term savings can be significant.*
- Automating complex DNA analysis or mass digital evidence review saves thousands of hours of specialized work.
- A more accurate profile reduces the time and resources spent on erroneous tracks.
- Automating repetitive tasks allows experts to focus on truly complex challenges.

In this context, gradual implementation is key, especially in countries with limited resources. Instead of adopting all the tools at once, it is advisable to start with a low-cost, high-impact pilot project. For example, starting with an AI to improve low-resolution videos, rather than expensive facial DNA phenotyping systems. Once the value has been demonstrated, larger investments can be justified.

Collaboration between forensic laboratories and academic or research centers, as promoted in the Sydney Declaration, is strategic in the face of budgetary and technological challenges. Partnering with supercomputer universities allows access to advanced technology without having to purchase it. In return, universities can use anonymized forensic data for their projects, generating a beneficial synergy: while academic experts develop and train basic AI models, forensics validate and ensure their scientific rigor.

This collaborative approach becomes relevant in the framework of international alliances, allowing laboratories in developing countries to integrate into global networks of good practices and validated models, benefiting from the learning of others and avoiding common mistakes. An illustrative case is that of a laboratory in Latin America or Africa that, faced with the challenge of analyzing large volumes of digital evidence, partners with a university department specialized in data science abroad. Instead of purchasing commercial software, they develop together an open-source tool for natural language processing, capable of filtering messages relevant to forensic review. Although less sophisticated, this tool reduces analysis time by up to 70%, optimizes human resources, and keeps technology under state control, avoiding costly licenses.

2.5 Ethical Risks and Challenges of Artificial Intelligence in Forensic Science

The use of AI in forensic science has generated significant advances and opportunities, as demonstrated in this chapter, but it also presents ethical and technical risks that demand immediate attention. When forensic systems operate in challenging environments, such as armed conflict, institutional collapse, or structural constraints, these risks are magnified. In addition to technical accuracy, transparency, accountability, and contextual sensitivity are essential when using AI for forensic reporting and decision-making.

The inability of forensic AI to be explained is one of its primary hazards. Many deep learning models function as "black boxes," producing results without fully understanding how they were arrived at, as noted by Stacey et al. (2025). This opacity undermines confidence in the findings, makes expert decisions difficult to defend in court, and jeopardizes their auditability. AI loses scientific and legal legitimacy even when it increases efficiency if its workings are incomprehensible to human experts.

According to the U.S. Department of Justice report from 2024,[6] automated forensic tools need to adhere to strict requirements for transparency, traceability, and validity. Algorithmic biases are created when models are frequently validated against small or unrepresentative databases. An AI runs the risk of making systematic mistakes if it is trained on data that does not accurately represent reality or particular realities. The reality of genetic interbreeding, for instance, is unknown in some populations worldwide, mainly in Africa, so we can at least attempt to create genetic processes that aid in the identification process; the frequency of toxic substances contaminating food or water; specific toxins that are causing mutations and then their methylation, which results in heart problems that cause sudden death; and a long list of conditions that are poorly understood in these regions or difficult environments.

If AI models are not sensitive to biocultural and social variability, they may increase human error rather than decrease it. Because they reproduce ambiguous patterns and explanations that the forensic expert himself is unable to provide, errors thus take on an ethical dimension in addition to being purely technical.

The erroneous belief that AI systems are infallible is another ethically troubling feature. Overestimating algorithmic accuracy can result in automated or inadequately reviewed forensic decisions, which can lead to errors in the justice system and its proper administration, as Stacey et al. (2025) caution. In actuality, forensic AI systems ought to be viewed as complementary instruments rather than as a replacement for human expert judgment. Combining forensic and machine experts is crucial; it is currently relevant but should be used with caution.

Forensic AI raises concerns about data control, model generation, and result access from the standpoints of quality and transparency. In order to guarantee the appropriate, accurate, responsible, and audited use of these technologies, the Department of Justice (DOJ, 2024) report highlights the necessity of establishing governance structures. Since it establishes safety, explainability, fairness, and accountability as prerequisites for the adoption of AI in forensic science, the adoption of ethical frameworks like the RAIF (Responsible AI Framework) put forth

[6] See https://www.justice.gov/olp/media/1381796/dl

by Stacey et al. (2025) is a significant step. Therefore, it is ethically necessary for forensic science to have access to AI. Automated tools need to be built and modified to work even under less-than-ideal circumstances. Before implementing AI-based solutions, processes for ongoing assessment, independent monitoring, and contextual adaptation must be put in place, as the Department of Justice report highlights. Importing models created in privileged environments is insufficient; they also need to have their parameters changed, be trained using local data, and have their use not cause more harm than good.

AI can help with expert report preparation by streamlining procedures, cutting down on time, and enhancing the way results are displayed visually. The reports must, however, be comprehensible, auditable, and tailored to the recipient's technical level (victims, judges, and attorneys). Explainability is a prerequisite for procedural justice as well as a technical necessity. Because its judgments must be critically assessed by human peers, AI is not an automatic tool that provides answers, as noted by Stacey et al. (2025) AI must answer to the scientific community and the legal system.

In forensic science, AI is a technological revolution, but if it is applied without careful ethical consideration, it may create new kinds of opacity and uncertainty. Public policy recommendations and technical and regulatory frameworks like the RAIF provide helpful direction for risk management. The biggest obstacle, though, is making sure that forensic AI is appropriately regulated and that expert witnesses are sufficiently trained in its use. This will stop AI "hallucinations" from entering the human brain and escalating our already dangerous cognitive biases. Without a doubt, AI must help safeguard human rights, fight impunity, and increase confidence in scientific data in difficult situations.

2.5.1 The Black Box in Forensic Artificial Intelligence: Balancing Technical Effectiveness with Epistemological Vulnerability

A paradigm shift in the processing, interpretation, and presentation of evidence-related data has been brought about by the introduction of AI in forensic science. Significant promises have been brought about by this new technological horizon, including increased efficiency in repetitive tasks, time optimization, human error reduction, and data analysis. But these advantages come with a host of ethical and epistemic problems, one of which is particularly prominent and the focus of much discussion: the opaque operation of many AI models, sometimes referred to as "black boxes."

Systems that produce outcomes without explicitly disclosing the steps that led to them are referred to as "black boxes." This means that in the context of forensics, an algorithm may generate a classification, a probabilistic value, or an expert conclusion, but neither the human operator nor the judicial recipient will be able to fully comprehend how that output was arrived at. This trait is not just technical; it has a direct bearing on forensic science's dependability, transparency, reproducibility, and culture of quality – all of which are essential to maintaining its legitimacy in the legal system.

Among many other factors currently under development, the need to automate complex processes like image pattern recognition, fingerprint comparison, voice profile evaluation, or even statistical interpretation of evidence frequently drives the use of AI systems in the forensic scenario. However, the traceability of the reasoning is lost when using extremely complex models, like deep learning. What started out as an expert's logical series of analytical steps has evolved into a series of imperceptible mathematical operations. Even though the findings seem compelling, their incomprehensibility makes it difficult to conduct scientific review and provide a defense in court.

Given the importance of forensic science to the criminal justice system, this phenomenon is especially concerning. The evidence that is offered in court needs to be unambiguous, intelligible, and subject to discussion by the parties. The process becomes asymmetrical when black boxes are present because algorithms generate answers but not justifications. In this way, an over-reliance on the machine's authority runs the risk of diluting the crucial role of the human expert. Due process may be undermined by the logic of automated precision if explainability mechanisms are not included.

The perception of AI systems in the legal system is another issue. There is a deeply rooted cultural inclination to believe that computer-generated content is more trustworthy or objective. Even when algorithms' internal workings are unclear or their models have been trained using skewed data, this illusion of infallibility can give them undue weight. In this situation, the black box takes the place of human accountability and critical analysis as a technical legitimation tool.

Given these dangers, forensic AI must be responsibly governed. The first step in using this strategy is to acknowledge that AI systems are not neutral. All algorithms are based on human choices about which variables to prioritize, how to preprocess the data, what error metrics to accept, and what data to include. The second requirement is that models be created in a way that can be explained by their architecture, meaning that the expert can at least partially reconstruct the underlying logic. Explainability is now a necessity for ethics and epistemology rather than a technical luxury.

Protocols that guarantee AI's validation, traceability, and auditability must also be implemented alongside it. This means creating institutional oversight and accountability systems in addition to meticulously recording training data, evaluation standards, and test scenarios. The black box should be viewed as a problem that needs to be resolved via responsible design, structural transparency, and continual professional training rather than as a justification for normalizing operator ignorance.

The reaffirmation of the human expert's position as the ultimate arbiter of forensic judgment is another crucial component. AI should never be used in place of expert judgment; rather, it should be considered an auxiliary tool. This suggests that professionals must have a critical mindset, be aware of the limitations of the system, and be able to articulate the outcomes in order to avoid blindly giving interpretation to the machine. Instead of promoting automated delegation, the existence of black boxes must promote a professional culture founded on reasonable skepticism.

Incorporating these factors into an institutional architecture that encourages participation, equity, and transparency is also crucial. The existence of black boxes can exacerbate the gaps in access to expert knowledge in diverse forensic environments with multiple actors and unequal resources. As a result, creating tools that are easy to understand and use is also crucial because they can only serve the forensic scientist's primary purpose of making their job easier if all parties involved in the process comprehend the evidence and the traceable tracking of its development.

Finally, the black box symbolizes a conflict between the potential for technical effectiveness and the vulnerability of epistemology. The urgent challenge is to domesticate AI and make it a responsible, comprehensible, and reliable tool, rather than to reject it. This means reconsidering not just its design but also professional practices, legal frameworks, and forensic science training. Progress cannot come at the expense of opacity. Forensic science at the service of justice and humanitarian action must continue to be based on transparency, human judgment, and critical deliberation.

2.5.2 Ethical Crossroads in Forensic Science: Navigating the AI Revolution and the Future of the Forensic Professional

In the forensic field, the arrival of AI is not a simple improvement; it poses a profound dilemma and an unprecedented crossroads in the context of the future need for the participation of forensic professionals in the various stages of analysis, as robots and algorithms take over tasks that were previously exclusively human. This conflict, which manifests itself as a social, scientific, and ethical problem, demands careful analysis and a framework for action for the future. Automation using AI aims to reduce human error, increase case processing speed, and free professionals from repetitive tasks. However, this same scientific advance confronts us with the possibility of massive job losses, which generates a profound social and ethical problem regarding the use of AI.

In the case of AI automation of forensic analysis, for example, through the use of AI and machine learning tools, the analysis of DNA profiles can be simplified and improved, especially in complex cases with genetic mixtures from several people (de Wit et al., 2025). Traditionally, the interpretation of these mixed profiles is a laborious process susceptible to the subjective variability of human analysts, which can lead to discrepancies. However, with the use of AI to analyze raw DNA profile data, patterns can be identified and profiles assigned to individuals more quickly and objectively than conventional forensic software. This creates the potential to democratize the analysis of complex genetic profiles, making it accessible even to laboratories with limited resources through automated and accessible interpretation. This could eliminate the need for forensic experts at this stage of the process.

Therefore, the loss of jobs in the forensic field, while an economic concern, extends to a much deeper level. The replacement of forensic scientists with AI presents several ethical and social dilemmas:

- *Responsibility and accountability:* If an algorithm makes an error in interpreting a genetic profile that leads to a wrongful conviction, who is responsible? The programmer, the analyst who blindly trusted the AI's output, or the laboratory that implemented the technology? The chain of responsibility becomes diffuse and complex, undermining public confidence in the justice system.
- *Bias and fairness:* AI algorithms learn from historical data. As mentioned in Section 2.5.1, if the training data contains inherent biases (for example, if it comes from populations overrepresented in criminal databases), the model could perpetuate and amplify these biases, which could lead to discriminatory results. AI may be objective with the data, but it is not inherently impartial if the data it processes is not.
- *Dehumanization of the profession:* The interpretation of forensic information, such as a genetic profile, is more than simple data analysis; it involves professional judgment, experience, and a narrative context. AI, no matter how advanced, lacks the intuition and critical thinking that a forensic expert brings to a case. Reducing the forensic expert's role to a mere "validator" of a machine's results can lead to deprofessionalization and a loss of the human essence of the work.
- *Distributive justice:* Automation benefits institutions (greater efficiency, lower long-term costs) but harms individuals (job loss, skills obsolescence). A distributive justice conflict arises in which the benefits of innovation are not distributed equitably.

However, the key to addressing this ethical and social conflict is not to halt technological progress, but to manage it intelligently and ethically. The solution is not to avoid AI, but to integrate it as an ally, not a substitute.

- *Refocusing the practitioner's role:* Instead of viewing AI as a replacement, we must consider it an augmentation tool. Forensic scientists of the future will not need to perform routine genetic analysis, but will focus on higher value tasks: contextual interpretation of results, validation of algorithm reliability, development of new methodologies, and expert testimony in court, where human judgment is irreplaceable. AI frees experts to do what machines cannot do.
- *Continuous training and adaptation:* Job loss can be mitigated by reorienting education and professional training. Forensic science programs must evolve to

include data analysis, basic programming, and AI principles. Today's forensic scientists must be trained to oversee, audit, and, when necessary, challenge the results generated by algorithms.

- *Regulatory framework and ethical standards:* It is crucial to establish an ethical and legal framework governing the use of AI in forensics. Regulations should require transparency and auditability of algorithms (knowing how and why they make decisions), as well as shared responsibility among developers, users, and institutions. It should establish clear guidelines on the validation and ethical deployment of these technologies.

2.6 Forensic Quality, Operational Skepticism, and Artificial Intelligence as a Bridge Between Standards and Innovation

A profound, almost philosophical conflict between two seemingly incompatible worlds – that of normative standardization and that of creative scientific practice – lies at the core of modern forensic science. Although this tension is not new, it has gotten worse in recent decades as a result of laws like ISO 17025 requiring the use of quality management systems, which guarantee institutional oversight, traceability, and reproducibility. But despite these assurances, there is a lingering wave of skepticism led by forensic experts who see these frameworks as constraints that restrict their capacity for creative problem-solving, expert judgment, and handling complex cases. Therefore, it is inevitable to ask: will these two paths ever intersect? Is it possible for the manager's institutional trust and the expert's methodological flexibility to come together? Perhaps the responsible integration of AI holds the key to the solution.

The foundation of forensic laboratories' quality systems, ISO 17025, establishes a framework to guarantee that the company manages its people, processes, and outputs appropriately rather than dictating individual professional competence or imposing particular techniques. However, in reality, a lot of organizations have converted this standard into strict operating procedures, or SOPs, that describe every stage of the analysis. When a forensic expert is presented with a unique, non-repeatable, multidisciplinary, or experimental case, these protocols are insufficient and even detrimental, even though they are helpful and even necessary for routine tasks like DNA typing or the detection of controlled substances. The forensic expert now requires a specific action plan, a case-specific roadmap that has been developed with judgment, expertise, and consideration rather than a prefabricated guide.

Quality in these intricate situations cannot be reduced to a checkbox; rather, it must be founded on the openness of scientific reasoning, the precision of expert opinion, and the documented rationale behind every choice. Thankfully, this reality is addressed by the standard itself in its section on non-conforming work, which permits the creation of ad hoc procedures as long as they are appropriately recorded, assessed, and justified. It's about extending the system's reach responsibly and rigorously, not about working outside of it.

AI may be very important in this situation: As a versatile instrument that acts as a mediator between institutional order and scientific adaptability and not as a replacement for the expert or as a new regulatory framework. An AI system that is well-designed can help with automated action plan documentation, make recommendations based on previous analysis, evaluate the consistency of outcomes, or spot irregularities that are invisible to the human eye. Additionally, it can support forensic reasoning in ambiguous situations by modeling, simulating, and defending alternative scenarios.

AI can also convert the technical reasoning of the expert into formal structures that satisfy the quality manager's requirements. Standards skeptics and compliance watchdogs can develop mutual understanding through explainable, non-opaque systems. In order to satisfy both institutional traceability and scientific creativity, an AI-generated or AI-supported action plan can create automatic internal audits, evaluate the validity of non-routine methods, and incorporate cross-references with current SOPs.

The design is crucial: forensic AI that is trustworthy, practical, and moral must honor the practitioner's autonomy rather than take its place. It must help, not control. Above all, it needs to be continuously validated, reviewed, and monitored by humans. Transferring the strictness of SOPs to opaque algorithmic systems carries the risk of making the same mistake under a different name. The goal is to give the standard contextual intelligence rather than digitize it.

Instead of being replaced in this new scenario, the forensic practitioner would be repositioned as a decision architect who is in charge of the crucial use of digital tools. In a similar vein, the quality manager would have access to real-time metrics, computational traceability, and dynamic indicators to track performance without needless constraints. As a result, forensic science would become more integrated, transparent, and agile.

However, this potential necessitates a change in institutional perspective. By acknowledging that both normative adoption and operational skepticism stem from justifiable concerns, the need to maintain scientific integrity and to ensure fairness – the argument between them will not be settled by imposing one hegemony over the other. AI can only act as a mediator if both sides are prepared to make concessions.

What now seems to be a contradiction between innovation and standards may actually work in concert. Forensic AI that is transparent, explicable, validated, and contextualized would enable managers to maintain quality without compromising flexibility and professionals to use their judgment with more assistance. Instead of being a rigid framework, the standard would evolve into a dynamic, flexible ecosystem that is results-driven but mindful of the scientific method.

In the end, the question of whether these two worlds can coexist should be framed as an opportunity to rethink forensic culture rather than as an intractable conundrum. Standardization and creativity are not mutually exclusive, nor is quality the enemy of science. If AI is applied with critical awareness, ethical responsibility, and a dedication to justice, it can serve as the tool that bridges the gap between the two.

2.7 Conclusion

A bright future is created by the fusion of the fundamental ideas of forensic science with the potential of AI. Reviving the discipline's core mission to resolve ambiguity through trace, reason, and context is more important than merely implementing new technologies. AI can act as both a technical ally and an epistemological mediator between the pursuit of justice and the complexity of the world in unfavorable situations where traditional frameworks fail. AI is becoming an essential tool in forensic science, especially in resource-limited countries, improving evidence identification, automating processes, and optimizing the analysis of results. Furthermore, its integration will enable more efficient collaboration between forensic experts from different disciplines and locations around the world, thereby reducing errors and biases and consolidating forensic reports of the highest quality.

The full automation of forensic laboratories and, for example, the use of AI for genetic profiling are promising scientific advances that inevitably pose the threat of job losses. However, this challenge can be approached not as a struggle between humans and machines, but as an opportunity for symbiotic collaboration, where the human brain will always have reflexive supremacy. The future of forensic science is not a laboratory without people, but one in which AI provides speed and objectivity, while the forensic professional contributes the wisdom, critical judgment, and ethical rigor essential to the pursuit of justice and the fight against impunity. The responsibility of forensic professionals and institutional systems is to lead this transition consciously and ethically, ensuring that technological advancement ultimately contributes to the well-being of societies.

References

Barash, M., McNevin, D., Fedorenko, V., and Givets, P. (2024) Machine learning applications in forensic DNA profiling: A critical review. *Forensic Science International: Genetics*, **69**, 102994. https://doi.org/10.1016/j.fsigen.2023.102994. PMID: 38086200.

Cărcăle, V.-A. (2025, April) The future of artificial intelligence (AI) applications in forensics. *Research Association for Interdisciplinary*, RAIN (pp. 250–255). Studies. https://doi.org/10.5281/zenodo.15481632.

Cawley, G.C. and Talbot, N.L.C. (2010) On over-fitting in model selection and subsequent selection bias in performance evaluation. *Journal of Machine Learning Research,* **11**, 2079–2107.

Chango, X., Flor-Unda, O., Gil-Jiménez, P., and Gómez-Moreno, H. (2024) Technology in forensic sciences: innovation and precision. *Technologies,* **12**, 120. https://doi.org/10.3390/technologies12080120.

Di Maggio, L.G., Gastaldi, C., Renzo, D.A., *et al.* (2025). https://doi.org/10.1007/s00366-025-02139-7) A robust methodology for dataset preparation and algorithm performance assessment in machine learning prediction of the fatigue life of additive manufactured components. *Engineering with Computers,* **41**, 2937–2952.

Dror, I.E. (2020) Cognitive and human factors in expert decision making: Six fallacies and the eight sources of bias. *Analytical Chemistry,* **92**(12), 7998–8004. https://doi.org/10.1021/acs.analchem.0c00704.

Dror, I.E. (2023) The most consistent finding in forensic science is inconsistency. *Journal of Forensic Sciences.,* **68**(6), 1851–1855. 10.1111.1556-4029.15369.

Dror, I.E. (2025) Biased and biasing: The hidden bias cascade and bias snowball effects. *Behavioral Sciences,* **15**(4), 490. https://doi.org/10.3390/bs15040490.

Dror, I.E. and Kukucka, J. (2021) Linear Sequential Unmasking–Expanded (LSU-E): A general approach for improving decision making as well as minimizing noise and bias. *Forensic Science International: Synergy,* **3**, 100161. 10\ignorespaces.1016/j.fsisyn.2021.100161.

Dror, I.E., Morgan, R., Rando, C., and Nakhaeizadeh, S. (2017) The bias snowball and the bias cascade effects: Two distinct biases that may impact forensic decision making. *Journal of Forensic Sciences,* **62**(3), 832–833. https://doi.org/10.1111/1556-4029.13496.

Eurojust. (2024) Artificial Intelligence Supporting Crossborder Cooperation in Criminal Justice.

Farber, S. (2025 https://doi.org/10.1111/1556-4029.70035. PMID: 40186399) AI as a decision support tool in forensic image analysis: A pilot study on integrating large language models into crime scene investigation workflows. *Journal of Forensic Sciences,* **70**, 932–943.

Fatima, S. K., Farooq, U., and Abid, A. (2025) AutoGen-driven multi-agent framework for iterative crime data analysis and prediction. arXiv preprint arXiv:2506.11475.

Geradts, Z. and Franke, K. (2023) *Artificial Intelligence (AI) in Forensic Sciences [Forensic Science in Focus].* Wiley.

Hassija, V., Chamola, V., Mahapatra, A., Singal, A., Goel, D., Huang, K., *et al.* (2024) Interpreting black-box models: A review on explainable artificial intelligence. *Cognitive Computation,* **16**, 45–74. https://doi.org/10.1007/s12559-023-10179-8.

Kayser, M., Branicki, W., Parson, W., and Phillips, C. (2023) Recent advances in forensic DNA phenotyping of appearance, ancestry and age. *Forensic Science International: Genetics,* **65**, 102870. https://doi.org/10.1016/j.fsigen.2023.102870. PMID: 37084623.

Ketsekioulafis, I., Filandrianos, G., Katsos, K., Thomas, K., Spiliopoulou, C., Stamou, G., *et al.* (2024) Artificial intelligence in forensic sciences: A systematic review of past and current applications and future perspectives. *Cureus,* **16**(9), e70363. https://doi.org/10.7759/cureus.70363. PMID: 39469392; PMCID: PMC11513614.

Kosta, S., Jain, S., and Suwalka, I. (2024) AI revolutionizing forensic analysis: Enhancing efficiency and accuracy in crime investigation. *International Advanced Research Journal in Science, Engineering and Technology,* **11**(S2).

Kowalski, G., Maciaś, M., and Wołoszczuk, A. (2014) Selected issues of collecting forensic evidence with a mobile robot. In: *Recent Advances in Automation, Robotics and Measuring*

Techniques (eds. R. Szewczyk, C. Zieliński, and M. Kaliczyńska). *Advances in Intelligent Systems and Computing*, Vol. **267**. Springer, Cham. https://doi.org/10.1007/978-3-319-05353-0_41.

Parmar, P. (2023) The integration of artificial intelligence in the forensic medicine and its applications in medico-legal autopsy, forensic toxicology, and disaster victim identification. *International Journal of Forensic Sciences*, **8**(4), 000331.

Parra, R.C., Condori, L.A., and Ubelaker, D.H. (2024) Forensic anthropology and the mitigation of cognitive biases in the investigation of human rights violations: Operationalization of a comprehensive theoretical model. *Forensic Anthropology*, **7**(1). https://doi.org/10.5744/fa.2023.0024.

Piraianu, A.-I., Fulga, A., Musat, C.L., Ciobotaru, O.-R., Poalelungi, D.G., Stamate, E., *et al.* (2023) Enhancing the evidence with algorithms: How artificial intelligence is transforming forensic medicine. *Diagnostics*, **13**(18), 2992.

Prince, S.J.D. (2023) *Understanding Deep Learning* (544 pp. MIT Press.

Ramchandra, M., Pravin, H., and Pravin, S. (2024) Digital forensics in the age of AI and ML: Evidence handling, validation and reporting. *Journal of Data Science & Artificial Intelligence*, **2**(1), 132.

RTI (2025) https://forensicrti.org/harnessing-ai-forensics/#1753739696384-2edd5496-48a4.

Sanna, S.L., Regano, L., Maiorca, D., and Giacinto, G. (2024) Exploring the robustness of AI-driven tools in digital forensics: A preliminary study. *arXiv*. https://doi.org/10.48550/arXiv.2412.01363.

Sehrawat, S., Najafian, K., and Jin, L. (2023) Predicting phenotypes from novel genomic markers using deep learning. *Bioinformatics Advances*, **3**(1), vbad028. https://doi.org/10.1093/bioadv/vbad028.

Shenoy, S.U., Nagar, V., and Akhith (2023) Artificial intelligence-based techniques for crime scene reconstruction and investigation: An overview. *Journal of Forensic Research*, **14**, 557.

Solanke, A.A. and Biasiotti, M.A. (2022) Digital forensics AI: Evaluating, standardizing and optimizing digital evidence mining techniques. *KI – Künstliche Intelligenz*, **36**(2), 143–161.

Stacey, J., Fleming, R., Sheppard, D., Sheppard, J., Dobbie, G., and Karunakaran, D. (2025) A responsible artificial intelligence framework for forensic science. *Forensic Science International*, **375**, 112548. https://doi.org/10.1016/j.forsciint.2025.112548. Epub 2025 Jun 26. PMID: 40633280.

Tiwari, P. (2024) Challenges and solutions in DNA fingerprinting: Sample quality, data analysis, and interpretation. *International Journal of Advanced Biochemistry Research*, **8**(1), 247–252.

Tynan, P. (2024) The integration and implications of artificial intelligence in forensic science. *Forensic Science, Medicine, and Pathology*, **20**, 1103–1105. https://doi.org/10.1007/s12024-023-00772-6.

U.S. Department of Justice. (2024, December) Artificial intelligence and criminal justice: Final report. https://www.justice.gov/olp/media/1381796/dl.

Wickramasekara, A., and Scanlon, M. (2024, April) A framework for integrated digital forensic investigation employing AutoGen AI agents. Proceedings of the 12th International Symposium on Digital Forensics and Security. IEEE. https://doi.org/10.1109/ISDFS60797.2024.10527235.

Wickramasekara, A., Breitinger, F., and Scanlon, M. (2025) Exploring the potential of large language models for improving digital forensic investigation efficiency. *arXiv*. https://doi.org/10.48550/arXiv.2402.19366.

de Wit, A.K.J.G., Wagenaar, C.D., Janssen, N.A.C., Hoegen, B., van de Wetering, J., Hoofs, H., *et al.* (2025) Making AI accessible for forensic DNA profile analysis. *Forensic Science International: Genetics*. Advance online publication. https://doi.org/10.1016/j.fsigen.2025.103345.

Xiao, T., and Zhu, J. (2025) *Foundations of Large Language Models, [Preprint]*. arXiv. https://arxiv.org/pdf/2501.09223v2. https://doi.org/10.48550/arXiv.2501.09223.

Yang, M., Li, S., and Zeng, J. (2024) The effects of AI-driven face restoration on forensic face recognition. *Applied Sciences*, **14**(9), 3783. https://doi.org/10.3390/app14093783.

CHAPTER 3

A Universal Guidance Model: The Minnesota Protocol in Challenging Environments

Roberto C. Parra[1,*], Pierre Perich[2], Allan G. Alvarez-Godoy[3], Michael Pollanen[4], Daouda Traore[1,*], Jorge L. Vasquez-Guerrero[5], Omer O. Adjibode[1,*], John Mbewu-Bodji[6], and Sami El Jundi[7]

[1] *The Specialized Forensic Team of the United Nations Joint Human Rights Office (UNJHRO) in the Democratic Republic of the Congo*

[2] *International Forensic Consultant, Marseille, France*

[3] *International Forensic Consultant, The Hague, Netherlands*

[4] *Ontario Forensic Pathology Service, Ontario, Canada*

[5] *Institute of Legal Medicine and Forensic Sciences of Peru, Lima, Peru*

[6] *Center of Forensic Medicine and Criminalistics of Kananga, DRCongo*

[7] *International Forensic Consultant, Coimbra, Portugal*

3.1 Introduction

The unalienable foundation of the international human rights system is the right to life. Its protection goes beyond the state's refusal to commit arbitrary killings; rather, it includes an active duty to prevent, protect, and, most importantly, investigate when there is a plausible suspicion that a death was caused illegally. Investigating is required; it is a logical and inevitable extension of respect for life. In this regard, the 2016 revision of the Minnesota Protocol[1] on the Investigation of Potentially Unlawful Deaths shows itself as a vital instrument that has moved beyond its technical aspect to become a global standard.

Above all, the Minnesota Protocol is a guide that aims to put international law into practical application.[2] It offers an operational framework based

*The views expressed herein are those authors and do not necessarily reflect the views of the United Nations.

[1] See https://www.ohchr.org/en/special-procedures/sr-executions/minnesota-protocol

[2] The obligation of states to investigate suspicious deaths using forensic science procedures. See https://docs.un.org/en/A/HRC/50/34

Forensic Science and Quality Management: Addressing the Era of Standardization in Challenging Environments, First Edition. Edited by Roberto C. Parra and Allan G. Alvarez-Godoy.

on principles that can be applied flexibly according to the institutional and contextual realities of each setting, rather than attempting to impose a strict universal model (Heyns et al., 2019). This feature makes it especially pertinent in situations where resources, political will, security, or institutional conditions are jeopardized. The Protocol's transformative potential is most evident in these difficult situations: where other standards fall short because of excessive technicality or regulatory rigidity, the Protocol provides a forward-thinking, flexible, ethical, and legally sound route.

The fact that the updated Protocol was developed from practice rather than a legal ivory tower is among its most important features. According to Heyns et al. (2019), the updated Protocol drew on decades of cumulative experience in challenging situations, ranging from urban investigations in cases of institutional collapse to the exhumation of mass graves during armed conflicts. It has unique credibility because of this empirical component. This is a tool created on the ground, where access to justice is not a given but rather an aspiration that is continuously threatened, rather than an idealistic document divorced from reality.

In this way, the Protocol lays out the essential rules that ought to guide every investigation: impartiality, independence, efficacy, timeliness, and transparency. However, it does more than just identify them as ideals. Instead, it provides specific instructions on how to put these ideas into practice, even in the face of adverse circumstances. The Protocol permits the establishment of reasonable minimum procedures that ensure investigative integrity without compromising its legitimacy in settings where access to crime scenes is restricted, where adequate forensic laboratories are unavailable, or where communities are paralyzed by fear.

Additionally, there is no one-size-fits-all formula suggested by the Protocol. It acknowledges that different contexts call for different approaches to the application of standards. It is not a matter of "comply or not comply," but rather of gradually approaching the international standard as closely as possible while taking current constraints into consideration. This forward-thinking strategy is particularly helpful in nations with legal systems that are not in line with international law or where forensic expertise and judicial independence are still developing.

The Protocol includes a basic ethical component in addition to its technical content. It declares that the dignity of victims, their families, and the impacted communities must be respected throughout every investigation. In addition to being required by law, the duty to tell the truth is also a moral obligation to those whose lives have been taken in unjustifiable ways. This ethical mindset is translated into particular actions, like the duty to notify relatives, safeguard witnesses, respectfully preserve human remains, and make sure they are properly identified. This viewpoint gives the investigation a human face in situations where human life has been reduced to a statistic or a political threat.

Furthermore, international tribunals, truth commissions, and independent forensic organizations on various continents have all used and cited the Protocol in addition to United Nations human rights bodies (Heyns et al., 2019). Even though it is not legally binding, its legitimacy as a reference standard is strengthened by this normative and practical reception. Its impact has been so great that it has evolved into a document that unites fields as disparate as humanitarian work, forensic anthropology, forensic medicine, international criminal law, and investigative journalism.

The specific goal of this chapter is to examine the Minnesota Protocol's applicability and relevance in challenging environments, that is, situations where complete adherence to international standards appears to be impractical. In addition to showcasing its technical prowess, the goal is to show how its design enables the gradual and contextualized application of policies that, despite their limitations, provide the genuine potential for recording infractions, safeguarding evidence, providing assurances of non-repetition, and, most importantly, honoring victims. This adaptability is a tactic to preserve rigor when circumstances make it challenging, not a sign of giving it up.

There is also a political and symbolic component to the Protocol's implementation in these settings. Its application can break cycles of impunity, bring systematic acts of violence to light, and even spark practice-based institutional transformation processes. Every recorded death with subpar investigative standards signifies a breach in the system of impunity. Furthermore, in the face of circumstances that seek to deny it, every procedure that involves the community, upholds family rights, and appropriately preserves human remains is an affirmation of the right to life.

The Minnesota Protocol has thus established itself as a guide that enables us to move forward, with realism but with firmness, toward the shared goal of ensuring justice for unlawful death, rather than an abstract document or one reserved for established judicial systems. This chapter will therefore begin with the assumption that the Protocol is a tool to support those who, from hostile contexts, continue to insist that every life matters and that every death merits an explanation, documentation, and, when necessary, punishment, rather than an end in and of itself.

3.2 Foundations of the Minnesota Protocol (2016)

The Minnesota Protocol is based on a basic idea of international human rights law: that every death that might be against the law needs to be thoroughly, fairly, and effectively investigated. The United Nations Handbook on the Prevention and Effective Investigation of Extrajudicial, Arbitrary and Summary Executions was first published in 1991 as a technical manual. It was completely rewritten in 2016 to include new developments in international law, forensic practice, and accountability mechanisms. Christof Heyns, who was the Special Rapporteur on extrajudicial, summary, or arbitrary executions at the time, led this revision effort with help from the Office of the High Commissioner for Human Rights and a group of experts from around the world (Heyns et al., 2019). The outcome was a more resilient and advanced methodological instrument, yet more adaptable and able to adjust to diverse institutional and operational environments.

The legal foundation of the Protocol is predicated on the principle that States' duty to safeguard the right to life extends beyond merely preventing arbitrary deaths; it encompasses a positive obligation to investigate any death potentially resulting from unlawful circumstances. This obligation encompasses a substantive aspect, safeguarding the right to life and limiting the lawful application of lethal force, and a procedural aspect, guaranteeing thorough investigations in instances where that right may have been infringed. Not looking into something is a violation of the right to life in and of itself. This shows how important investigation is as an essential part of legal protection.

The 1989 UN Principles on the Prevention and Investigation of Extrajudicial Executions were the basis for the first Protocol in 1991 and are still used in the new version. The 2016 update was not just technical; it also tried to explain all the legal, operational, and scientific parts that are needed for a good investigation. The Protocol not only lays out the basic requirements for a legitimate investigation, one that is quick, effective, independent, fair, and open, but it also gives suggestions for how to put these requirements into practice in different situations.

The 2016 version is distinguished by the integration of the most sophisticated forensic knowledge available at that time. This is clear from how thoroughly it covers things like managing a crime scene, interviewing witnesses, collecting and preserving evidence, recovering and identifying human remains, following international standards for autopsy procedures, and documenting findings in a technical way. The Protocol serves as an operational compendium for state investigators, international missions, independent experts, human rights organizations, and victims or their representatives.

The Protocol is different from other documents because it focuses on professional ethics. This aspect, frequently overlooked in technical manuals, serves as the foundational principle of the proposed methodological approach. It understands that the investigation's integrity depends on both standardized procedures and the behavior of the professionals who do it. The Protocol sets up ethical rules for professional independence, honesty in reports, respect for victims and their families, keeping information private, and standing up to outside pressures that could change the course of truth.

The Minnesota Protocol was designed from the start to be a useful guide that turns international legal standards into useful tools for conducting investigations. But its role as a teacher is just as important. The document is set up in a way that makes it useful for training lawyers, forensic experts, prosecutors, judges, and people who work for international organizations or in civil society. This training goal comes from the fact that many of the problems that make it hard to do good investigations aren't because of a lack of political will, but because of a lack of technical and regulatory knowledge. It also reflects the multidisciplinary nature of the actors involved in investigations.

The Protocol does not require one way to investigate. In fact, its nature is to guide and change. It makes it clear that contexts are different. Some have strong institutions and working judicial systems, while others have weak institutions, armed conflict, structural impunity, or the breakdown of the rule of law. In all of these situations, the Protocol serves as a normative compass that helps people follow international standards, even when not all of the technical details are there. This flexibility is not a flaw; in fact, it is one of the Protocol's best features, making it useful even in the most difficult situations.

The historical progression of the Protocol also signifies a transformation in the understanding of the relationship between law and science within international law. The increasing use of forensic science in human rights investigations in the 1980s, especially in Latin America, showed how technical knowledge can help find the truth in situations where people are not held accountable (Ubelaker et al., 2019). The groundbreaking efforts of the Argentine Forensic Anthropology Team (EAAF) serve as a quintessential illustration. The Minnesota Protocol represents a normative synthesis of the convergence between science and human rights, proposing standards that acknowledge the significance of scientific evidence and the necessity of its validation in accordance with ethical and legal principles. Morris Tidball-Binz, the Special Rapporteur on extrajudicial, summary, or arbitrary executions,[3] presented Report A/HRC/50/34 to the Human Rights Council during its fiftieth session (June–July 2022),[4] which examines Forensic death investigation systems and the difficulties they face today. The text emphasizes that states have an obligation to look into any death that may be illegal because doing otherwise would be a violation of the right to life. International guidelines like the Minnesota Protocol and the Principles on the Effective Prevention and Investigation of Arbitrary Executions must be followed in order to achieve this.

The report emphasizes how important autopsies and forensic scientists are in elucidating the circumstances and causes of death, which benefits public health and justice. It does, however, point out some significant flaws, including a lack of qualified personnel, a lack of autonomy from law enforcement or prosecutors, a lack of funding, subpar facilities, and a lack of a gender perspective. The effectiveness and impartiality of investigations are jeopardized by these restrictions. In addition, the report highlights best practices from nations that value independence, openness, and thorough training, including South Africa, Colombia, Chile, and Costa Rica. The Special Rapporteur comes to the conclusion that in order to preserve justice, save lives, and respect human rights, forensic science must be strengthened.

---

[3] See https://www.ohchr.org/en/special-procedures/sr-executions

[4] See report https://docs.un.org/en/A/HRC/50/34

The Minnesota Protocol of 2016 is a big step toward making investigations into possible unlawful deaths more consistent around the world. Its legal basis, scientific importance, and moral, ethical, and practical nature make it an important guide to making sure that investigations follow not only the rules but also the basic ideas of truth, justice, and respect. It is a strategic tool for defending the right to life in situations where this right is most vulnerable and, therefore, most valuable because it can be used in many different ways.

3.3 The Duty to Investigate in Challenging Environments

The Minnesota Protocol is based on one unchanging idea: every death that could be against the law must be looked into in a way that is thorough, independent, fair, quick, and open. This obligation is activated irrespective of the alleged responsible party and, crucially, regardless of the presence or absence of operational state structures.[5] To put it another way, the duty to investigate doesn't go away when things are bad; in fact, it becomes even more important when the institutional environment is weak, violent, or immune to punishment.

"Challenging environments" are situations where the conditions for a normal forensic investigation, which are usually peace, stable institutions, and access to technical resources, are not fully or partially present. This encompasses nations engaged in armed conflict, authoritarian regimes characterized by systematic evasion of accountability, failed states, areas devoid of state presence or under the dominion of non-state armed groups, and societies where judicial institutions lack autonomy or are co-opted by political agendas.

The situation in the eastern Democratic Republic of the Congo is a clear example of this. The armed conflict between the M23 rebel group and the state has led to many serious violations of international humanitarian and human rights law. In these areas, military operations, civilian massacres, forced displacement, and the presence of many armed groups make it hard not only to keep track of deaths but also to safely get to the scenes, protect witnesses, and keep physical evidence safe.[6] Even so, the Minnesota Protocol says that the State still has to investigate even if the conditions aren't perfect. This duty, on the other hand, is heightened as part of the commitment to the principle of non-impunity. For instance, United Nations Human Rights (OHCHR) and Congolese national

[5] Torture, discriminatory violence, excessive force, and deaths in custody are examples of ongoing violations of the right to life. Systemic obstacles to investigations include institutional bias, conflicts of interest, fear of retaliation, and a lack of independent complaint procedures. Accountability is further weakened by political meddling and inadequate forensic capabilities. Nevertheless, resolving these problems is essential to guaranteeing justice, avoiding impunity, and enhancing public confidence in law enforcement. See https://www.ohchr.org/en/calls-for-input/2025/call-input-special-rapporteur-summary-extrajudicial-or-arbitrary-executions

[6] See https://news.un.org/en/story/2025/06/1164466

agencies have recorded deaths in North and South Kivu many times.[7,8] Despite limited infrastructure, mobility, and personnel protection, the information gathered can reconstruct events, identify patterns of systematic violence, and set precedents for future legal action. The Protocol's essence is to strive for truth even under challenging circumstances.

Neighboring the Democratic Republic of the Congo (DRC) to the south, Angola regained its institutional stability after 27 years of civil war (1975–2002). However, it continues to face areas of instability along the border with the DRC, where human rights violations and the use of sexual violence as a weapon of war are not uncommon. Additionally, the significant social gap within Angola fuels high levels of violence, while the country has yet to develop a robust police and forensic structure capable of investigating violent crimes in general and human rights violations in particular. Recent initiatives by the country's Attorney General's Office reflect a political will to address these structural deficiencies and better fulfill its democratic commitments under international law, leading to efforts in human resource training based on the Minnesota Protocol.

The Protocol also covers deaths that happen during social protests in democratic countries. For example, in Peru,[9] dozens of people died in 2022 and 2023 as a result of citizen protests against decisions made by the government and Congress. The Peruvian State is required to conduct investigations in accordance with the principles of the Protocol because of these deaths, which are often blamed on security forces using too much force. Opening administrative or criminal proceedings is not enough; the investigation must be done in a way that is legally, technically, and ethically sound. Having judicial structures in place does not mean that standards will be followed. Independence, fairness, and institutional will are the most important things.

In cases of large-scale social protests, like those in Chile,[10] Colombia,[11] Iran,[12] Angola,[13] and many other environments, the Protocol serves as a reminder that deadly force can only be used in very limited circumstances. If someone dies, the act itself must be looked into, as well as the chain of command, the orders given, institutional failures, and patterns of systematic repression. Investigating deaths

---

[7] See https://www.ohchr.org/en/press-releases/2025/02/democratic-republic-congo-parties-conflict-must-treat-dead-bodies-dignity

[8] See https://news.un.org/en/story/2025/02/1160231

[9] See https://www.ohchr.org/en/press-releases/2023/10/peru-un-human-rights-office-calls-meaningful-reforms-guarantee-right

[10] See https://www.ohchr.org/en/press-releases/2019/12/un-human-rights-office-report-chile-crisis-describes-multiple-police

[11] See https://www.un.org/sexualviolenceinconflict/wp-content/uploads/2025/02/report/situation-of-human-rights-in-colombia-report-of-the-united-nations-high-commissioner-for-human-rights/g2500325.pdf

[12] See https://news.un.org/en/story/2022/11/1130927

[13] See https://www.ohchr.org/en/press-releases/2025/07/comment-un-human-rights-office-spokesperson-thameen-al-kheetan-deaths-during

during protests enables us not only to comprehend the specifics of individual incidents but also to elucidate the systemic dynamics of state violence.

The Protocol can link various forms of documentation, typically created by journalists, activists, or international missions, with upcoming legal accountability procedures in regions like Sudan, Palestine, Myanmar, or Ukraine, where a large number of people are killed in conflicts or under authoritarian governments. The ability to gather satellite evidence, credible testimonies, minimal dossiers supporting the chain of custody, and other forensic evidence can make the difference between ongoing impunity and the possibility of future justice. In this sense, the Protocol is a means to difficult situations where legal proceedings can succeed rather than an end in and of themselves.

Finally, another example that warrants attention is Brazil. More than three decades after the end of its dictatorship and the implementation of a robust democratic federal constitution, Brazil has an organized forensic structure spread across 27 federal units (26 states and the Federal District) and a federal unit, of these 18 operate independently from the police. Despite having sophisticated laboratories that serve as regional and even international references, the country continues to struggle with endemic police violence, reaching epidemic levels in some regions (particularly in the states of São Paulo and Rio de Janeiro), and significant quality issues, especially the lack of standardization, including in procedures for maintaining the chain of custody, both in police investigations and forensic operations. This combination of institutional violence and the absence of standardized forensic practices contributes significantly to the country's impunity, which has led to multiple convictions by the Inter-American Court of Human Rights (IACHR/CIDH)[14] for failing to meet its obligations to protect life.

Some judgments by the IACHR/CIDH explicitly reference the Minnesota Protocol as a standard in investigating police violence, which prompted Brazil's National Justice Council to produce Portuguese versions of this and other protocols.[15] However, the country still lacks initiatives that ensure the efficacy and effectiveness of this effort beyond merely providing a document in Portuguese.

One of the Protocol's most important contributions is that it understands that justice doesn't always happen right away. In numerous complex situations, investigations commenced today may yield tangible consequences in the future. This does not lessen their significance; rather, it converts inquiries into forms of resistance against erasure and denial. Even if it doesn't have immediate legal effects, strict documentation creates memory archives, helps establish historical truth, and makes the social demand for justice stronger.

---

[14] See https://www.cnj.jus.br/poder-judiciario/relacoes-internacionais/monitoramento-e-fiscalizacao-das-decisoes-da-corte-idh/casos-contenciosos-brasileiros/

[15] See https://www.cnj.jus.br/wp-content/uploads/2024/08/protocolo-minnesota-por.pdf

The duty to investigate in difficult situations also means that secondary international mechanisms must be used.[16] The Protocol acknowledges that when the State is either unable or unwilling to conduct an investigation, the international community, via commissions of inquiry, specialized mechanisms, or international tribunals, can play a supplementary role. This has been evident in the international investigative mechanisms concerning Syria,[17] Iraq,[18] and many other environments[19] where the Protocol has functioned as a technical framework for the gathering of forensic and testimonial evidence.

The obligation to investigate does not rest exclusively with the judicial system. Communities that are affected, civil society groups, journalists, and human rights defenders also have a big part to play. The Protocol acknowledges them as valid stakeholders in the process, contingent upon their adherence to ethical and methodological standards. In many cases, these people are the ones who start the documentation process in very dangerous situations, and their work is then used in official or international investigations.

The obligation to investigate does not lessen in difficult situations. Instead, it is made stronger to fight against invisibility, stop repetition, and bring back the legal and social value of each life lost. The Minnesota Protocol is a complete guide to dealing with these problems and making the truth even at the edges of the law. The Protocol provides a plan that makes the possible necessary at every crime scene without experts, every secret grave without a laboratory, and every witness who is afraid to speak. Its strict enforcement, even if only in part or in small steps, is a sign of respect for those who died unfairly and a sign that justice has the right to enter even in times of chaos.

3.4 Implementation Strategies Adapted to Challenging Contexts

One of the most powerful and unique things about the Minnesota Protocol is that it can be put into action and changed as needed. The Protocol was designed to be a practical guide for action in real-life situations, which are often unstable, unsafe, or disorganized by institutions. This is different from other international legal instruments that set out ideal frameworks without ways to put them into practice. It is not a strict guide or a technical recipe that only works in very complicated forensic laboratories. Instead, it is a flexible strategic platform that can be

[16] See https://www.ohchr.org/sites/default/files/Documents/Publications/CoI_Guidance_and_Practice.pdf

[17] See https://www.ohchr.org/en/press-releases/2024/12/syria-evidence-gross-human-rights-violations-and-international-crimes-must?utm_source=chatgpt.com

[18] See https://www.ohchr.org/sites/default/files/UNAMI_Report_Accountability_for_Human_Rights_Violations_and_Abuses_ENG.pdf?utm_source=chatgpt.com

[19] See https://www.ohchr.org/en/meeting-summaries/2023/06/human-rights-council-holds-interactive-dialogue-extrajudicial-summary-or?utm_source=chatgpt.com

used in many different situations, even (and especially) in situations that would normally not be good for regular forensic investigation.

This methodological flexibility does not imply a decrease in rigor. The Protocol, on the other hand, says that the investigation of possibly illegal deaths must stay within certain ethical and technical limits that ensure the results are reliable, even if that means changing the way things are done. So, it suggests what we could call a "operational gradation," where actions are prioritized that, while basic, can keep evidence, make records, and help with the first documentation of the events. For example, community interviews with important witnesses, basic photos of scenes or bodies, participatory mapping to mark graves, temporary burials with georeferenced markers, and collecting little information when there are no qualified experts are all examples.

These practices are not made up on the spot; they are based on knowledge gained over decades of fieldwork, mostly by civil society groups, independent forensic teams, international organizations, and human rights missions. In nations where the governmental framework is deficient in forensic laboratories or specialized prosecutors, particularly in numerous rural areas of eastern Congo, these modified strategies are the sole means to guarantee that fatalities do not remain entirely obscured. In fact, their worth goes beyond just being records; they also serve as a way to symbolically fight against impunity.

The Protocol's design, which is based on principles instead of strict rules, makes this possible. Investigations must meet five basic requirements: they must be effective, independent, fair, quick, and open. The methods for meeting these standards may differ based on the resources at hand, but the standards themselves should not be changed. For instance, a complete autopsy by forensic doctors is recommended; however, in its absence, a detailed external examination with photographic documentation may be utilized, contingent upon the assurance of the chain of custody and the preservation of the corpse's dignity.

Another important part of this adapted implementation is that local actors are involved. The Protocol does not see communities as just people who get technical help; it sees them as important parts of the investigation process. For instance, this could mean teaching community leaders how to find mass graves, how to use participatory tools to record testimonies, or how to teach paramedics and rural health workers how to collect postmortem data. These actions not only improve the quality of investigations but also help institutions grow by strengthening local processes of memory, the demand for justice, and forensic governance.

The principles set forth by the Sydney Declaration on Forensic Science (2022) now offer an additional conceptual framework. An international group of experts led by Claude Roux wrote this declaration, which sets out a broad and strategic vision for forensic science (See Chapter 1). It acknowledges that strict standardization isn't always possible in every situation. The Declaration suggests a principles-based approach that encourages scientific integrity, the contextualization of forensic knowledge, and methodological flexibility without lowering the quality of the results. The spirit of the Declaration supports and makes the operational logic of the Minnesota Protocol more official in many ways.

Both documents have a practical but moral view of forensic science: it's not enough to just follow the rules; you also need to understand the situation, weigh the risks, think about the limits, and act with careful thought. This way of thinking about knowledge is very important when things are hard. It's not about "doing what you can," but about doing what's necessary within your limits, knowing that even small actions can have big legal, social, and symbolic effects.

In settings like Sudan, Gaza, eastern parts of the Democratic Republic of Congo, or the Tigray region of Ethiopia, where access is blocked, bodies are being buried in locations that are still unknown or secret, and international teams are unable to reach them for security reasons, the only way to initiate an investigation is to use specific methods such as interviewing displaced people, obtaining information through satellite imagery, using open-source intelligence, and working with community networks. If these methods are based on the Minnesota Protocol, the results can be used to start international court cases, set up truth commissions, or add to historical memory archives.

Another important part of this plan is training on the job. Many international forensic teams have created fast-track training programs for local staff. This allows them to quickly develop a basic operational capacity to record finds, exhume bodies, and preserve evidence or document testimonies, as has been demonstrated in certain post-conflict regions of the Democratic Republic of the Congo.[20] This decentralized training model has been effectively implemented in Colombia, Peru, Angola, Guatemala, Iraq, Ecuador, among other environments.[21] The training is not just technical; it also covers forensic ethics, human rights, and international standards. Through the development of technical expertise and improved investigative capabilities, this process fortifies the local justice system. Local authorities acquire real-world experience, embrace international best practices, and build long-term capacities that enhance accountability, credibility, and the efficiency of administering justice under the direction of international experts during real-time investigations.

There are some problems with adaptive implementation. One of the biggest problems is that standards could be lowered in the name of adversity. So, both the Minnesota Protocol and the Sydney Declaration say that being flexible doesn't mean being random. Every methodological choice must be recorded, explained, and assessed in accordance with established norms. This makes sure that the investigation stays legally valid, technically sound, and socially acceptable.

[20] See https://www.ohchr.org/en/stories/2022/11/forensic-investigators-bring-dr-congo-victims-closer-justice

[21] Personal communication (2025) with Dr. Morris Tidball-Binz, United Nations Special Rapporteur on extrajudicial, summary or arbitrary executions (https://www.ohchr.org/en/special-procedures/sr-executions/mr-morris-tidball-binz).

Implementation strategies adapted or coached by local professionals are a valid, technically, and rigorously sound way to fulfill the duty to investigate potential human rights violations, not a backup or replacement option. In situations where forensic laboratories or forensic investigation systems are unavailable, inaccessible, or simply nonexistent, the Minnesota Protocol remains a useful framework. However, its implementation requires strong dedication, sociocultural adaptation, political commitment, working under high levels of stress, protecting victims' dignity, and pursuing minimum standards where resources do not exist. The Protocol presents enormous potential to develop forensic science in transformative and contextually relevant ways both on its own and when combined with the guiding principles set out in the Sydney Declaration; both tools create levels of quality management that cannot be replaced by other mechanisms. Through this integration, the scope of justice-oriented forensic investigation is expanded and adherence to international human rights standards is ensured, even in situations where other quality assurance frameworks may be impractical or ineffective.

3.5 Best Practices and Relevant Experiences

The empirical application of the Minnesota Protocol in diverse global contexts has significantly validated its efficacy as a technical and regulatory instrument. Even though it was meant to be a universal guide, its legitimacy comes not only from the principles it lays out, but also from the fact that it has been shown to work in places where institutions are unstable, violence is systemic, and there are no established forensic structures. The experiences gathered in Latin America, Africa, the Middle East, and Asia illustrate that, even in highly unfavorable circumstances, the Protocol can serve as a catalyst for justice, a means of documentation, and a foundation for institutional empowerment.

The Argentine Forensic Anthropology Team (EAAF), which was started in 1984 in response to crimes committed during the military dictatorship, is a good example of this in Latin America (Ubelaker et al., 2019). The EAAF created a method based on the principles that would later be organized into the Minnesota Protocol: independence, scientific rigor, putting the victim first, and working with affected communities. They did this without any institutional support or initial state support. Its interventions in Argentina, Peru, Guatemala, El Salvador, Colombia, and Mexico, among other nations, have shown that rights-based forensic practice can be established from the ground up, tailored to specific contexts, and can produce internationally acknowledged technical standards.

In Colombia, the Search Unit for Missing Persons (UBPD) has partially institutionalized the use of these principles. The UBPD works under the rules of the Peace Agreement and has worked closely with groups of victims, independent forensic experts, and international organizations. The UBPD has modified practices from the Minnesota Protocol to suit the Colombian context, which is marked by the ongoing presence of armed actors, territorial fragmentation, and a fundamental distrust of the State. Using participatory methods, respectful burials, georeferencing of graves, and community interviews, it has made a lot of progress in finding missing people. It has also created a hybrid model of forensic investigation and transitional justice.

In Africa, there have been many responses to war crimes, political violence, and government repression. For instance, in the Democratic Republic of the Congo, both UN missions and local groups have used the Minnesota Protocol to keep track of mass killings, secret burials, and summary executions and many other applications. The UN Joint Human Rights Office (UNJHRO) has helped with forensic investigations after conflicts between the state and groups like the Kamuina Nsapu militia, among others.[22,23] This shows how international standards can be put into action with the help of local actors, even when there aren't any fancy laboratories or forensic tools available. Forensic reports have been created that help the courts and truth-telling systems by using interviews, mapping mass graves, and collecting basic remains.

A common thread in these experiences has been the need to adjust to the fact that the state is not very strong. The document, "*Addressing the Lack of Forensic Scientific Evidence and Expertise in the 'Trigger Mechanisms'* of Genocide Investigations" (Komar et al., 2020), shows exactly how the lack of expert evidence and forensic scientific expertise makes it harder to use international mechanisms to stop and punish genocide. Empirical research indicates that the absence of initial data collection, even in minimal form, significantly reduces the likelihood of eliciting an international response (Komar et al., 2020). The document therefore recommends strategies for developing fundamental capabilities and states that field training, the use of cost-effective technologies (such as the implementation of the Berkeley Protocol[24]), and interdisciplinary collaboration can partially compensate for the lack of sophisticated laboratories. This vision strengthens the Minnesota Protocol's operational logic and makes it okay to use in situations where justice seems far away.

In the Middle East, international teams or civil society groups have mostly been in charge of keeping track of crimes in Syria and Iraq because it is impossible to do so in working judicial systems. Organizations like the Independent International

[22] See https://www.ohchr.org/en/stories/2022/11/forensic-investigators-bring-dr-congo-victims-closer-justice

[23] The UN Joint Human Rights Office in Congo (UNJHRO) supported 19 mobile courts and 13 joint investigation teams between January 2023 and November 2024. As a result of these efforts, 1,010 people were charged with grave violations of international humanitarian and human rights law, and 777 of them were found guilty. See https://www.ohchr.org/en/stories/2025/01/drc-mobile-courts-fight-impunity-and-bring-dignity-victims

[24] See https://www.ohchr.org/en/publications/policy-and-methodological-publications/berkeley-protocol-digital-open-source

Investigation Team on Syria have shown that the Minnesota Protocol can be used even when there is open war.[25] In these situations, technologies like satellite imagery analysis, remote interviews, social media data mining, and digital reconstructions have been used to get around the fact that it is impossible to get to crime scenes in person.[26,27] These strategies do not supplant a comprehensive in-person investigation; however, they can produce contextualized and credible evidence, beneficial for historical documentation and prospective judicial proceedings.

Countries in Asia, like the Philippines[28] and Myanmar,[29] have had similar problems: the government not wanting to help, threats to witnesses, co-opted courts, and the repression of people who defend human rights. Still, community groups have been able to use the Minnesota Protocol to put into place some basic investigative methods. In Myanmar, for instance, the documentation of atrocities against the Rohingya people has mostly come from testimonies taken in refugee camps in Bangladesh, as well as pictures, personal items, and maps made by the people who had to leave their homes.[30,31] This documentation has been very important for holding people accountable in the International Criminal Court and the global justice system.

A significant characteristic of these practices is their formative quality. The Minnesota Protocol is not only a guide for investigations, but it has also been used to train people. International organizations, universities, forensic teams, and human rights defenders have used its principles to teach police officers, doctors, humanitarian workers, and whole communities how to do their jobs better. This ability to teach makes it more legitimate as a tool that can be used for both immediate action and for creating a culture of human rights. This builds up local skills that make it less necessary to rely on outside experts and help truth and justice processes last.

These experiences show that the Minnesota Protocol has gone beyond being just a set of rules. It has turned into a place where people can take action, work together, learn, and keep records. Its strengths are that it can be changed to fit different situations, it is based on ethics, and it can be activated by many people, even when the State is not working. It is not just a tool for established

[25] See https://www.ohchr.org/en/press-releases/2024/12/syria-evidence-gross-human-rights-violations-and-international-crimes-must

[26] See https://carnegieendowment.org/research/2025/01/international-crimes-accountability-matters-in-post-assad-syria?lang=en&utm_source=chatgpt.com

[27] See https://www.hrw.org/topic/technology-and-rights/digital-investigations-lab?utm_source=chatgpt.com

[28] See https://www.ohchr.org/en/press-releases/2020/06/philippines-un-report-details-widespread-human-rights-violations-and

[29] See https://www.ohchr.org/en/documents/country-reports/ahrc5756-situation-human-rights-myanmar-report-united-nations-high

[30] See https://today.usc.edu/human-rights-abuses-rohingya-refugees-usc-parveen-parmar/?utm_source=chatgpt.com

[31] See https://www.ohchr.org/en/hr-bodies/hrc/myanmar-ffm/reportofthe-myanmar-ffm?utm_source=chatgpt.com

judicial systems; it has been especially useful in places where justice is missing or disputed.

So, these best practices not only prove that the Protocol works, but they also make it more useful. Every forensic intervention in a dangerous setting, every body identified through rudimentary techniques, and every community empowered to safeguard memory signify an affirmation of the right to life and a repudiation of impunity. In light of present adversities – wars, oppression, disappearances, and coerced migrations – these experiences provide not only motivation but also proof that dignity can be preserved even amidst institutional voids. People who believe that justice is a group effort are still writing the Minnesota Protocol.

3.6 Recurring Challenges

Using the Minnesota Protocol in difficult situations is not easy, and it faces many challenges that test its ability to adapt. In many situations, the problems are not just technical; they are also structural, political, and related to security. These restrictions make it harder to do good investigations and protect the people who do them and the people who work with them.

One of the most common problems is that witnesses, experts, and community members who are involved in the documentation process don't have enough protection. In places where armed groups are active or where the State is actively or passively involved in violations, people who try to tell the truth are threatened, punished, or even killed. This not only stops people from getting involved, but it also stops ongoing investigations, silences important witnesses, and makes it harder to get important information.

Another common problem is when armed groups or government forces get in the way. In some places, like Syria, Myanmar, Colombia, Mexico, and the eastern Democratic Republic of the Congo, crime scenes are controlled by people who put limits on investigations or change the locations on purpose to get rid of evidence. The inability to access sites or the need to negotiate with those who control them makes the proceedings less independent and safe.

Furthermore, it is common for people in conflict zones to intentionally destroy, alter, or contaminate physical evidence. Disturbed graves, burned bodies, forged documents, or altered crime scenes are all ways to cover up crimes.[32] In these situations, the chain of custody is very weak, and conclusions may be unreliable. Still, the Minnesota Protocol, in conjunction with the Berkeley Protocol,[33] can allow investigators to record the circumstances of deaths and violence in

[32] https://www.ohchr.org/en/press-releases/2021/11/tigray-conflict-report-calls-accountability-violations-and-abuses-all

[33] https://www.ohchr.org/en/publications/policy-and-methodological-publications/berkeley-protocol-digital-open-source

general, even in these cases, providing them with important information about how impunity operates.

Institutional deficiencies, on the other hand, are always a problem. Investigations are hard to move forward with a clear legal framework because there are no records, prosecutors are careless, staff members leave, training is lacking, and internal rules are not followed. Even when individuals want to, the government may not have the basic tools it needs to do investigations with the least amount of effort.

In many cases, the state itself is the biggest problem. Denying access, making victims or investigators criminals, changing expert reports, and blocking the courts all make it harder to do the duty to investigate. They also make it easier for victims to be victimized again and make the culture of impunity stronger.

The Minnesota Protocol is a tool that helps with forensic work and lets people write down the structural problems that make it hard to get justice. It records not just the crime itself, but also how people try to cover it up and keep it quiet. Being able to name the unnamed is a way of resisting and building truth.

3.7 Value of the Protocol as a Universal Standard in the Fight Against Impunity

The Minnesota Protocol has become a universal minimum standard for looking into deaths that may have been illegal, even though it is not legally binding. Its authority does not stem from formal legal power, but rather from its epistemic legitimacy, meticulous technical construction, and widespread acceptance by diverse stakeholders within the international human rights framework. The Protocol has, in practice, gained an informal normative status that makes it an unavoidable reference in both judicial and extrajudicial contexts. Its value has grown in situations where institutional guarantees are weak.

The Protocol has been cited by several regional human rights courts since it was revised and adopted in 2016. The Inter-American Court of Human Rights has used it as a technical standard to judge how well Member States' investigations are done, especially in cases of police violence, enforced disappearances, and extrajudicial killings. Its usefulness comes from the fact that it gives objective, not just legal, standards for figuring out if an investigation was done independently, quickly, effectively, fairly, and openly. The Protocol lays out these five principles in such a way that they can be used by courts to check the quality of state actions that go beyond just existing in name only.

The Protocol has also been used by groups like the UN Human Rights Committee and Special Rapporteurs on extrajudicial killings. In their final comments and suggestions, these mechanisms have told States to make sure that their investigations follow the Protocol's standards, which they see as a reliable and technically sound guide for state action within the framework of the right to life. This legitimacy has been bolstered by its consistent application in reports from international fact-finding missions, particularly in Myanmar, Syria, South Sudan, and Venezuela, where the Protocol has served as the methodological foundation for documenting crimes against humanity in situations of repression or armed conflict.[34]

The Protocol's precise technical language is one of its best features. It makes it possible for many different people, including forensic experts, prosecutors, human rights defenders, police officers, judges, and community representatives, to understand and use it. This clarity does not mean that the document is easier to understand. In fact, its modular and progressive structure makes it easier to use at different levels of training and institutional sophistication. It has been used as a teaching tool in training manuals, university courses, and operational guides for groups like the International Committee of the Red Cross (ICRC), Amnesty International, and the United Nations High Commissioner for Human Rights (OHCHR).

The Protocol is a set of rules that forensic scientists must follow when doing autopsies, collecting evidence, handling human remains, taking pictures, interviewing witnesses, and keeping track of evidence. This has enabled forensic teams with constrained resources in regions such as Africa, Latin America, and the Middle East to organize their methodologies in accordance with internationally accepted standards, even in the absence of specific national regulations or fully operational judicial systems. Even if the Protocol is only partially or slightly changed, using it in investigations makes them more valuable legally and gives them more power as evidence in international situations.

The Protocol has a lot of political and symbolic value, in addition to its technical value. Truth commissions in places like Guatemala, Colombia, Peru, and Sierra Leone have used it, showing that it can also be used to rebuild history, honor victims, and make memory processes more legitimate. In these instances, the Protocol has facilitated the establishment of objective criteria to ascertain patterns of violence, identify institutional responsibilities, and distinguish between combat fatalities and extrajudicial executions. This aspect is especially significant in transitional justice processes, as the formulation of an accurate narrative regarding the past is largely contingent upon the thoroughness of forensic investigations.

The Protocol's universal value is also shown by how well it can cut across institutions. Judicial systems, international organizations, NGOs, forensic groups, and governments at all levels have all used it. Because it can work with many different legal systems and in different situations, this tool is very useful. The fact that it was created through a wide-ranging consultation process with experts in human rights, forensic medicine, forensic anthropology, international criminal law, and civil society groups has made it more legitimate.

[34] See https://docs.un.org/en/A/HRC/50/34

One of the most important things about the Protocol is that it doesn't compete with other legal systems; instead, it works with them. In particular, its compatibility with the Rome Statute and the jurisprudence of the International Criminal Court (ICC) has made it easier to use in the documentation of international crimes.[35] The Protocol serves as a bridge between forensic science and the building of complicated legal cases by giving a technical framework that can be checked. This makes the chain of evidence stronger when testimonial evidence is weak or limited.

The Protocol has been adopted as a teaching guide in many universities and training centers for justice officials at the pedagogical level. Its structure makes it easy to use in classes on human rights, forensic medicine, forensic anthropology, and criminalistics. Also, the fact that it is available in many languages and is easy to access makes it even more global, letting local actors use it without having to rely on institutional translations or expensive middlemen.

Finally, one of the things that makes the Protocol a good universal minimum standard is that it is epistemologically strong. The Protocol offers a principles-based rationale rather than rigid ISO standards or context-free automated procedures, which would "industrialize" forensic science. Its ability to adapt to challenging circumstances while maintaining rigor illustrates that quality depends not only on infrastructure but also on scientific and ethical rigor. In this way, the Minnesota Protocol anticipated modern debates on forensic epistemology, endorsed by the Sydney Declaration, by proposing a forensic science based on people, places, and justice.

The Minnesota Protocol is more than just a list of recommendations; it is a strategic tool that has worked, been proven to be real, and changed things. As a universal minimum standard, it is valuable because it can be used in many different situations, is technically sound, is open to different methods, and can bring together people from different backgrounds to work toward a common goal: making sure that every death that could be illegal is looked into with the respect, seriousness, and humanity it deserves. In a world full of violence, unfairness, and lack of consequences, the Protocol is a moral and practical guide that helps people keep their focus on dignity.

3.8 Conclusions

In difficult or extremely unfavorable situations, the Minnesota Protocol is not only a technically sound tool but also a moral/ethic requirement. In situations where formal justice systems have been suppressed by violence, institutional structures have collapsed, and the examination of bodies becomes crucial for identifying serious human rights violations, it serves as an essential framework

[35] See https://www.icj.org/wp-content/uploads/2019/09/Universal-PG-14-Unlawful-death-Publications-Reports-Practitioners-Guides-series-2019-ENG.pdf?utm_source=chatgpt.com

for forensic investigation and Human Rights Investigations. Its value lies in the ethical principles it upholds as well as the investigative standards it recommends: a forensic practice dedicated to protecting the right to life and recognizing victims as individuals with rights that continue to exist after death.

This chapter has demonstrated that the Minnesota Protocol constitutes significantly more than merely a compilation of best practices. It is a flexible platform that can be used in a variety of situations, from war to structural violence. It can be used in difficult situations because of its clear technical language, flexible methods, and focus on principles. This doesn't mean giving up quality or legality. It has been used by civilian teams, truth commissions, humanitarian groups, and international organizations in places as different as Latin America, Africa, and the Middle East, which shows how popular it is around the world.

The Minnesota Protocol has proven to be extremely relevant and useful over time. It improves the efficacy of forensic interventions when needed and fortifies local capacities through ongoing, specialized training. However, its purview goes beyond the purely forensic realm, establishing itself as a political tool for upholding human rights and advancing peacebuilding initiatives. The Protocol expressly opposes disciplinary reductionism in the recording and analysis of forensic evidence by encouraging a thorough approach to investigations. Rather, it highlights how crucial it is to incorporate various viewpoints in order to completely comprehend the social, political, and cultural circumstances that surround each case. By doing this, it emphasizes that forensic practice must integrate more comprehensive analytical frameworks and cannot be limited to a purely technical exercise. In the end, the Protocol emphasizes how important it is to handle each case with contextual sensitivity in order to guarantee a more comprehensive and morally sound search for justice and the truth.

One of the Protocol's main benefits is that it can make not only death, but also the circumstances around it, visible. These include institutional inaction, the denial of mourning, the criminalization of victims, and cover-up strategies. In light of these difficulties, its methodology provides a means to recover the truth through scientific practice, without compromising sensitivity or contextualization. This tool is one of a kind in the world of international standards because it combines technical rigor with a commitment to humanism.

The Minnesota Protocol's adoption and execution represent a deep dedication to justice and the international movement to end impunity, going beyond a merely technical decision. In order to guarantee that forensic and Human Rights investigations meet the highest international standards, their efficacy depends on a meticulously planned implementation, ongoing training, methodical practice, and ongoing improvement. The Protocol is a crucial first step in reestablishing public confidence in truth and accountability processes in situations characterized by institutional weakness or the lack of conventional justice mechanisms. Furthermore, its applicability is increased in situations involving forensic inequality, where access to justice is frequently restricted due to factors like geography, financial capability, or infrastructure. Its uniform and widespread use is therefore essential, not only in highly specialized morgues with cutting-edge equipment but also in smaller mortuary or thanatology units, especially in environments where issues with justice and openness are most noticeable.

References

Heyns, C., Casey-Maslen, S., Fisher, T., Knuckey S., Probert, T. and Tidball-Binz, M. (2019) Investigating Potentially Unlawful Death under International Law: *The 2016 Minnesota Protocol,* 52 Int'l. Law. 47. https://scholarship.law.columbia.edu/faculty_scholarship/4194.

Komar, D., Parra, R.C., and El Jundi, S. (2020) Addressing the lack of forensic scientific evidence and expertise in the "trigger mechanisms" of genocide investigations. *Forensic Science International,* **317**, 110499. https://doi.org/10.1016/j.forsciint.2020.110499.

Office of the United Nations High Commissioner for Human Rights. (2016) The Minnesota Protocol on the Investigation of Potentially Unlawful Death (2016): *The Revised United Nations Manual on the Effective Prevention and Investigation of Extra-Legal,* Arbitrary and Summary Executions. United Nations. https://www.ohchr.org/sites/default/files/Documents/Publications/MinnesotaProtocol.pdf.

Ubelaker, D.H., Shamlou, A., and Kunkle, A.E. (2019) Forensic anthropology in the global investigation of humanitarian and human rights abuse: Perspective from the published record. *Science & Justice,* **59**(2), 203–209. https://doi.org/10.1016/j.scijus.2018.10.008. PMID: 30798870.

CHAPTER 4

Deaths in Custody Are a Silent Global Tragedy: An Analysis of Burkina Faso's Challenging Environment in Dialogue with International Experiences

Daouda Traore[1,*], Roberto C. Parra[1,*], Norbert W. Ramde[2], Bérаré Doudoulgou[2], Ratouissamda Kagambega[2], Omer O. Adjibode[1,*], and Jorge L. Vasquez-Guerrero[3]

[1] *The Specialized Forensic Team of the United Nations Joint Human Rights Office (UNJHRO) in the Democratic Republic of the Congo*

[2] *Forensic Physician at the University Hospital Center (CHU) of Bogodogo, Ouagadougou, Burkina Faso*

[3] *Institute of Legal Medicine and Forensic Sciences of Peru, Lima, Peru*

4.1 Introduction

Deaths in state custody constitute one of the most serious expressions of institutional vulnerability in contexts where deprivation of liberty implies not only a regime of control but also a reinforced obligation of the State to protect the life and integrity of detainees. The paradox that those under state surveillance, apparently in "safe" spaces, can die from violent, preventable, or poorly treated causes reveals serious structural flaws in the criminal justice, prison health, and human rights monitoring systems. The implications of these deaths are not limited to the individual; they constitute warning signs regarding the general functioning of the rule of law and the effective enforcement of the fundamental principles of international humanitarian law and human rights. This chapter is based on a retrospective study conducted in Burkina Faso of 20 deaths that occurred in "garde à vue" (deprivation of liberty taken as part of a judicial investigation), all examined by the country's sole forensic medicine service between 2016 and 2020. The analysis reveals a worrying combination of a lack of forensic examination of compatibility with the detention cell, use

*The views expressed herein are those authors and do not necessarily reflect the views of the United Nations.

Forensic Science and Quality Management: Addressing the Era of Standardization in Challenging Environments, First Edition. Edited by Roberto C. Parra and Allan G. Alvarez-Godoy.

of violence, and precarious detention conditions. None of the deceased had been evaluated by a doctor during detention; most had traumatic injuries; and in no case was the forensic team involved in the removal of the body. The scene of death was inspected on one occasion only. Most of the deaths occurred in police cells in extremely hot, overcrowded conditions. The lack of autopsies in some cases of deaths in custody, the scarcity of additional studies (e.g., forensic toxicology), and limited forensic capacities reveal a system that does not facilitate the determination of the circumstances of deaths in custody. This study exemplifies and is part of a broader phenomenon. Globally, deaths in custody remain poorly documented, often poorly defined, and frequently poorly investigated, as revealed by the recent report by Morris Tidball-Binz (report A/HRC/53/29), who is the Special Rapporteur on extrajudicial, summary, or arbitrary executions, an independent human rights expert appointed by the United Nations Human Rights Council.

Despite the existence of international frameworks such as the Minnesota Protocol for the Legal Investigation of Extrajudicial, Arbitrary, or Summary Executions OHCHR (2016), as well as the International Committee of the Red Cross (ICRC) good practice guidelines on deaths in custody (2013), significant gaps persist between principles and practices. These instruments establish essential parameters for a proper investigation, including thoroughness, impartiality, promptness, protection, monitoring, independence, and participation of family members. Furthermore, they emphasize the State's obligation to act ex officio in the event of any death in custody, whether or not formally reported, and to guarantee access to justice, truth, and reparation.

The contribution of Ruiz et al. (2014) is essential in this context, as it proposes a comprehensive redefinition of the concept of death in custody. Rather than focusing exclusively on the physical location of death, the authors argue that the causal link between the structural conditions of confinement and the occurrence of death should be considered. This dynamic perspective makes it possible to integrate into the analysis deaths that occur after "strategic transfers" to the hospital or after immediate release, common practices in many contexts to evade the official classification of "death in custody" and its legal consequences. Furthermore, they underscore the need to critically assess whether so-called "natural deaths" are not, in fact, preventable deaths aggravated by medical negligence, institutional violence, or inhumane conditions of detention.

In addition, the retrospective study by Wu et al. (2019) on 172 deaths in custody in China provides a valuable comparative basis. Despite an accredited forensic system with established protocols and formal medical coverage, the pattern reveals a high incidence of deaths from cardiovascular disease and suicide, especially in short-term detention centers. This data raises the question of whether institutional infrastructure alone is sufficient to prevent deaths, or whether it should be accompanied by deeper cultural, ethical, structural, and even conceptual reforms.

When someone in custody dies, it directly calls into question the State's duty. From a forensic and human rights standpoint, these fatalities necessitate prompt investigation as purported infringements of the right to life, in accordance with the criteria set forth by the Minnesota Protocol and ICRC guidelines. Not doing so is not only a technical mistake, but it also shows that the institution is not accountable. In difficult African settings like Burkina Faso, and by extension, in various contexts of the Global South, resource scarcity cannot excuse negligence, nor can the lack of systematic data justify neglect and impunity.

This chapter seeks to examine deaths in custody through a comparative and interpretive lens, correlating data from the study in Burkina Faso with international standards and analogous experiences in other global regions. From this analysis, we will endeavor to pinpoint institutional constraints, recommend reforms, and enhance the integrity of forensic practice that ensures truth, justice, and dignity, even within the most obscure aspects of the criminal justice system. When custody and structural violence become silent, forensic science and ethical commitment must be the voices that break it.

4.2 Death in Custody and Limits on Institutions in Burkina Faso

4.2.1 The Rules and Structure of Detention in Burkina Faso

The Burkinabe Code of Criminal Procedure (CPP) says that preventive police custody (GAV) is a form of coercion. It lets a person be held in a police station or gendarmerie brigade under the watchful eye of the courts for a set amount of time. Even though this practice was meant to help with criminal investigations, it makes the State even more responsible for protecting the lives, health, and safety of detainees.

The 2018 Statistical Security Yearbook says that in Burkina Faso, more than 12,000 adults and almost 4,000 minors were put under GAV measures. However, there are no national rules that require regular medical checks on people who are being held, and there are no standard procedures in place to stop abuse or neglect in institutions. Article 515-15 of the Criminal Code allows the prosecutor to appoint a doctor to examine the detainee, but does not require an initial or periodic medical evaluation. Because of this gap in the law, medical exams are only done rarely, which puts the detainee at risk of bad health, abuse, or even torture that may go unnoticed.

4.2.2 Design of Forensic Study

The Forensic Medicine Service of the Bogodogo University Hospital (CHU) conducted a study over five years, from 2016 to 2020, examining 20 cases of deaths that occurred during the GAV and were subject to a forensic examination requested by the Public Prosecutor's Office. This retrospective study encompassed only cases officially referred to the forensic department, indicating a potential underestimation of the phenomenon.

Data collection relied on autopsy reports, court orders, and visits to detention facilities, utilizing individual files that encompassed variables such as age, sex, profession, type of injury, cause of death, and conditions of detention. The selection comprised solely individuals who perished during detention or at the moment of arrest, contingent upon a court's request for a forensic evaluation. Cases that did not involve the Public Prosecutor's Office were not included, which is a big problem.

4.2.3 Profile of the Victim

The 20 cases studied were all men, and their average age was 37.05 years (range, 18 to 49 years). Fifty percent of the victims worked in the informal sector (trades like mechanics, carpentry, and masonry), 25% worked in the formal sector, and the other 25% were unemployed. This profile shows how socially and economically weak the detainees are, which could affect their access to justice, legal defense, and medical care.

In total, 60% of the deaths occurred in 2019, suggesting an anomalous increase or an unspecified structural crisis. Also, 90% of the cases happened in Ouagadougou, the capital of the country. This could mean that there are more arrests in cities or that the cases are more visible in institutions.

4.2.4 Structural Problems and Conditions of Detention

In three cases, the conditions of detention were examined. In one case, the cell was overcrowded (approximately 30 people), the temperature inside was between 33 and 41°C, there was no adequate air circulation, and the cells were only 9.12 m^2. There was no air conditioning in any of the cells. This situation may have made people with preexisting conditions worse physically.

During their incarceration, none of the detainees received a forensic examination. This discovery is especially troubling because the law says that the prosecutor can decide when to have medical exams. The absence of this practice in any instance signifies a systematic, rather than a mere incidental, omission. The forensic service also didn't take part in any of the body recovery procedures, which constitutes a shortfall in the search for and preservation of evidence.

4.2.5 Forensic Findings and Circumstances of Death

Seventy-five percent of the bodies (15 of 20) exhibited discernible traumatic injuries, encompassing blunt force trauma, stab wounds, and ballistic injuries. In 16 of the 20 cases (80%), autopsies were done. The other four had external examinations. There was only one body that had imaging done after death. Qualitative toxicological analyses were conducted in 11 instances (55%), while pathological examinations were performed in 15 instances (75%). Nonetheless, toxicological tests were restricted to identifying the presence of psychoactive substances, without evaluating concentrations or lethal effects.

Seventy percent of the deaths happened in police facilities, 15% in hospitals (where the detainees had already been transferred), 10% in gendarmerie units, and 5% at the place of arrest. In 50% of the cases, the cause of death was determined to be asphyxiation due to suffocation. The evidence suggests a rare mechanism linked to detention conditions (confinement), although the lack of a reconstruction of the scene prevents definitive conclusions from being drawn.

4.2.6 Critical Analysis

The study's results reveal a lack of forensic examinations to ensure compatibility with the police custody cell, a lack of forensic body removal, and limited use of full autopsies and toxicological analyses, which may limit access to truth-telling. The high number of traumatic injuries and deaths by asphyxiation supports the idea that some of these deaths may be linked to excessive force, cruel treatment, or inhumane conditions.

Moreover, the fact that all of the dead were young men from disadvantaged backgrounds raises the issue of banditry and drug use in this environment. The GAV is a deadly trap for detainees in a country where not all procedural provisions are enforced. Ette et al. (2012) in Abidjan, Ivory Coast, in a retrospective study on deaths in police custody, recorded 33 cases over an eight-year period (January 2001 to December 2008). Violence was involved in 24 cases. This result once again shows that places of detention, which are supposed to be secure, can quickly become dangerous for detainees.

Deaths in custody are not rare; they are a structural problem caused by a lack of protection, the use of force, unsafe detention conditions, and a lack of proper forensic procedures. This situation presents an immediate challenge to justice and human rights policies both nationally and regionally.

It is very important to use international standards like those suggested by the Minnesota Protocol and the ICRC Guidelines. It is not only a legal requirement for countries to make sure that investigations are thorough, independent, quick, and open, but it is also a basic ethical requirement to protect the right to the truth and stop more deaths from happening. Burkina Faso, with only one forensic service and limited institutional coverage, is a clear example of why forensic science needs to be improved as a way to make sure justice is done, not just as a tool for finding out what happened after someone dies. Institutional coverage represents a critical example of why forensic science must be strengthened as a guarantee of justice and not as a residual instrument after death.

4.3 Considerations of International Good Practices that Land in the Practice of Challenging Environments

The inquiry into fatalities in custody is not an optional action; it is an international duty upheld by human rights law, international humanitarian law, and forensic ethical standards. This obligation is based on the State's duty to protect life and make sure that when someone dies in a situation where the State has full control over the person, it is held accountable. Different tools have set up rules and guidelines to help with these investigations. This chapter examines the following pivotal documents: the ICRC Guidelines on Deaths in Custody (2013), the conceptual analysis by Ruiz et al. (2014), the retrospective study by Wu et al. (2019), the UN Human Rights Council report A/HRC/53/29 UN (2023), and the handbook by Payne-James et al. (2017) on forensic monitoring and torture prevention. These instruments enable the evaluation of the extent of adherence to or divergence from international standards in contexts like Burkina Faso.

4.3.1 The ICRC Approach: Essential Elements that Should be Known Regarding Forensic Work

The ICRC has five basic rules for how to look into deaths in custody: every investigation must be quick, complete, fair, separate, and open to reasonable public scrutiny. The right to life and the duty of States to stop systematic violations of human rights and international humanitarian law are the sources of these principles.

The ICRC says that the death of any person in custody should be seen as suspicious, and an institutional investigation mechanism should be started right away. To do this, the crime scene must be protected, a forensic doctor must be called in right away, a full autopsy must be done according to international standards (like the Minnesota Protocol), witnesses must be interviewed, and evidence must be carefully documented and kept safe.

In the context of Burkina Faso, it is evident that none of these principles are consistently fulfilled. The absence of forensic personnel to remove the body, the absence of an autopsy in some cases, the lack of rigorous surveillance during detention, and the neglect of documentation protocols constitute a failure to meet minimum standards of care.

4.3.2 Broadening the Definition

The article by Ruiz et al. (2014) presents a bioethical and structural viewpoint on deaths in custody, proposing that such incidents should not be confined to fatalities occurring within the physical confines of a cell. They highlight the necessity to examine the continuum of state custody, encompassing fatalities in hospitals subsequent to arrest or immediately following release. In the trimodal behavior in which death usually occurs after trauma, either immediately or due to early or late complications, it is necessary to consider its direct relationship with the trauma, which in these circumstances initiates the pathophysiological cascade that determines the death of the person.

This procedure makes it possible to find common ways that officers "institutionally evade" their duties, such as when they move a seriously ill detainee to a hospital to avoid the death happening in their custody. It also questions the use of the "natural death" category, which often hides deaths that could have been avoided because of carelessness or cruel treatment. This structural view is especially important in the study conducted in Burkina Faso, where three inmates died in the hospital after their transfer.

4.3.3 Comparative Evidence: The Chinese Case

Wu et al. (2019) examined 172 fatalities in custody within Chinese detention facilities from 1999 to 2016. The system has accredited infrastructure and formally established protocols, but the results show that most of the deaths were caused by things that were thought to be natural, like heart, liver, and respiratory diseases. Suicides and homicides were next. The average age of the dead was 38.6 years, which is similar to the age range of people who die in Burkina Faso.

The study demonstrates systematic deficiencies in medical surveillance, response to preexisting symptoms, and the identification of signs of violence, despite formal autopsies and a more technically sound chain of custody. This case illustrates that accreditation or formal protocols alone do not ensure the effective prevention of deaths in custody; rather, structural and ethical factors are paramount, as emphatically emphasized in the Sydney Declaration (Roux et al., 2022).

4.3.4 United Nations Observations: Report A/HRC/53/29

The Human Rights Council's report A/HRC/53/29 UN (2023) reinforces the State's obligation to guarantee the independent, prompt, and effective investigation of all deaths in custody and warns of patterns of impunity when these conditions are not met. The document emphasizes the need for autopsies to be conducted by independent experts, in a transparent manner, and with the participation of family members or their legal representatives.

It emphasizes that the denial or delay in investigation violates not only the right to the truth but also the right to an effective remedy. Furthermore, it insists that causes of death cannot be presumed to be natural without an independent scientific assessment. This statement is crucial in the context of Burkina Faso, where some deaths were attributed to natural causes.

4.3.5 Documentation to Prevent

This landmark practical guide edited by Payne-James et al., 2017, "Monitoring Detention, Custody, Torture and Ill-treatment," provides a pragmatic framework for averting fatalities in custody, integrating forensic medicine, human rights oversight, and medical ethics. It suggests rules for independent and consistent forensic medical examinations, interviews with detainees, reviews of prison records, and analyses of the material conditions.

The manual's integrated approach is built on one main idea: you can't stop something from happening without outside supervision and thorough record-keeping. It also says that autopsies must follow international technical standards, like those in the Minnesota Protocol, and that all forensic professionals must work independently of their institutions. In the study conducted in Burkina Faso, these principles were not fully respected, due to the lack of involvement of forensic pathologists in forensic body removals, and the absence of autopsies and forensic toxicology in some cases.

4.4 The Debate About What It Means to Death in Custody: Bioethical and Structural Aspects

4.4.1 Beyond the Physical Location: The Continuum of State Custody

From a forensic and human rights point of view, one of the biggest problems with looking into deaths in custody is the definition of the term "death in custody." This idea has always been connected to the place where the death happens, like a prison cell, police station, or detention center. But Ruiz et al. (2014) say that this definition is not enough and can be used to avoid institutional responsibilities. Indeed, many deaths directly or indirectly associated with detention do not occur in the place of confinement, but in hospitals, during transfers, or immediately after release, although they are still causally related to the conditions of custody or abusive practices.

This structural approach suggests a more comprehensive interpretive framework, viewing custody as a continuum of state control rather than a distinct location. Consequently, any death occurring while an individual is in the custody or surveillance of the State, or resulting from State actions or omissions during that time, must be classified as a death in custody and, hence, subjected to heightened due-diligence standards in the investigation. The United Nations Human Rights Council's report A/HRC/53/29 UN (2023) backs up this view by saying that deaths that happen in hospitals or after release must be looked at as if the State is responsible if there is reasonable evidence of prior malpractice, negligence, or institutional violence.

4.4.2 Strategies for Institutional Evasion and Dispersed Accountability

In different situations, states or their representatives have come up with ways to lessen or shift blame for deaths in custody. One of the most common things that happens, as shown in the study by Ruiz et al. (2014), is that some detainees are taken to a hospital when their health is already very bad. This late seeking of medical attention, which seems to be meant to protect life, is often based on an institutional logic of avoidance: if someone dies in a medical facility instead of a prison cell, it may not be included in the official record of deaths in custody, which means it won't be looked at by the public or the courts. Three detainees died in the hospital in the study conducted in Burkina Faso.

Another common tactic is to let people who are in serious condition go right away, without telling anyone or registering them, so that the police don't have to investigate. These actions go against the ideas of openness, accountability, and due process. Payne-James et al. (2017) say that the integrity of documentation and monitoring processes is important for stopping these sneaky strategies. Custody does not conclude with the mere administrative act of release; it terminates only when the repercussions and obligations arising from state authority over the individual are extinguished.

4.4.3 Natural Death vs. Preventable Death: Ethical and Forensic Consequences

Wu et al. (2019) conducted a study in China that indicates a substantial percentage of deaths in custody are categorized as "natural," primarily attributable to cardiovascular, hepatic, and respiratory diseases. However, a critical evaluation indicates that numerous fatalities may have been averted through prompt medical intervention, suitable detention conditions, and effective monitoring. In the study conducted in Burkina Faso, poor detention conditions were implicated in the occurrence of death in several cases. As a result, these deaths would have been preventable.

The difference between a "natural" death and a "preventable" death is very important from a bioethical point of view. If something is classified as "natural" without an independent medical assessment, a full autopsy, or toxicological tests, it means that it is assumed to be normal, which could hide negligence, omission, or even institutional violence. The ICRC guidelines (2013) and the Minnesota Protocol say that every death in custody should be treated as suspicious until a thorough investigation shows otherwise. Medical ethics necessitates that the forensic professional operate autonomously, ensuring their analysis encompasses not only the immediate cause of death but also the contextual and structural factors that may have impacted it. Payne-James et al. (2017) assert that the forensic physician must not merely delineate injuries or illnesses but should also elucidate their implications concerning the detention environment, accessibility to treatment, and the potential occurrence of cruel or inhumane treatment. The forensic doctor must answer the question of whether the death could have been prevented, and in cases where the prisoner suffered from illnesses that required medical attention and treatment, they must conduct the forensic investigation to determine whether such care was provided and the required treatment administered.

4.4.4 Invisibility, Underreporting, and Access to the Truth

Underreporting is one of the worst things that can happen when you have a narrow definition of death in custody. Official statistics often leave out deaths that happen outside the detention center's physical boundaries or that aren't reported in a formal way. This creates an institutional invisibility that makes it hard to understand how big the problem really is and makes it hard to come up with ways to stop it from happening.

The lack of data disaggregated by sex, age, cause of death, underlying medical condition, and length of detention reinforces this opacity. Burkina Faso has national statistics on deaths in custody. The forensic medicine service has only examined cases that occurred during police custody and are subject to a judicial investigation.

The right to the truth, according to international human rights law, means not only knowing the facts but also understanding the patterns in society that create them. There can be no accountability or compensation for the families of victims without accurate and accessible information. So, redefining the idea of death in custody is not just a matter of semantics; it is an act of epistemic and political justice. The lack of awareness among legal authorities, whether judges or prosecutors, regarding deaths in custody often translates into a lack of interest in human rights, a failure to put due effort into preventing and investigating such deaths, thereby perpetuating impunity and the existence of aggressive criminal rehabilitation systems.

4.4.5 Last Reflections

Taking a bioethical and structural view of deaths in custody lets us change the focus from where the death happened to the conditions that made it possible. This viewpoint acknowledges the presence of institutional patterns that promote impunity, invisibility, and re-victimization. The ICRC principles (2013), the Human Rights Council report UN (2023), the empirical studies by Ruiz et al. (2014) and Wu et al. (2019), and the recommendations of the document by Payne-James et al. (2017) all agree that the analytical and normative framework for custody needs to be broadened.

This redefinition is very important in several countries, including Burkina Faso, where forensic medicine is developing, in order to ensure that people can get to the truth, justice, and non-repetition. We can only move toward effective prevention and a detention model that is in line with the basic principles of human dignity and state accountability if we understand how complicated deaths in custody are. Forensic investigation of deaths in custody is essential for safeguarding the right to life and ensuring State accountability. Although the right to humane treatment during detention is universally recognized, deficient conditions and institutional violence continue to undermine it. In this context, the independence and technical quality of forensic experts become critical, as their conclusions guide criminal proceedings and determine whether negligence, abuse, or torture occurred. However, the custodial environment itself generates ethical and practical tensions that can compromise expert objectivity, particularly when they depend on the very institutions potentially implicated. For this reason, solutions must be structural: establishing binding standards of practice and strengthening existing national procedures, while avoiding prescriptive models that are unfeasible in resource-limited settings.

Only through such measures investigations can be impartial, effective, and consistent with international human rights obligations (Wangmo et al., 2014). Binding yet nonrigid standards establish essential obligations without imposing unrealistic procedures. As Wangmo et al. highlight, such flexible frameworks enable context-appropriate investigations while preserving independence and rigor. By focusing on principles and verifiable outcomes, they strengthen credibility, fairness, and alignment with international norms in custodial medico-legal investigations.

In our forensic experience and through the documentation of multiple contexts of deprivation of liberty, we strongly endorse the arguments advanced by Tomczak and Mulgrew (2023), who demonstrate that current systems for recording and classifying deaths in custody present profound epistemological limitations that contribute to the persistent structural invisibility of these deaths. The authors show that internationally used categories—"natural," "suicide," "homicide," "accident," or "other causes"—are not only heterogeneous and difficult to compare but also obscure recurrent mechanisms of risk, institutional negligence, and systemic health inequalities. From our practice, this observation aligns closely with patterns documented across various countries: deaths classified as "natural" that stem from architectural barriers and delayed medical attention; suicides recorded without rigorous assessment of environmental and historical risk factors; or deaths resulting from excessive use of force that are subsequently diluted into ambiguous classifications. We concur with Tomczak and Mulgrew (2023) that the absence of disaggregated data by gender, age, legal status, ethnic identity, or migratory condition prevents the identification of disproportionately affected groups and reproduces longstanding inequities. Likewise, we share their call for an alternative epistemological approach that conceives deaths as complex and contextual phenomena rather than merely administrative events to be placed into rigid and mutually exclusive categories. Field evidence confirms that only an approach capable of recording who dies, where they die, how they die, and under which institutional circumstances can effectively guide prevention policies and ensure the fulfillment of states' obligations of due diligence, transparency, and accountability. We fully support the authors' proposal to develop more precise, digitalized, contextualized information systems aligned with human rights standards, as they represent an essential step toward making these deaths visible and transforming institutional management of life and dignity in custodial settings.

4.5 Comparison with China: A Proven System Faces Persistent Structural Challenges

When comparing the dynamics of deaths in custody between Burkina Faso and China, we are faced with two very different situations. In Burkina Faso, the system is less developed and lacks the technical resources it needs. In China, on the other hand, there is an institutional framework with formalized protocols, accredited technical resources, and advanced forensic infrastructure. Nonetheless, this technical distance does not inherently signify a substantive disparity regarding effective prevention or material justice for victims. The study by Wu et al. (2019) on deaths in custody in China between 1999 and 2016 reveals that, despite structural progress, critical challenges persist that limit full compliance with state obligations regarding the protection of the right to life.

4.5.1 Comparative Profile: Quantity, Age, and Etiologies of Mortality

The Chinese study examined 172 instances of fatalities in custody. The average age was 38.6 years, which is similar to what was found in the Burkina Faso study, where most of the dead were young men of working age. This demographic overlap indicates that, irrespective of the degree of institutional advancement, the principal victims of these fatalities are predominantly young individuals and pretrial detainees.

The Chinese report says that cardiovascular, liver, and respiratory diseases are the most common "natural" causes of death, followed by suicides and some homicides. In Burkina Faso, while fatalities from pathologies were documented, a considerable number exhibited visible trauma.

4.5.2 The Contradiction of Accreditation Devoid of Reflexive Transformation

The Chinese case exemplifies a significant paradox: possessing an accredited system does not inherently ensure the elimination of negligent practices or the complete discharge of the duty of care. Despite established procedures, regular autopsies, and formal protocols, deaths persisted from preventable causes and in situations indicative of inadequate oversight.

This shows that technical accreditation, while useful, doesn't automatically change the way institutions work. Standards can be superficially enforced, failing to alter cultural norms of impunity, negligence, or structural violence. Ruiz et al. (2014) refer to this as structures of institutional irresponsibility, where there are rules but they don't change the things that cause deaths that could have been avoided.

4.5.3 The Function of Forensic Medicine in Both Scenarios

In China, the study by Wu et al. (2019) reveals that all deaths underwent forensic examination and autopsies, apparently meeting the minimum standard required by the Minnesota Protocol. In Burkina Faso, on the other hand, some deaths were not autopsied and no expert was assigned to perform a forensic examination of the body at the crime scene. This difference is important and shows how important it is to make protocols official and give forensic work the resources it needs.

But just following the rules isn't enough. In the Chinese case, mistakes were found in the first classification of the cause of death, missed signs of previous violence, and problems with cross-referencing medical information. This shows that forensic analysis needs to be done by professionals who are not connected to the case, have access to clinical information, and can work together with other institutions. In both cases, forensic science has trouble being a transformative force: in one case because of material limitations, and in the other because of institutional and cultural constraints.

4.5.4 Mechanisms for External Control and Oversight

One of the most important differences between the two situations is how much outside supervision there is. China has set up systems for oversight, but they are very centralized and don't involve many independent groups or civil society. In Burkina Faso, surveillance is carried out by judicial and health authorities.

They agree with what Payne-James et al. (2017) said and say that effective prevention needs outside observers, easy ways to report problems, and regular independent audits. The absence of these components, in both structurally deficient and technically validated systems, constrains the State's actual ability to discern patterns of abuse or neglect.

4.5.5 The Weight of Political and Cultural Contexts

In both Burkina Faso and China, fatalities in custody must be analyzed from a political perspective. In the first case, insufficient forensic infrastructure and personnel limit any investigation into human rights violations. In the second case, the centralization of power, the control of information, and the lack of judicial independence make it harder to find the truth and limit the chances of strategic litigation or compensation.

Both examples show that stopping deaths in custody needs more than just better buildings. It needs political will, openness, citizen involvement, and a culture of respect for human rights in the institutions. In this way, forensic science must be more than just a technical tool; it must also be a way to keep an eye on things, speak out against them, and change them.

4.5.6 Last Reflections

The juxtaposition of Burkina Faso and China illustrates that the issues surrounding fatalities in custody cannot be addressed merely through technical accreditation or formal regulatory frameworks. Although these conditions are essential, they are inadequate in the presence of institutional frameworks that normalize negligence, condone violence, or evade accountability.

A complete approach needs to combine technical skills with ideas like independence, outside oversight, community involvement, and structural prevention. Deaths in custody are not just a one-time event; they are a sign of how well the criminal justice system is working in terms of democracy and morality. Therefore, addressing them requires looking beyond document compliance and committing to a real, ethical, and political transformation of the justice system.

4.6 Recommendations for Action in Challenging Environments

The ongoing occurrence of deaths in custody in varied and complex contexts such as Burkina Faso (and Africa generally), China (or Asia generally), or Latin America illustrates that the resolution of this issue is not confined to the establishment of legal frameworks or attempts at accreditation with impractically stringent standards; rather, it necessitates a comprehensive and context-specific approach. From the main documents reviewed (the ICRC guidelines (2013), the conceptual study by Ruiz et al. (2014), the retrospective analysis by Wu et al. (2019), the report A/HRC/53/29 UN (2023), and the forensic document by Payne-James et al. (2017), we can make a number of recommendations that could work in both Africa and Latin America or Asia. These recommendations are based on the idea of the Global South as a world order and are based on similar structural characteristics, institutional limitations, and patterns of impunity.

4.6.1 Changing the Idea of State Custody

In global contexts, a major barrier to achieving justice in cases of deaths in custody is a narrow and constricted interpretation of the term "state custody." Historically, this term has been solely associated with physical confinement within an institution, such as a police station, prison, or detention center. However, this definition is insufficient given the multiple scenarios in which state power can exercise control over an individual.

The Human Rights Council report (A/HRC/53/29) suggests a wider definition of custody, which sees it as a situation of functional control and institutional responsibility. This perspective maintains that the state's duty to safeguard life persists even when an individual is transferred to a hospital, discharged in critical condition, or placed under the oversight of another governmental entity. Any death that happens while someone is in custody must be looked at in terms of state responsibility, and automatic investigative processes must be set in motion.

This change in how we think about things makes it possible to close the gaps that have historically allowed people to get away with crimes. It also requires a review of legal frameworks, institutional practices, and operational protocols, ensuring that the State's duty of care is effectively exercised, even beyond formal confinement. Taking this wider view is an important step toward stopping these deaths from happening in the first place.

4.6.2 Treat all Deaths in Custody as Potentially Suspicious

The ICRC and the Minnesota Protocol both say that every death in custody should be treated as suspicious. This presumption has an ethical and legal basis:

since the State is in a position to guarantee life, any loss of life under its control implies, at the very least, a possible dereliction of its duty of care. This presumption is especially important in many African and Latin American countries, where the courts are weak and there isn't much oversight of institutions.

It is not always the case that State agents acted maliciously when every death is treated as suspicious. However, it does mean that immediate, impartial, and thorough investigative mechanisms must be put in place. This logic shifts the burden of proof: the family no longer has to prove that violence happened; instead, the State has to make sure that the death was investigated to the highest standards. This procedure also protects honest officials by making it clear what is their fault and what is the fault of the system.

In practice, this presumption must be translated into concrete measures: crime scene preservation, the involvement of independent forensic personnel, photographic records of bodies, immediate interviews with detainees and custodians, and the performance of full autopsies that include relevant forensic laboratory studies, medical history reviews, and documentation of any history of abuse or previous illnesses. These actions must be commenced immediately, even in instances where a natural cause is initially presumed, such as preexisting conditions.

Wu et al. (2019) demonstrated that several deaths in custody in China, initially deemed natural, revealed factors indicative of negligence, insufficient medical care, or inadequate confinement conditions. In Burkina Faso, there are also documented cases that show the absence of autopsies and forensic body removal in some cases.

Taking suspicion as a rule is, therefore, an important part of breaking the cycle of impunity that has historically surrounded deaths in custody. This presumption starts a chain of events that leads to prevention and institutional accountability. This chain must be maintained through clear laws, enough forensic resources, and strong political will.

4.6.3 Ensuring the Independence of Experts and the Integrity of the Forensic Process

The independence of the forensic personnel tasked with establishing the cause of death is a fundamental aspect of ensuring a credible and effective investigation into a death in custody. When forensic services are directly subordinate to security or justice institutions, the likelihood of bias, omissions, or manipulation escalates considerably. The process's credibility is hurt not only by the chance of a cover-up, but also by the public's belief that there is no line between those doing the investigation and those who could be investigated. Therefore, the autonomy of the institutes of legal medicine and forensic sciences is a necessity.

The integrity of the forensic process commences with the expert's functional autonomy. They need to be able to look at, understand, and write down their findings without being pressured by politics, hierarchy, or institutions. In numerous instances, forensic reports represent the sole objective evidence capable of refuting official narratives or initiating alternative investigative pathways. So, any kind of interference hurts both the truth of the facts and the victims' right to justice.

This independence must be shown not only in the way the organization is set up, but also in the way it works. The chain of custody, documentation of the discovery site, application of international protocols, access to medical records, and the possibility of performing additional tests are all elements that reinforce the validity of the results. A forensic process that is dedicated to the truth should also be open about its findings and willing to be checked by outside experts.

4.6.4 Create National Registries and External Oversight Mechanisms

The UN report (A/HRC/53/29) makes it very clear that the lack of systematic data leads to impunity. The absence of aggregated data on deaths in custody hinders precise evaluation of the issue and undermines efforts for effective prevention. Many countries in the Global South, if not the vast majority, do not have official public registries that allow for the identification of patterns, risk institutions, or recurring circumstances. Because there isn't any organized information about this, the phenomenon stays hidden, people get away with it, and victims and their families are left unprotected.

It should be a top priority for institutions to set up unified national registries for deaths in custody. These registries should have basic information like the name of the deceased, where they were held, when they died, what likely caused their death, if they had any visible injuries, if they had any previous medical conditions, if they had ever complained of abuse, and whether or not an autopsy was done. This database must be available to human rights defenders, oversight bodies, and, in some cases, the general public, as long as it protects personal information.

It is also important to set up external and independent monitoring systems to check on the conditions of detention and the investigations into deaths in custody on a regular basis. These mechanisms can include national observatories, specialized rapporteurships, or joint committees that include people from civil society. Their role should not only be to respond to problems, but also to prevent them. They should be able to make suggestions, ask for reports, and suggest changes to the way things are done.

There are both registries and outside systems that can help break down institutional walls and create a culture of openness and responsibility. They are important tools for turning a long-term structural problem into a public issue that has real consequences and legal consequences when the state fails to protect life.

4.6.5 Training Prison and Judicial Officials

It is important to train officials who work in the state custody system and judicial police officers to stop deaths in custody and make sure that investigations are done properly. In many African and Latin American contexts, prison officers, police officers, and judicial officials do not receive sufficient training in human rights, international detention standards, or forensic protocols. This lack not only makes it harder for them to deal with emergencies, but it can also lead to careless or abusive behavior, either directly or indirectly.

Training is more than just holding one-time workshops; it needs to be a long-term effort by the institution that includes technical knowledge, ethical awareness, and critical thinking about the State's role as the protector of life. It should include things like how to spot signs of torture or mistreatment, how to handle deaths in custody, how to keep the scene safe, how to respect the chain of custody, detainees' rights, and the basic rules for using force in a fair way. It is also important to teach legal authorities how to use the Minnesota Protocol so that they know how to use it as evidence and what procedures to follow.

Also, training needs to be done in a way that cuts across different institutions. It is essential that police forces, prosecutors, judges, prison staff, and forensic experts share common learning spaces to foster a coherent institutional culture based on prevention, accountability, and respect for human dignity. At the same time, institutions need to improve their own abilities so that they can keep using these training methods for a long time. This way, knowledge won't depend on outside people or staff changes. Training is not just a technical tool; it is also a way to change the structure of the state custody system.

4.6.6 Guarantee Participation and Reparation for Victims and their Families

The right to truth, justice, and reparations should be the main focus of all government policies about deaths in custody. Family members must be able to read forensic reports, choose their own experts, take legal action without fear of retaliation, and get help from mental health and legal professionals.

The report A/HRC/53/29 says that not giving someone information is a form of re-victimization, especially when the courts don't act fairly. So, there needs to be safe and effective ways to share information, as well as special funds to pay for independent expert reports and lawsuits for human rights abuses.

4.7 Conclusion: Protecting Life on the Margins of the System

Deaths in custody constitute one of the most common yet least visible forms of institutional violence. In the Global South, where judicial systems are constrained, and detention conditions are harsh, these deaths reveal profound failures in protecting fundamental rights. This chapter has argued that state responses must move beyond reactive and fragmented measures toward a comprehensive strategy grounded in prevention, independent investigation, and meaningful reparation. Reevaluating the very notion of state custody is essential, as the authority exercised by state agents carries a nondelegable duty to safeguard life. Accordingly, every death in custody should be treated as potentially suspicious to prevent negligence, institutional inertia, and concealment. The independence of forensic expertise, the preservation of reliable records, robust external oversight, and sustained professional training are foundational to dismantling patterns of impunity. These elements must not be understood as a technical checklist but as interdependent components of a broader cultural and institutional transformation that affirms the dignity of all persons deprived of liberty and guarantees that no death is ignored or inadequately explained.

The experiences examined in Burkina Faso and China demonstrate that the effectiveness of investigations depends not only on international protocols, adequate resources, and the operational autonomy of experts but also on the political will to uphold them. Importantly, these challenges are not confined to the Global South; they manifest across regions and systems worldwide though they become especially visible—and devastating—in resource-limited or otherwise challenging environments.

From this perspective, states operating in such contexts face a dual obligation: to strengthen institutional capacities in line with instruments such as the Minnesota Protocol, and to adapt these principles to their own social, historical, and political realities. Improving autopsies or refining procedures is necessary but insufficient; what is required is a reorientation of how the State understands and engages with the lives and deaths of individuals under its custody. These deaths are not administrative anomalies. In many instances, they represent unnoticed or uninvestigated crimes that demand the same urgency, rigor, and ethical commitment as other forms of structural violence.

Recognition, investigation, prevention, and reparation are not only legal imperatives, but they are also moral ones. Even in under-resourced settings, as seen in the documentation from Burkina Faso, it is possible to identify actionable pathways. Yet the existence of international standards or accredited protocols, as illustrated by the examples from China, does not itself guarantee effective protection. What are indispensable are voluntary adherence, independent monitoring mechanisms, and an active citizenry capable of demanding transparency and dignity.

The magnitude of the challenge is considerable, but so too is our collective capacity to address it. Reorienting state priorities toward those most vulnerable, often nameless in the records and without legal representation, can help restore institutional legitimacy. Ultimately, no penitentiary or judicial reform can endure unless it begins by recognizing the full humanity of those in custody. Protecting life on the margins is not merely a legal or forensic task; it is an act of memory, justice, and collective future-building.

The magnitude of the challenge is substantial, but equally significant is our ability to respond effectively. Reorienting the state's focus toward the most vulnerable, those lacking names in the records or legal representation, can serve as a means to restore lost legitimacy. No penitentiary or judicial reform can be sustained unless it begins with the recognition of the full humanity of those in custody. In the end, protecting life on the margins is not just a job for the law or forensic science; it is a way to create memory, justice, and the future.

References

Etté, H.Y., Djodjo, M., Botti, K., and Ebouat, K.M.E.V. (2012) Qu ' en est-il des décès en garde à vue à Abidjan ? Étude rétrospective sur 8 ans (2001–2008). *La Rev médecine légale*, **3**, 27–33. https://doi.org/10.1016/j.medleg.2011.11.004.

International Committee of the Red Cross. (2013) Guidelines for investigating deaths in custody. *ICRC*. https://www.icrc.org/en/doc/assets/files/publications/icrc-002-4126.pdf.

Office of the United Nations High Commissioner for Human Rights (OHCHR). (2016) The Minnesota Protocol on the Investigation of Potentially Unlawful Death (2016): *The Revised United Nations Manual on the Effective Prevention and Investigation of Extra-Legal, Arbitrary and Summary Executions*. https://www.ohchr.org/sites/default/files/Documents/Publications/MinnesotaProtocol.pdf.

Payne-James, J., Beynon, J., and Vieira, D. (eds.) (2017) *Monitoring Detention, Custody, Torture and Ill-treatment: A Practical Approach to Prevention and Documentation*. 1st edn. CRC Press. https://doi.org/10.1201/9781315211459.

Roux, C., Bucht, R., Crispino, F., De Forest, P., Lennard, C., Margot, P., *et al.* (2022) The Sydney Declaration – Revisiting the essence of forensic science through its fundamental principles. *Forensic Science International*, **332**, 111182. https://doi.org/10.1016/j.forsciint.2022.111182.

Ruiz, G., Wangmo, T., Mutzenberg, P., Sinclair, J., Elger, B.S. (2014) Understanding death in custody: A case for a comprehensive definition. *Journal of Bioethical Inquiry*, **11**(3), 387–398. https://doi.org/10.1007/s11673-014-9545-0.

Tomczak, P. and Mulgrew, R. (2023) Making prisoner deaths visible: Towards a new epistemological approach. *Incarceration: An International Journal of Imprisonment, Detention and Coercive Confinement*, **4**. https://doi.org/10.1177/26326663231160344 (Original work published 2023).

UN (2023) Deaths in prisons: Report of the Special Rapporteur on extrajudicial, summary or arbitrary executions. *United Nations Human Rights Council*, 53rd Session. A/HRC/53/29. https://undocs.org/en/A/HRC/53/29.

Wangmo, T., Ruiz, G., Sinclair, J., Mangin, P., and Elger, B.S. (2014) The investigation of deaths in custody: A qualitative analysis of problems and prospects. *Journal of Forensic and Legal Medicine*, **25**, 30–37. https://doi.org/10.1016/j.jflm.2014.04.009.

Wu, S., Ren, L., Pan, M., Qiu, X., Ding, Z., Wang, Y., *et al.* (2019) Retrospective analysis of 172 cases of custodial deaths in China between 1999 and 2016: forensic experience in China. *International Journal of Legal Medicine*, **134**(4), 1487–1493. https://doi.org/10.1007/s00414-019-02209-8. Epub 2019 Dec 4. PMID: 31802193.

CHAPTER 5

From Conflict to Cooperation: ICRC's Forensic Humanitarian Efforts in Challenging Contexts

Denise Abboud[1], Vincent Mazraani[2], Rafael De Abreu E Souza[1], Maria Dolores Morcillo Mendez[1], Jane Taylor[1], and Pierre Guyomarc'h[1]

[1] *International Committee of the Red Cross (ICRC), Geneva, Switzerland*

[2] *International consultant with the International Committee of the Red Cross (ICRC), Geneva, Switzerland*

5.1 Introduction

The International Committee of the Red Cross (ICRC) stands as a crucial entity in the sphere of humanitarian aid, recognized for its unwavering commitment to impartiality, neutrality, and independence. Founded in 1863, the ICRC operates under a mandate from the international community to safeguard the lives and dignity of those affected by armed conflict and violence. Its core mission is to provide protection and assistance to affected populations while promoting the prevention of human rights and humanitarian law violations. This includes addressing protection risks and advocating for adherence to international humanitarian law (IHL).

The ICRC's humanitarian efforts can be categorized into three main areas:

1. *Protection in war:* This includes safeguarding civilians from the ravages of conflict, ensuring the humane treatment of prisoners of war and detainees, and working to restore family connections severed by violence.
2. *Assistance for victims of armed conflict:* The organization provides essential support to those impacted by violence, focusing on economic security, access to clean water and sanitation, and health services.
3. *Preventive action:* The ICRC actively promotes IHL and works with national authorities to enhance the implementation of these laws, ensuring that the principles of humanity are upheld even in times of war.

Forensic Science and Quality Management: Addressing the Era of Standardization in Challenging Environments, First Edition. Edited by Roberto C. Parra and Allan G. Alvarez-Godoy.

With operations extending across more than 90 countries, the ICRC plays a vital role in responding to the needs of the most vulnerable populations, continually adapting its strategies to meet the challenges posed by modern conflicts.

Henry Dunant (1828–1910), a pivotal figure in the founding of the ICRC, profoundly shaped the landscape of humanitarianism. His experiences during the brutal Battle of Solferino in 1859, where he witnessed the horrific aftermath of the conflict between French/Piedmontese forces and the Austrian army, compelled him to take action. In 1862, Dunant published his seminal work, A Memory of Solferino, advocating for the establishment of societies dedicated to the care of wounded soldiers. Supported by General Dufour, who later chaired the diplomatic conference that adopted the original Geneva Conventions, and together with jurist Gustave Moynier and surgeons Louis Appia and Théodore Maunoir, they founded the "Committee of Five." Their vision laid the groundwork for the ICRC and the global movement of humanitarian assistance that followed.

The commitment of the Committee of Five to alleviating human suffering resonates deeply with the ICRC's contemporary work, particularly in addressing the needs of missing and deceased persons in the wake of mass fatalities resulting from conflict, disasters, and migration. Properly handling the remains of individuals who have lost their lives due to hostilities or other humanitarian crises is not merely a matter of respect; it is fundamental to the healing process for communities grappling with loss, trauma, and fear. The emotional burden of unresolved grief can haunt societies long after the physical scars of violence have faded.

5.2 The Establishment of the Forensic Unit: An ICRC Commitment to Forensic Humanitarian Action

Historical examples highlighting the need for forensic humanitarian and human rights action have always existed. The mass execution of approximately 22,000 Polish soldiers in 1940 at Katyn Forest is just one such example. The German authorities' creation of the Katyn Commission in 1943, comprising 12 forensic experts through the Polish Red Cross, aimed to investigate these war crimes, revealing the vital role that forensic science plays in achieving justice and closure (Zalewski, 2000).

In Argentina, the transition to democracy in December 1983 saw the establishment of the National Commission on the Disappearance of Persons (CONADEP) to address the tragic legacy of enforced disappearances during the military regime from 1976 to 1983, a period in which an estimated 30,000 individuals went missing. The creation of the Equipo Argentino de Antropología Forense (EAAF) in 1984 was a crucial development in the quest for truth, focusing on locating and identifying the victims of the regime. This effort was significantly supported by Dr. Clyde Snow, a renowned forensic anthropologist from the American Association for the Advancement of Science, who brought his expertise to help uncover the truth behind these disappearances (Meyer, 2011). The work of EAAF has been instrumental in identifying remains and providing families with much-needed closure, culminating in the prosecution of nine generals in 1985, showcasing how forensic investigations can illuminate the truth and foster accountability. Similar efforts were conducted by Snow and specialists from the United States and Germany in 1985 for the identification of Nazi fugitive Josef Mengele, the "angel of death", whose body was exhumed from a cemetery in Brazil in 1979; the process was used as an example to establish less confession-based and more evidence-based forensic protocols on war crimes and crimes against humanity (Keenan and Weizman, 2012).

The conflicts in the Balkans during the early 1990s further underscored the necessity of forensic humanitarian and human rights efforts. The establishment of the International Criminal Tribunal for the Former Yugoslavia (ICTY) in 1993 and the subsequent creation of the International Commission on Missing Persons (ICMP) in 1996 addressed the issue of over 40,000 missing individuals, highlighting the importance of forensic science in the aftermath of war (ICMP, 2017).

These historical instances illustrate that forensic humanitarian actions, which apply the knowledge and skills of forensic sciences to humanitarian and human rights contexts, are crucial in supporting affected populations. Humanitarian aid encompasses a broad definition, aiming to provide essential support to those in need, save lives, alleviate suffering, and maintain human dignity. The ICRC's dedication to these principles underscores the enduring relevance of Dunant's vision in today's world, as the organization continues to navigate the complexities of modern conflicts and their aftermaths, ensuring that the rights and dignity of all individuals are upheld, even in the most challenging circumstances.

5.3 The ICRC Forensic Unit

In 2003, the ICRC took a significant step in enhancing its humanitarian response by establishing a dedicated forensic unit. This initiative arose from the recognition that the needs of families affected by armed conflict and disasters extend beyond understanding the causes and manner of deaths. From October 29 to November 1, 2002, a regional conference on the missing was organized by the ICRC in Lima, bringing together human rights organizations, forensic experts, and international bodies to discuss strategies to address the humanitarian consequences of disappearances. The regional collaboration on the issue of missing persons in Latin America was a preparatory effort for broader conversations, held in February 2003, in Geneva. The discussions at this international conference highlighted the critical importance of not only investigating deaths for accountability purposes but also prioritizing the identification of remains for humanitarian reasons (ICRC, 2003).

The ICRC's report on the missing and their families emphasized that forensic specialists operating in contexts involving missing persons bear an ethical obligation to advocate for a comprehensive identification process. This obligation extends to meticulously observing and documenting all information relevant to the identification of remains. Forensic experts must prioritize the rights and needs of families throughout the process of exhumation and identification, ensuring that their dignity is upheld during this profoundly sensitive time. Furthermore, they are required to be well-versed in the pertinent provisions of international humanitarian and human rights laws, reinforcing the notion that the identification of the deceased is not merely a technical task but a humanitarian imperative.

Subsequent to this conference, the establishment of the ICRC forensic unit began with the hiring of Australian forensic pathologist Stephen Cordner as its first forensic expert. Alongside British war surgeon Robin Coupland, Cordner drew from their 2003 mission to Iraq to propose the main pillar of the forensic unit: supporting families in need amidst severe security challenges, endangered forensic care, lack of capacity in specific forensic disciplines, and destroyed infrastructure incapable of handling overwhelming workloads (Cordner, Coupland, 2003). In Autumn 2003, Cordner and Coupland invited Morris Tidball-Binz, a founding member of the Argentine Forensic Anthropology Team (EAAF) to become the unit's first forensic coordinator (Tidball-Binz, 2017).

The Forensic Unit of the ICRC is dedicated to upholding the dignity and rights of deceased individuals and their families. It operates under principles that guide its humanitarian efforts in armed conflicts, violence, and natural disasters, where people may go missing, become separated from their families, or suffer ill-treatment and sexual violence. Medico-legal systems and forensic institutions play a crucial role in addressing these humanitarian concerns. Central to this system, medico-legal institutions are key players in responding to and preventing violations of the physical and moral integrity of victims of conflict, thereby safeguarding their right to life. This central role justifies the inclusion of forensics as a protection service within the ICRC structure.

The ICRC applies forensic science exclusively for humanitarian purposes. Treating the dead with respect is paramount, ensuring bodies are handled with dignity and unidentified remains are properly identified. This process adheres to strict forensic principles and standards to prevent the deceased from going missing and to bring solace to grieving families.

To strengthen local responses, the ICRC supports medico-legal systems in developing policies, implementing best practices, and improving working conditions. This involves providing high-quality forensic programs that meet professional standards, either through direct action or by advising states and relevant entities. The ICRC also advocates for the rights of the deceased under IHL, reminding states of their obligations to treat the dead with dignity.

In its quest to support the provision of answers, the ICRC assists authorities and other actors in effective search and identification processes for missing or deceased persons. It promotes a multidisciplinary approach, ensuring data protection and providing tools for information management. The ICRC engages with parties to conflict, working with armed forces, non-state armed groups and communities to ensure the deceased are properly searched for, recovered, identified, and returned to their families for final disposal according to cultural and religious beliefs. Often the ICRC acts as a neutral intermediary to help families reclaim the remains of their loved ones.

The forensic unit of the ICRC is also involved in emergency preparedness, promoting planning for mass fatalities and training on the proper management of the dead in emergencies. This includes providing forensic equipment and addressing the risks posed by migration and people dying on migratory routes.

Respect for social, cultural, and religious diversity is integral to the ICRC's work: the organization collaborates with communities, religious groups, and other experts to ensure that emergency responses and international protocols respect specific religious practices and cultural traditions.

Through its comprehensive initiatives, the ICRC enhances forensic practices in some of the most challenging environments worldwide. In regions ravaged by conflict, forensic specialists often flee leaving a void in human resources, while forensic facilities and infrastructure are frequently destroyed. Additionally, these areas may suffer from inadequate legal frameworks, lack of essential equipment, and disrupted communication networks, all of which hinder effective forensic work. By integrating adapted and fit-for-local-communities forensic services with humanitarian principles, the ICRC promotes the dignified treatment of the deceased and supports families searching for their missing loved ones. Their work in strengthening local medico-legal systems, advocating for the rights of the deceased and their families, and preparing for emergencies exemplifies their commitment to addressing complex humanitarian issues. The ICRC's role in forensic diplomacy, partnerships, and direct action not only aids in the immediate aftermath of crises but also helps in building resilient systems capable of managing future challenges. As we explore the concept of forensic humanitarian action, we will delve deeper into how the ICRC's unique approach continues to evolve, ensuring that forensic science remains a crucial tool in humanitarian response.

5.4 Forensic Humanitarian Action by ICRC

In times of armed conflict, other situations of violence, natural disasters, and migration, many individuals go missing, some tragically lose their lives, and numerous human remains remain unclaimed either within forensic institutions following examination or outside of them without any examination. Both international human rights law (IHRL) and IHL place clear legal and humanitarian obligations on states to ensure dignified management of human remains, including the search, recovery, identification, and return of deceased individuals to their families. National laws should reinforce these obligations, although their implementation may vary.

The lack of reliable identification procedures affects many aspects of human life. The effectiveness of these obligations hinges significantly on the strength of medico-legal and death investigation systems, which are responsible for conducting thorough death investigations and certifying the cause and manner of deaths that are unnatural, violent, or suspicious; sudden or unexpected; unusual; or pose a potential threat to public health and safety, as well as confirm identities through multiagency and multidisciplinary processes of identification for the living and the deceased.

Forensic humanitarian action represents a crucial intersection between forensic science and humanitarian principles, aiming to address the needs of families and communities affected by loss and uncertainty in the aftermath of conflict, violence, natural disasters, or migration crises. This is accomplished by applying forensic expertise to recover and identify the deceased, as well as ensure a dignified treatment of all remains. It builds upon established frameworks in IHRL and IHL to protect individuals – both living and deceased – while honoring the dignity of those affected and strengthening the efforts to provide answers, closure, and support to families during times of crisis.

5.5 Strengthening of Medico Legal Systems in Challenging Environments: Medico-legal Systems and their Role in the Response to Issues of Humanitarian Concern

Effective governance and resilient infrastructure are essential for a state's response to emergencies and the prevention of humanitarian issues. The medico-legal system, which varies by country, includes judiciary, law enforcement, and forensic institutions and can involve other entities such as emergency services, volunteer organizations, and National Red Cross and Red Crescent Societies during emergencies. The primary role of the medico-legal system is to support justice, human rights, and the rule of law. It also informs policy-making, crime prevention, and public health and safety through data that aids in evaluating healthcare and research and in developing prevention programs. In post-conflict scenarios, it is vital for truth, justice, memory, reparation, and non-repetition efforts. Recognizing the role, gaps, and challenges of the medico-legal system is essential for humanitarian and development actors. By understanding these elements, they can devise and implement sustainable strategies to strengthen the system, from political advocacy to operational assistance.

Strengthening medico-legal systems is essential for effective humanitarian responses, particularly in environments where conflict, resource limitations, and political instability present significant obstacles. By building robust forensic capacities, states can improve investigations, safeguard rights, and support affected communities. Dysfunctional medico-legal systems face numerous challenges that impede their proper functioning. Key requirements for an effective medico-legal system include robust policies and legal frameworks, defined procedures and roles, adequate human resources, proper infrastructure and equipment, engagement with families and target communities, efficient information management, and quality control and assurance. However, in conflict, many systems struggle with issues such as poor management of the deceased, unidentified bodies, numerous missing persons, and inadequate investigations of human rights violations.

In contexts with significant humanitarian concerns, even strong judicial and law enforcement entities may be undermined by weak or nonexistent forensic institutions. Overwhelmed workloads, lack of government support, and inadequate quality assurance often lead to mistakes, mistrust from families, and diminished credibility of state authorities. Overall, despite some regions having proper regulations and structured systems, the sheer volume of cases can overwhelm institutional capacities. This highlights the need for stronger support and resources to improve the functionality of medico-legal systems in addressing humanitarian needs.

Medico-legal systems face numerous challenges that impact effectiveness and the ability of states to respond to emergencies and meet international legal obligations. Key issues identified by ICRC operational forensic teams over the last 20 years of operations include a lack of policies, regulations and procedures; a lack of resources; inadequate involvement of beneficiaries and families; a lack of information and Information Management Systems; a fragmented approach to humanitarian programmes; and poor emergency preparedness and responses.

Overall, the functionality of medico-legal systems is compromised by gaps in policies, procedures, resources, information management, and coordination. A more integrated, systemic approach is necessary to strengthen these systems and ensure they fulfill their roles effectively in responding to humanitarian needs.

This section explores the importance of strengthened medico-legal structures and highlights a regional example from the Arab world, where leadership, collaborative strategies, and active local involvement can lead to advancing forensic science capacity in response to complex humanitarian challenges faced in this region.

Forensic sciences constitute a foundation in criminal investigations, judicial systems, and humanitarian actions worldwide. Yet, within the Arab world, the advancement of forensic science capacity encounters distinct obstacles.

This section explores the status, challenges, and prospects of capacity building in forensic sciences across Arab nations from a practical rather than theoretical standpoint.

Al-Ahdal et al. (2013) underscored the imperative for increased investment in training, infrastructure, and research to surmount barriers hindering progress in forensic science. Hassan et al. (2018) identified challenges such as scarce resources, antiquated technologies, and the absence of standardized practices, urging strategic improvements. In parallel, Taff and Butt (2010) emphasized the key role of bolstering forensic science in the Middle East and North Africa to strengthen justice and security, proposing measures like instituting training programs and fostering collaboration between forensic scientists and legal professionals. Additionally, Fareed and Al-Ahdal (2017) examined forensic science education in Arab universities, pinpointing gaps in curriculum, resources, and faculty expertise, and offering actionable recommendations for enhancement.

When delving into the concept of capacity building, it becomes evident that its multifaceted nature involves individual, organizational, and systemic levels of development. It is defined as a process that strengthens the ability of individuals, organizations, and communities to identify and resolve their own challenges (The UNDP Capacity Development Resource Center). Capacity building functions on principles of empowerment, participation, sustainability, and flexibility. Its effective implementation necessitates diverse strategies including training, organizational development, networking, resource mobilization, and policy advocacy, all accentuated by an integrated approach addressing both individual and systemic factors.

The forensic humanitarian action of the ICRC stresses the significance of adaptive and context-specific approaches to capacity building, advocating for interventions tailored to the distinct needs, priorities, and capacities of the identified populations while remaining responsive to evolving circumstances and contexts. El-Zoghbi and Abdelmegeid's (2016) paper further emphasizes the necessity of tailoring capacity-building initiatives to the unique challenges and opportunities within the Arab region, considering factors such as political instability, economic development, and social cohesion.

5.5.1 Gaps and Challenges

Drawing from the ICRC expertise in forensic sciences capacity building and over 20 years of work in forensic humanitarian action including across the Arab nations, several pivotal gaps and challenges in the Arab world can be identified, though they could very well fit many other contexts worldwide:

1. *Lack of standardization and a regional accreditation body:* Despite the presence of local accreditation bodies tied to ministries for domestic accreditation of forensic curricula and laboratories, there is a notable absence of a regional body for accrediting or auditing forensic laboratories. This gap necessitates

laboratories aspiring for accreditation to translate all standard operating procedures (SOPs) and quality management system (QMS) manuals into a foreign language (usually English) to meet international standards and guidelines, adding an unnecessary layer of complexity and resource requirement. Consequently, many laboratories and universities often abandon their pursuit of standardization and accreditation, opting instead to adhere solely to the local requirements of their auditing bodies, which are frequently either lacking or subpar.

2. *Impact of conflict on forensic and medico-legal systems:* Countries plagued by conflict experience daily emigration of skilled experts and often witness the collapse of their medico-legal systems. Strengthening these systems during conflicts and disasters is crucial not only to fulfill international law obligations but also to address humanitarian issues, uphold human rights, and facilitate recovery and reconstruction efforts in affected regions.
3. *Imbalance in academic curricula availability:* There exists a significant disparity between the availability of academic curricula and the actual needs in various countries. Some nations with higher caseloads lack adequate academic programs, relying heavily on practical experience gained on the job, while others with more advanced academic systems face a shortage of practical training opportunities. There remain countries where neither practical experience nor academic curricula exist.
4. *Reliance on foreign data in forensic studies:* There is a notable lack of scientific studies focusing on Arabic populations, particularly evident in forensic anthropology. This reliance on foreign data hinders the accuracy and applicability of forensic techniques within the region.
5. *Limited peer-to-peer exchanges:* The forensic community in the Arab world displays a weak network, resulting in fewer peer-to-peer exchanges and collaborations within Arabic countries, particularly for individuals lacking proficiency in foreign languages, thereby constraining opportunities for fruitful exchange and mutual learning.
6. *Focus on individual training over systems strengthening:* Current capacity-building efforts predominantly focus on individual training rather than on strengthening and building local systems. This approach fails to address underlying systemic issues and impedes the retention of competent individuals within the local context.
7. *Insufficient local leadership in capacity-building projects:* Many capacity-building projects are led by nonlocal teams who often lack a deep understanding of the root causes of issues and fail to implement proper monitoring and evaluation processes post-implementation. Despite some Arab countries facing economic challenges, they possess advanced expertise in forensic sciences. There is a need to recognize and leverage this expertise by mapping existing capacities and fostering cross-border collaboration to enhance forensic science capabilities across the region.

8. *Challenges in identifying change drivers:* It is often challenging to pinpoint individuals who are genuinely motivated to drive change for the betterment of society. There is observable evidence of individuals utilizing development projects primarily for personal career advancement rather than for the collective progress of their communities. Consequently, this dynamic results in a talent drain, where skilled professionals, nurtured by capacity-building initiatives, pursue international opportunities, thereby hindering local development efforts.
9. *Neglect of basic science and essential forensic practices:* In politically and economically stable Arabic countries, there is a tendency to prioritize the adoption of high-cost technologies and equipment over fundamental scientific techniques and essential forensic practices. This inclination often overlooks cost-effective methods that are universally applicable. In essence, despite the availability of resources, their utilization lacks prudent decision-making, resulting in missed opportunities for more efficient and widespread implementation of forensic methodologies. Furthermore, numerous capacity-building projects contribute to this trend by investing in expensive equipment and new technologies that may not be essential. Consequently, once these projects conclude, beneficiaries may struggle to afford maintenance or software updates, rendering the acquired resources underutilized or obsolete.
10. *Limited focus on forensic humanitarian action:* There exists an imbalance in the prioritization of forensic services, with a notable emphasis on those serving justice and security objectives, in contrast to the essential role of forensic humanitarian action. This disparity overlooks the imperative of addressing the multifaceted consequences of conflict, violence, migration, disasters, and ill-treatment in detention settings. For instance, it is evident that forensic systems in Arab countries often fail to allocate adequate resources to address humanitarian concerns. These include critical tasks such as the search and identification of missing persons, the identification of unidentified human remains stored in medico-legal and forensic facilities, and the identification of deceased migrants following shipwrecks or incidents leading to their demise. This imbalance underscores the urgent need for greater attention and investment in forensic humanitarian action to mitigate the humanitarian consequences of various crises and ensure the dignity and rights of affected individuals are defended.

5.6 Implementation of Quality Management Systems

In conflict-affected countries, forensic departments and units face a myriad of challenges when it comes to adopting international standards in forensic operations. The realities on the ground are stark and often daunting: limited resources, inadequate infrastructure, and the constant threat of ongoing violence severely hinder the capacity to perform forensic investigations to international standards. Additionally, these countries often suffer from a lack of trained personnel, insufficient access to updated technologies, and the absence of robust legal and institutional frameworks that support forensic activities. The tumultuous environment exacerbates issues such as chain of custody breaches, contamination of evidence, and the inability to secure and protect investigation scenes. Furthermore, the psychosocial toll on forensic professionals working in such high-stress environments cannot be understated, often leading to burnout and high turnover rates. Despite these formidable obstacles, the ICRC plays a crucial role in supporting local forensic actors, helping them to build and implement QMSs that align to the extent possible with international standards. Through coaching, training, technical assistance, and capacity-building initiatives, the ICRC strives to enhance the operational capabilities of forensic institutions, ensuring that they can provide accurate and reliable forensic services even in the most challenging circumstances.

Establishing an effective QMS in forensic science in humanitarian practices is essential to ensure reliable, ethical, and standardized approaches in complex and high-stakes contexts. This section explores the framework and methods for implementing a QMS to improve the governance, quality, and resilience of forensic practices.

5.6.1 Good Governance in Forensic Practices

The effective implementation of a QMS is based on the principles of good governance, which prioritize transparency, accountability, integrity and ethical responsibility. These principles are particularly vital in contexts where the accurate identification of the deceased and the dignified treatment of remains are fundamental not only to justice, but also to community healing and closure. Good governance also fosters trust in forensic and medico-legal institutions, which is essential for the cooperation of affected families and communities and for compliance with international standards. In conflict-affected regions, the ICRC supports local forensic actors in the process of establishing clear governance frameworks that ensure accountability and transparency, despite the challenging operating environments.

5.6.2 Total Quality Management (TQM) Principles Applied to Forensic Practices

TQM principles, such as continuous improvement, families (customer) orientation, and stakeholder engagement, create a framework that emphasizes the need to ensure quality at every stage of forensic processes.

Continuous improvement is particularly relevant as forensic technologies and methodologies evolve; it ensures that procedures remain up-to-date, meet humanitarian needs, and comply with international standards. In addition, a focus on the needs of families and communities ensures that forensic processes remain sensitive to the cultural and social implications of caring for and identifying the deceased. The ICRC integrates TQM principles into its coaching endeavors and training programs, helping local forensic units to continuously enhance their processes and better serve their communities.

5.6.3 Process-based Approach to Quality Management System

To effectively implement a QMS, the ICRC forensic Quality Management specialists adopt a process-based approach, mapping and optimizing key, support, and management processes. This approach helps define how each activity contributes to the overall forensic mission objectives of the forensic entity that ICRC is supporting, thereby promoting workflow efficiency and accountability.

a. *Key processes:* Core forensic processes include search and recovery, identification, data collection and documentation, and the return of remains to families. Each step must be meticulously managed to standards, from handling remains to producing reliable, evidence-based documentation.
b. *Support processes:* These include the administrative, logistical, and technological support essential to forensic operations, such as data management systems and forensic equipment maintenance. Support processes ensure that key activities can be conducted smoothly and efficiently, even in challenging environments.
c. *Management processes:* Management oversight is crucial to ensuring adherence to QMS policies, risk management, and continuous improvement. This includes governance and review systems that maintain accountability, transparency and quality in all judicial activities.

5.6.4 Six Mandatory Factors for Effective Forensic Process Management

To effectively manage forensic processes, a QMS in this area must focus on six fundamental factors:

a. The operating environment encompasses the physical, cultural, and legal conditions in which forensic processes are carried out. In forensic practice, a controlled, secure, and compliant environment is essential to prevent contamination, ensure confidentiality, and maintain the chain of custody. A clean, well-organized, and properly equipped laboratory space, as well as clear protocols for handling evidence, is essential. The environment also extends to the socio-political context, where understanding local laws, cultural practices, and ethical considerations is fundamental to obtaining reliable and respected results.

b. Objectives are the defined goals that guide forensic services, ensuring that they contribute to the organization's mission and the needs of stakeholders. In a forensic context, objectives may include accuracy, timeliness, objectivity, and reliability of analyses. Objectives are set based on client expectations, legal requirements, and ethical responsibilities. For example, objectives could include achieving accurate turnaround times for reports, increasing human remains identification rates, or improving transparency in the forensic reporting process.
c. Metrics are quantitative indicators used to measure performance and quality. Effective indicators allow investigative organizations to monitor the effectiveness of processes, detect deviations, and implement corrective actions quickly. Common investigative indicators include analytical accuracy rates, turnaround times, case backlogs, and error-related reanalysis rates. These indicators help forensic laboratories and units assess their performance and ensure they are meeting required standards.
d. Methods refer to the standardized procedures and scientific techniques used in forensic analysis. These ensure the consistency, accuracy, and reproducibility of forensic examinations. In forensic laboratories, validated methods are essential to maintain reliability and credibility. These may include DNA analysis protocols, fingerprint examination procedures, or evidence handling and processing protocols.
e. Resources include the financial, technological, material and human resources needed to support forensic processes. The availability of sufficient resources is essential to maintain high-quality standards and to efficiently process the demands of forensic cases. Adequate resources include state-of-the-art equipment, appropriate testing materials, and a trained workforce. Investment in technology, such as updating data analysis software, improves the speed and accuracy of results.
f. Competencies refer to the skills, knowledge, and expertise that forensic personnel need to perform their duties effectively. Competence ensures that staff members are qualified and able to provide reliable, ethical and scientifically sound results. Competence in forensic sciences encompasses specialist knowledge in techniques, as well as mastery of the ethical and legal aspects of evidence handling. Continuing education and aptitude testing ensure that staff remain competent and up-to-date in their field.

5.6.5 Implementation Steps

Implementing a QMS requires a step-by-step approach, tailored to the local environment and organizational resources. Key steps include:

- Conduct an initial assessment of forensic practices, infrastructure, and current challenges in the region.

- Establish clear policies and objectives aligned with international standards and organizational values.
- Develop documented workflows for each investigation process to ensure clarity and consistency.
- Provide comprehensive training on QMS principles and forensic techniques.
- Regular audits and assessments to identify areas for improvement and ensure continued compliance with QMS standards.
- Consider feedback from staff and stakeholders to improve processes and adapt to emerging needs.

5.7 Maintaining Quality Management in Forensics

To support QMS, organizations must prioritize continuous improvement, adaptability, and responsiveness to local needs. Partnering with local forensic systems, conducting regular training, and promoting a culture of quality and ethics are essential to ensure long-term success. Collaboration with international organizations and governments can also support resource sharing, technical assistance, and policy advocacy, thereby strengthening the QMS and improving forensic capacity at scale. The ICRC's approach emphasizes ongoing support and capacity building to help local actors sustain high standards in their forensic practices, even in the face of ongoing conflict and resource limitations.

With a well-defined and resilient QMS, forensic humanitarian actors can uphold high standards of practice, ensuring reliable, respectful, and effective support to affected families and communities. Through the ICRC's comprehensive support, local forensic institutions can overcome the challenges of conflict environments and build systems that are both robust and sensitive to the needs of those they serve.

5.8 Challenges and Solutions in Forensic Operations

The ICRC forensic response, despite following the main directions mentioned above, needs to adapt to gaps diagnosed in the field. Establishing forensic operations varies in nature and process depending on access, acceptance, available resources and what would be the best possible practices to implement considering a challenging and volatile reality. In conflict zones, all those challenges tend to be exacerbated, and operations may necessitate difficult choices, especially considering that ICRC forensic services do not act in isolation from other departments and humanitarian needs.

A common challenge faced by practitioners in conflict zones is that many international standards were developed in ideal conditions where constraints put by conflict were not an issue. In this sense, implementing those standards has to come critically, and many forensic humanitarian action choices may have to be based on what is less bad to choose.

International standards for forensic science serve as benchmarks for best practices in medico-legal and forensic processes. Forensic sciences rely on scientific methodologies, which emphasize structured documentation and systematic procedures to reduce the risks of errors and uncertainties. However, in conflict zones, there is often a pressing need to adapt these practices, requiring flexibility, agility, and innovation to meet the demands of such challenging contexts. Striking a balance between the rigorous standards of forensic science and the nimble approaches required in humanitarian crises can mean the difference between achieving lasting outcomes or risking the loss of critical evidence and opportunities for humanitarian relief.

In active conflict areas, forensic specialists must carefully evaluate which parts of international standards are feasible to implement, weighing the potential risks and implications of deviations from these norms. Forensic sciences in humanitarian actions in such settings often involve sacrificing certain procedural elements while identifying a threshold below which compromises could hinder the provision of answers to families. For example, a forensic team might gain limited access to a territory controlled by non-state actors, where time, resources, and technological capabilities are restricted. In such cases, the team must prioritize the minimum data and procedures required to ensure that recovered remains are properly documented and identifiable, even if ideal conditions are absent. This could mean supporting non-state armed combatants to laminate a small paper they usually carry in their pocket with their pseudonym as the only way to somehow improve the prevention of their disappearance after death by allowing evidence to establish a hypothesis of identification to survive longer, in contexts where the majority of the population has neither birth certificates nor civil identification cards.

Operational limitations in conflict zones—such as prohibitions on georeferencing tool usage, restricted access to note-taking, and limitations on personnel and equipment—often necessitate a return to fundamental forensic practices without advanced technology. This may mean conducting recovery operations without basic supplies such as body bags or refrigerated transport, which, though far from ideal, enable the collection of essential data for later identification. Specialists must rely on their expertise to make adaptive decisions that preserve the possibility of identification in the future, balancing limited resources and logistical barriers.

Conflict-induced disruptions to supply chains may further complicate adherence to forensic standards. The destruction of infrastructure and local industries often impedes access to essential equipment and supplies, mandating creative adaptations that rely on minimal resources or local alternatives.

Forensic humanitarian work, therefore, requires a nuanced approach that involves engaging with local communities, non-state actors, and various levels of political and military structures. This includes adopting a contextually appropriate vocabulary and emphasizing neutrality and impartiality in all forensic actions. Developing a forensic humanitarian lexicon is often a critical first step. In such environments, forensic teams must also navigate perceptions and cultural sensitivities, including ensuring that their appearance, equipment, and methods are viewed as neutral and impartial by affected communities and parties to the conflict. Note-taking can be viewed as similar to criminal investigation approaches when sometimes the only solution would be using retrospective notes. Specific brands and colors of clothes and equipment also have to be carefully chosen, for example choosing between white and black body bags can be a matter of security.

The lack of trained forensic personnel, compounded by population displacement and limited infrastructure, often means that specialists must work with minimally trained volunteers or community members. These dynamics demand that forensic teams develop simplified, scalable processes that can maintain evidentiary integrity with the resources available. To this end, the forensic unit has, over the past 20 years, implemented innovative approaches to adapt its protocols for the unique challenges of conflict settings. It is not uncommon to support basic literacy training for grave diggers or morgue assistants when there is a need to help implement basic procedures to guarantee the traceability of bodies in cemeteries, often without formal administration.

In a global landscape where forensic sciences increasingly depend on advanced technology, conflict zones require a recalibration toward basic methodologies and equipment-independent solutions to achieve reliable results. That is because many technological tools used in forensic investigations are similar to those used in intelligence and counterintelligence and in the conduct of hostilities and may carry significant negative perceptions. Training first responders to use steps, arms and hands, shadow and the position of the sun, to estimate measures in a given space, or draw sketch plans by eye, using objects as relative scales or based on virtual grids, are solutions adopted by forensic specialists in many humanitarian settings when burial sites have to be somehow mapped. Nonetheless, when conditions permit, integrating advanced technologies—albeit in modified forms adapted to intermittent power supplies or infrastructural challenges—can enhance the accuracy and precision of forensic procedures, providing vital support for the identification and documentation of the deceased.

Conversely, there is an increasing need and demand for innovative solutions in the use of technology within forensic humanitarian operations. One such innovation is the use of geographic information systems (GIS) in the early stages of forensic investigations, particularly in understanding the circumstances of disappearances. GIS can assist in developing predictive models that not only help narrow down search areas but also improve identification efforts by correlating the locations of disappearances with areas where bodies have been found.

Remote sensing, in particular, holds significant potential. It can be used to safely access locations for humanitarian operations, thereby refining planning and reducing the risks to field workers. Additionally, remote sensing minimizes exposure to hazardous materials, such as weapon contamination in conflict zones. However, a major challenge lies in obtaining imagery, as satellite data are often controlled by the parties to the conflict, who may withhold or limit access to this information for strategic reasons, and aerial images are private, costly and also controlled by parties.

Forensic specialists working in humanitarian contexts can face complex ethical challenges, often influenced by cultural and religious sensitivities and by the party's pressure. These issues must be carefully considered when making decisions aimed at minimizing harm. Forensic practitioners must balance the long-term, medium-term, and short-term impacts of their choices, taking into account both the forensic needs of the population and the broader humanitarian context. This includes negotiating access to territories and considering providing responses that are not always only technical due to pressure from parties, but are strategic to allow continuity of some essential humanitarian services such as food distribution and medical care. In many occasions, forensics is a door opener to blocked dialogues with parties, however, putting forensic sciences in humanitarian actions in the forefront of difficult choices such as recovering a body not only to support a family but also more to open a dialogue with a non-armed state group who otherwise would not discuss any of the broader protection risks and would not listen to any broader IHL discussion. Such relationships must be approached responsibly, as forensic decisions can have wide-reaching impacts on humanitarian aid provision, community trust, and the safety of personnel.

Another challenge arises from cultural beliefs surrounding the handling of deceased individuals. In some communities, there is a strong belief that bodies of the deceased, particularly those who died in battle, must remain untainted. This belief may be at odds with the forensic requirement for personal protective equipment (PPE), such as gloves, which could be seen as desecrating the body. Similarly, there may be strict cultural protocols governing how bodies are touched or how forensic specialists interact with family members, often influenced by gender norms. In some areas, the very act of marking burial sites or identifying graves may be forbidden, leading to resistance or even violence against those attempting to keep records, which complicates efforts to maintain traceability.

Forensic specialists working in these humanitarian settings must therefore be prepared to develop protocols that respect cultural differences while ensuring consistency in forensic practice. This requires navigating a delicate balance between adhering to forensic standards and being flexible enough to accommodate local customs and practices. Nevertheless, in some cases, it may be necessary to impose a minimum level of forensic procedures to ensure that families receive answers, even if these practices conflict with cultural beliefs. The opposite is also true: sacrificing some standards of forensic practice to keep what is a minimum threshold under which nothing would be ever solved to be able to apply some actions that will do some good.

Building comprehensive training in forensic humanitarian action is a challenge faced by the ICRC and other organizations in the field. Benefits would come with the integration of universities to the complicated realities of emergency response and humanitarian aid in the field of forensics to allow new generations of forensic humanitarian workers to be prepared to face the challenges of resource limitations, cultural sensitivities, ethical dilemmas, operational constraints, training and capacity building, adapting to technological constraints, security concerns, coordination with other humanitarian efforts, documentation and data integrity, and dealing with constrained legal and political frameworks inherent to forensic humanitarian operations.

5.9 Future Directions and Recommendations

As the application of forensic sciences continues to evolve within humanitarian contexts, there is a growing need to address existing gaps and adapt to emerging challenges, particularly in regions facing complex political and social landscapes. Future directions should focus on strengthening frameworks, enhancing collaboration, and building sustainable local capacity to ensure effective, responsive forensic systems (Cheikhi et al., 2017).

Recognizing that state authorities are the primary agents for preparedness, response, and recovery, the following recommendations are proposed for humanitarian and development actors at the international, regional, and national levels. These recommendations aim to develop systemic and sustainable programs to address issues related to missing persons, family separation, mismanagement of the dead, and emergency preparedness and response. These actions will also impact other issues such as ill-treatment and sexual violence.

- *Elevate the need to strengthen medico-legal systems in political and diplomatic agendas:* Advocacy efforts should incorporate the importance of enhancing medico-legal systems, particularly forensic services, to help states prevent and respond to humanitarian issues. Raising awareness, engaging the public, and providing concrete advice on strengthening the system can improve state understanding and increase their commitment. Clear and actionable messaging is crucial for effective influence.
- *Incorporate this narrative in fundraising efforts:* While states work on policy improvements, international funding and partners can provide support through training, equipment, and infrastructure within a systemic approach.

- *Leverage national IHL committees:* Drawing on the success of these committees, specific efforts to strengthen medico-legal systems should be added to their agendas. This can promote concrete actions nationally and foster discussions on best practices regionally and internationally.
- *Develop strategies based on identified gaps and challenges:* Comprehensive assessments of medico-legal systems can highlight the obstacles preventing states from fulfilling their humanitarian obligations. This understanding aids in crafting effective strategies and communication efforts.
- *Decide between supporting local systems or establishing parallel mechanisms:* Depending on the situation, it may be better to strengthen existing local systems or establish parallel mechanisms. In either case, the medico-legal system, particularly forensic services, should be integral to these efforts.
- *Promote a multidisciplinary approach:* Engage all entities of the medico-legal system comprehensively to avoid duplication of efforts and integrate various approaches toward system strengthening.
- *Enhance professional skills and operational expertise:* Humanitarian and development organizations should improve their capabilities to implement robust strategies. Tools and assessments, including legislative checklists and model laws, can aid in understanding and resolving persistent problems despite existing regulations.
- *Establish operational partnerships:* Collaborate with UN agencies and other development actors to leverage development plans and investments. Synergies between humanitarian action, development, and peace efforts can enhance overall effectiveness, especially when preventive approaches are adopted.
- *Assess the feasibility of implementing international standards in conflict areas:* Forensic sciences in humanitarian actions in these settings may require adjustments to certain procedural elements. This is done after carefully considering the risks and implications of deviations from international standards. It is crucial to establish a threshold beyond which such compromises could hinder the ability to provide meaningful answers to families.

5.9.1 Recommendations for Advancing Forensic Science Capacity in the Arab World

Building on the identified gaps presented in section IV-1 and based on the ICRC experience in forensic science capacity building in the Arab nation, the following recommendations are presented:

1. *Establishment of a regional accreditation body:* Collaborative efforts should be made to establish a regional accreditation body for forensic laboratories. This body would ensure standardized practices and accreditation processes across Arabic countries.
2. *Strengthening medico-legal systems in conflict zones:* Special attention and resources should be directed toward strengthening medico-legal systems

in conflict-affected areas to meet international obligations, uphold human rights, and facilitate recovery efforts. This should involve regional cooperation and support to rebuild collapsed systems.

3. *Balancing academic curricula and practical experience:* Efforts should prioritize aligning academic curricula with the specific needs of countries, fostering a harmonious blend of theoretical knowledge and practical experience. Facilitating exchange programs and establishing partnerships between academic institutions and forensic practitioners can effectively bridge this gap. Additionally, the pivotal role of forensic science departments of universities in the region remains underutilized and should be maximized to enhance forensic science education and training, leveraging the potential to significantly impact capacity-building efforts in the region.
4. *Promoting research on Arabic populations:* Encouraging and funding scientific studies on Arabic populations, particularly in forensic anthropology, forensic archeology and other fields of forensic science is essential to reduce reliance on foreign data and ensure culturally relevant forensic practices.
5. *Enhancing peer-to-peer exchanges:* Measures need to be taken to cultivate robust networks and facilitate peer-to-peer interactions within the forensic community across the Arab world. This could involve establishing an Arab society of forensic practitioners or a center of expertise, alongside arranging conferences, workshops, and online platforms dedicated to knowledge dissemination, collaboration, and community building. Existing initiatives, such as regional Centers for Forensic Sciences, could be further bolstered with a specific focus on engaging Arabic practitioners and students.
6. *Shifting focus towards system strengthening:* Capacity building efforts should prioritize strengthening local forensic systems rather than overly focusing on individual training. This involves investing in organizational capacity to retain competent professionals and ensure sustainable development.
7. *Local-led development projects:* Capacity building initiatives must prioritize the integration of local and regional teams possessing comprehensive understanding of contextual challenges and needs, including considerations of religious and cultural sensitivities. Robust monitoring and evaluation mechanisms should be established to guarantee the efficacy and long-term sustainability of interventions, fostering greater ownership and impact within the communities served. Furthermore, identifying and utilizing existing regional expertise through assessing current capabilities and promoting collaboration across borders to improve forensic science capabilities throughout the region.
8. *Fostering gatekeeper commitment:* Strategies should be devised to incentivize gatekeepers to prioritize the greater good over personal interests. This could entail providing avenues for career progression and acknowledging their roles in fostering systemic enhancements.

9. *Emphasizing basic science and essential practices:* Policymakers and stakeholders should recognize the importance of basic scientific techniques and essential forensic practices. Investments should be made to ensure access to these fundamental resources alongside high-cost technologies. Encourage forensic institutions to prioritize evidence-based decision-making when accepting forensic technologies and equipment. This involves conducting thorough cost–benefit analyses to assess the value and necessity of high-cost technologies compared to fundamental scientific techniques. Emphasize the importance of selecting methods that are cost-effective, universally applicable, and align with international standards. Furthermore, incorporate sustainability planning into capacity-building projects focused on forensic science. Ensure that investments in equipment and technology are complemented by adequate provisions for maintenance, software updates, and staff training. Develop strategies to address long-term sustainability challenges, such as establishing partnerships with local industries or securing funding for ongoing operational expenses.
10. *Integrating forensic humanitarian action:* Ensure a systemic and continued engagement with government agencies, policymakers, and international organizations to prioritize funding and support forensic humanitarian action. It is important to advocate for the critical role of forensic services in addressing humanitarian crises, including the search and identification of missing persons and the dignified management of human remains. Equally, specialized training and capacity-building programs should ensure providing forensic practitioners with the skills and knowledge necessary to effectively respond to humanitarian crises, including mass fatality incidents, conflicts, and natural disasters. Through Fostering collaboration and knowledge-sharing among forensic professionals, working in humanitarian contexts to enhance preparedness and response capabilities and to incorporate humanitarian principles into forensic science education and training curricula. Emphasize the humanitarian dimension of forensic work, including the importance of preserving the dignity, rights, and cultural sensitivities of individuals affected by crises. Finally, promote a holistic approach to forensic practice that integrates humanitarian considerations into all aspects of forensic investigation and identification processes.

In conclusion, while challenges persist in advancing forensic science capacity in the Arab world, there exists a unique opportunity for developed and economically prosperous Arabic countries to spearhead regional efforts. By investing in and leading the enhancement of forensic science practices, these nations can drive transformative initiatives that address the identified gaps. Collaborative endeavors, such as establishing an Arabic disaster victim identification (DVI) team, creating a regional database for families of missing persons, and cultivating a network of Arabic community practitioners, can significantly bolster forensic science capabilities across the region.

Moreover, leveraging resources and expertise, including through partnerships with academic Arab organizations and forensic centers, the Arab countries can advance initiatives that promote justice, security, and humanitarian action. By embracing this leadership role and investing in collaborative endeavors, the Arab world can collectively elevate its forensic science capabilities, ensuring equitable access to justice, safeguarding human rights, and fostering societal resilience in the face of conflict, violence, and disasters.

However, at the intersection of foreign policy and capacity building lies a delicate balance of interdependence and mutual benefit, particularly concerning the well-being of communities in developing Arab states. It is crucial to ensure a continued focus on the best interests of these communities while also maintaining the engagement of states investing in their development. This requires ongoing dialogue, cooperation, and alignment of priorities to ensure that capacity-building efforts are effectively tailored to address the specific needs and challenges faced by communities in the region.

5.10 Conclusion

The ICRC remains committed to strengthening forensic systems through forensic sciences in humanitarian actions by designing and implementing humanitarian programs that are increasingly adopting a systemic approach focused on long-term impact and sustainability. While advocating for States' adherence to IHL and other relevant rules remains a crucial cornerstone in preventing humanitarian crises and protecting affected populations.

In contexts of armed conflict, other forms of violence, disasters, and large-scale migration and internal displacement, the medico-legal system—comprising judiciary, law enforcement (including the military when applicable), and forensic services—plays a vital role in fulfilling states' obligations under IHL and IHRL. These systems are essential in addressing humanitarian concerns, particularly those related to missing persons, the prevention of disappearances, and the proper management of deceased individuals and their families.

Effective advocacy, persuasion, mobilization, and influence remain key to promoting international law. Beyond reminding states of their legal obligations, there is a need for enhanced dialogue with high-level decision-makers, influencers, religious leaders, and academic circles in national, regional, and international forums. While international actors have provided extensive recommendations, the challenge lies in their implementation, often hindered by isolated, fragmented approaches and nonfunctional medico-legal systems with weak or nonexistent forensic services torn by conflict.

Incorporating innovative narratives and actionable content about the significance of well-structured and functional medico-legal systems can enhance the quality and impact of protection dialogues. Strengthening these systems ensures an effective response to long-term and chronic needs, mitigates risks, and prepares local authorities to manage crises. Moreover, it fosters trust among states, communities, humanitarian organizations, and donors, facilitating cooperation and effective humanitarian action.

Through our work on strengthening forensic systems and forensic sciences in humanitarian actions, the ICRC is committed to promoting comprehensive and sustainable solutions that bolster medico-legal systems, ensuring they are equipped to handle humanitarian challenges and uphold international law.

References

Al-Ahdal, N.M., Fareed, A.M., and Hassan, H.M. (2013) Capacity building in forensic science in the Arab world: Challenges and opportunities. *Journal of Forensic Sciences*, **58**(6), November.

Cordner, S. and Coupland, R. (2003) Missing people and mass graves in Iraq. *The Lancet*, **362**(9392), 1325–1326.

El-Zoghbi, M.A. and Abdelmegeid, F. (2016) Capacity building: A necessary and essential component for sustainable development. *The Journal of Development Communication*, **27**(1), January.

Fareed, A.M. and Al-Ahdal, N.M. (2017) Forensic science education in Arab world universities. *Journal of Forensic Sciences & Criminal Investigation*, **5**(2).

Hassan, H.M., Al-Ahdal, N.M., and Fareed, A.M. (2018) Forensic sciences in Arab countries: The current situation and future challenges. *Arab Journal of Forensic Sciences & Forensic Medicine*, **2**(2), December.

Keenan, T. and Weizman, E. (2012) *Mengele's Skull: The Advent of a Forensic Aesthetics*. Sternberg Press.

Meyer, D. (2011) *The Politics of Memory in Argentina: From the Disappeared to the Truth*. Palgrave Macmillan, New York.

Taff, M.A. and Butt, N. (2010) Strengthening forensic science in the Middle East and North Africa: A bridge between science and justice. *Forensic Science International*, **192**(1–3), January.

Tidball-Binz, M. (2017) Forensic humanitarian action: The ICRC forensic services. *International Review of the Red Cross*, **99**(905), 1–32. https://international-review.icrc.org/sites/default/files/irrc_99_905_12.pdf.

Zalewski, W. (2000) The Katyn Massacre: A historical perspective. In: *Katyn: The Untold Story of the Massacre*. Random House, New York, pp. 45–62.

CHAPTER 6

Sexual Violence in Armed Conflict: Promoting Forensic Evidence as a Humanitarian Action

Roberto C. Parra[1,*], Allan G. Alvarez-Godoy[2], Daouda Traore[1,*], Pierre Perich[3], Omer O. Adjibode[1,*], John Mbewu-Bodji[4], and Sami EL Jundi[5]

[1] *The Specialized Forensic Team of the United Nations Joint Human Rights Office (UNJHRO) in the Democratic Republic of the Congo*

[2] *International Forensic Consultant, The Hague, Netherlands*

[3] *International Forensic Consultant, Marseille, France*

[4] *Center of Forensic Medicine and Criminalistics of Kananga, DR Congo*

[5] *International Forensic Consultant, Coimbra, Portugal*

6.1 Introduction: Naming the Unspeakable, Preserving the Invaluable

Forensic science in humanitarian actions is not limited to preserving the posthumous dignity of the dead and their loved ones (Tidball-Binz, 2020; Ubelaker et al., 2020). On the margins of official history, where war not only destroys bodies but also senses and their social worldview (Anstett, 2023; Parra et al., 2020, 2023). Sexual violence in contexts of armed conflict persists as one of the most brutal expressions of power and dehumanization (Mukwege, 2024; OHCHR, 2024; Ali-Bitenga et al., 2021, 2025; Ali-Bitenga and Kitoka-Moke, 2022; Leatherman, 2011). It manifests itself not as a side effect but as a deliberate strategy to dominate, divide, and subjugate entire communities (UN, 2025). Often carried out by armed actors, state or non-state, this form of violence leaves traces that go beyond the physical, reaching the symbolic, the psychic, and the collective (UN, 2025). The practice continues to be used as a weapon of terrorism, a strategy of political repression, and a tactic of war according to the Secretary-General's Report on Conflict-Related Sexual Violence, which was presented to the Security Council in July 2025 (S/2025/389) *"Sexual violence*

*The views expressed herein are those authors and do not necessarily reflect the views of the United Nations.

Forensic Science and Quality Management: Addressing the Era of Standardization in Challenging Environments, First Edition. Edited by Roberto C. Parra and Allan G. Alvarez-Godoy.

continued to be used as a tactic of war, torture, terrorism and political repression, while multiple and overlapping political, security and humanitarian crises deepened." (UN, 2025: 4). Its impacts cut across national boundaries: they lead to widespread displacement, support trafficking organizations, stigmatize people, and erode social cohesion. According to the report, survivors' access to essential services is hampered by ongoing underfunding, and the decrease in peace operations has resulted in gaps in protection. Attacks on medical and humanitarian workers are another factor that makes it difficult to provide aid in urgent situations. Despite the existence of international legal frameworks, impunity is still a structural issue (UN, 2025). The report notably emphasizes the value of forensic science: its exacting application makes it possible to record infractions, guarantees the preservation of evidence, and facilitates efficient legal procedures, all of which contribute to justice, truth, and reparation (UN, 2025).

The harm inflicted does not end with the act itself: it continues in silence, in the stigmatization of survivors, in the lack of justice, and in forensic and legal systems that fail to recognize, record, and redress (Arrief, 2011; Latek, 2014). Naming this violence is already an act of ethical confrontation. It implies breaking with a tradition of invisibilization and trivialization. But beyond the discourse, technical and methodological tools capable of translating testimony into evidence and evidence into legal action are required (Rubini et al., 2024). A scoping review on forensic medical examinations following sexual violence related to conflicts is presented by Rubini et al. (2024). Its main conclusion is that there are incredibly few rigorous studies, and out of 2,800 original articles, only 17 met the requirements in less than 10 years. Most did not describe injuries specific to sexual violence, instead concentrating on the general physical and psychological effects. Forensic evidence was rarely incorporated into court proceedings, and almost all studies were carried out in host nations rather than conflict areas. The authors come to the conclusion that not much has been done over the years to address the problem using a methodical forensic approach, despite how serious it is. In this sense, forensic assistance is positioned as a crucial instrument, not only for criminal prosecution but also as a form of recognition, dignity, humanitarian action, and resistance in the face of impunity. Far from a neutral or merely expert practice, forensic intervention in cases of sexual violence in conflict becomes a profoundly political and humanitarian exercise.

The case of the Democratic Republic of Congo (DRC) starkly exemplifies this reality, as in several other countries across the globe (UN, 2025). In years, DRC has witnessed multiple episodes of mass violence, including campaigns of systematic rape against women and girls (UN, 2025).

In response to these serious problems, various international actors have promoted the implementation of standardized forensic protocols for the documentation of sexual violence in conflict contexts. One of the most relevant is the International Protocol on the Documentation and Investigation of Sexual Violence in Conflict: Best Practice in the Documentation of Sexual Violence as a Crime or Violation of International Law (Ferro Ribeiro and van der Straten Ponthoz, 2017), originally developed by the United Kingdom and adopted by various United Nations agencies. This protocol not only promotes technical rigor in data collection but also integrates ethical principles of respect, confidentiality, informed consent, and a victim-centered approach. Its application in the DRC made it possible to compare its effectiveness with clinic humanitarian forms previously used, revealing a clear superiority in the quality of the data collected, its potential judicial value, and its contextual sensitivity (Komar et al., 2021).

This chapter starts from that concrete experience to reflect on the value of forensic assistance during the protection of information (evidence) as a way to preserve the invaluable: the voice of the victims, the traceability of the crime, the manifestation of truth, and the possibility of future justice. Far from a purely technical approach, it is proposed to understand forensic documentation as a tool of applied humanity, which can, when properly designed and implemented, restore part of the dignity of survivors, guarantee their right to the truth, and strengthen judicial processes with international standards of evidence.

Preserving the priceless implies recognizing that the victim's body is a fragile and complex archive. That the evidence will not always be visible, but that it must still be sought with rigor, respect, and care (Ferro Ribeiro and van der Straten Ponthoz, 2017; UNODC, 2024; WHO, 2016). It also means that time, context, and the way in which forensic information is collected affect its value, not only legally but also symbolically and restoratively (Mukwege and Berg, 2016; Naimer et al., 2017). In this sense, forensic assistance cannot be detached from the broader frameworks of transitional justice, public health, and human rights. It must be integrated into them as a strategic and articulated component (UN, 2025).

Naming the unspeakable is, then, the first step to transform violence into judicial truth and evidence into collective memory. This chapter seeks to contribute to this transformation by articulating forensic knowledge with humanitarian principles and highlighting the urgent need to establish resilient documentation systems in adverse scenarios. Only in this way forensic science will cease to be an elite tool confined to distant laboratories, where the focus often lies on explaining technical and scientific terms to lawyers and judges and become what it should also be: a science at the service of life, communities, and relatives, even where death prevails (Mukwege and Berg, 2016).

6.2 Contemporary Approaches to Sexual Violence in Conflict

6.2.1 Sexual Violence as an International Crime and as Structural Violence

Sexual violence in conflict contexts has historically been minimized, treated as a collateral consequence of war or as an individual experience detached from the structural systems that make it possible. However, contemporary developments in international humanitarian law, international criminal law, and the social sciences have consolidated a new understanding: this violence constitutes a war crime, a crime against humanity, and can even be configured as genocide when it is committed with the intention of destroying, in whole or in part, an ethnic, religious or national group (ICC, 2013, 2021, UN, 2025). Rape, forced prostitution, forced pregnancy, forced abortion, forced sterilization, forced marriage, and any other type of sexual violence of comparable seriousness committed against women, men, girls, and boys that is either directly or indirectly connected to a conflict are all considered forms of "conflict-related sexual violence" as used in this chapter (UN, 2025).

The international tribunals for Rwanda and the former Yugoslavia played a key role in establishing this jurisprudence. In particular, the cases of Akayesu (ICTR)[1] and Kunarac (ICTY)[2] set precedents by recognizing sexual violence as an integral part of systematic campaigns of extermination and ethnic cleansing. These rulings not only redefined the legal nature of the crime, but exposed the deep connection between sexual violence, gender, and power. Instead of impulsive or spontaneous acts, rape was presented as a weapon of war, strategically planned to dehumanize, control, humiliate, and displace populations (Arrief, 2011; Latek, 2014).

However, beyond the legal level, sexual violence in conflict must also be understood as an extreme form of structural violence, rooted in patriarchal power relations, intersectional discrimination, and systematic dispossession (Arrief, 2011; Ferro Ribeiro and van der Straten Ponthoz, 2017). In many conflict-affected countries, previous social dynamics already tolerated or made invisible forms of gender-based violence (UN, 2025). Conflict, then, does not create new violence, but rather amplifies and legitimizes existing violence, facilitating its systematic and unpunished use (Médecins Sans Frontières, 2021). In this sense, any contemporary approach must integrate both the legal perspective and the critical reading of the structural determinants that enable this form of aggression (Médecins Sans Frontières, 2021; WHO, 2016, UN, 2025).

However, sexual violence as a weapon of war needs to be understood beyond the boundaries of gender, as men and boys are also systematic victims of this tool of individual and collective destruction (Garrido, 2021; Sivakumaran, 2007). This was acknowledged by the UN Security Council for the first time in 2019, through United Nations Security Council Resolution 2467 (2019), S/RES/2467 (2019).[3]

While recent reports have emerged of sexual torture against prisoners in the context of the Russo-Ukrainian conflict (OHCHR, 2024), instances involving Palestinians detained in Israeli prisons have been documented for over a decade (Weishut, 2015) and continue to occur, according to a report by the Independent International Commission of Inquiry on the Occupied Palestinian Territory,

---

[1] International Criminal Tribunal for Rwanda. (1998, September 2). The Prosecutor v. Jean-Paul Akayesu (Case No. ICTR-96-4-T). Trial Chamber I Judgment. Paragraphs 507–508, 688, 731.

[2] International Criminal Tribunal for the former Yugoslavia. (2002, June 12). The Prosecutor v. Kunarac et al. (Case No. IT-96-23-T & IT-96-23/1-T). Appeals Judgment. Paragraphs 127–130.

[3] See https://www.un.org/shestandsforpeace/sites/www.un.org.shestandsforpeace/files/unscr_2467_2019_on_wps_english.pdf

including East Jerusalem, and Israel to the 58th session of the Human Rights Council in 2025 (A/HRC/58/CRP.6).[4]

6.2.2 From Silence to Litigation: Evolution of the Forensic Approach

For decades, the institutional response to sexual violence in armed conflict was characterized by silence (UN, 2025). Victims rarely reported the facts, fearing reprisals, stigmatization, or lack of judicial response (Médecins Sans Frontières, 2021; Physicians for Human Rights, 2024; UN, 2025). Even when they did go to health services, records were minimal, and forensic medical information was rarely collected with an evidentiary logic (Mukwege and Nangini, 2009, UN, 2025). This disconnect between the humanitarian and legal worlds meant that crimes went unpunished and that the possibility of justice for victims was almost nonexistent (UN, 2025).

This panorama began to change through international initiatives that sought to close the gap between clinical assistance and legal documentation (UN, 2025). These efforts recognized that forensic evidence exists at the intersection of healthcare and legal processes and that its effective use depends on coordinated action among a diverse range of actors (UN, 2025). Such collaboration involves not only health assistance but also forensic practitioners, laboratory specialists, investigative authorities, law enforcement agencies, psychosocial services, and the judiciary, including both prosecutors and defense counsel (WHO, 2016). The Istanbul Protocol (OHCHR, 2022) introduced fundamental principles on the investigation of torture and ill-treatment and served as a methodological precedent for other, more specific protocols (OHCHR, 2022). In 2014, the United Kingdom, as part of its Initiative to Prevent Sexual Violence in Conflict (PSVI), launched the first edition of the International Protocol on the Documentation and Investigation of Sexual Violence in Conflict, with a second edition in 2017 (Ferro Ribeiro and van der Straten Ponthoz, 2017). This document proposes a comprehensive guide for forensic documentation of sexual violence in conflict contexts, based on international standards in human rights, forensics, clinical psychology, and criminal litigation.

The value of this protocol lies in its holistic approach: it is not limited to medical or expert aspects, but provides guidelines for interviewing victims with a trauma-focused approach, collects contextual and socio-political information, and articulates the collection of physical evidence with the principles of humanitarian ethics (Komar et al., 2021). In addition, it recognizes the future usefulness of the medical information collected, not only for national or international litigation but also as part of the processes of memory, truth, and reparation.

[4] See https://www.ohchr.org/sites/default/files/documents/hrbodies/hrcouncil/sessions-regular/session58/a-hrc-58-crp-6.pdf.

6.2.3 Emergence of the Forensic Science in Humanitarian Model

Given the inability of national justice systems to adequately document sexual violence in crisis situations, a new trend has emerged that vindicates the role of forensic science from a humanitarian perspective (Wells 2017, Tidball-Binz, 2020). This approach recognizes that forensic intervention should not be limited to criminal prosecution but can be an essential tool to protect victims, support families and communities, and preserve historical memory, as well as contribute to policy development, strengthen public health systems, uphold human rights, and inform transitional justice processes.

One of the distinctive axes of this forensic humanitarian model is its emphasis on preservation, informed consent, confidentiality, and protection of the victim are central principles that govern any intervention (Kurner and Marelli, 2020; Wells, 2017). In contexts where justice can take years, or even never at all, rigorous documentation of the facts acquires a strategic value. Preserving evidence, even if it cannot be used immediately, is to guarantee the possibility of truth and justice in the future (UN, 2025). This act of recording is not neutral: it becomes a gesture of recognition toward the victims and their stories, and an affirmation that the crime will not be forgotten. The various structures of armed actors must know and understand that this is a humanitarian act in itself; this can be transformed into a persuasive and powerfully dissuasive message for those who commit these attacks.

In the DRC, the implementation of the International Protocol allowed for full and detailed examinations, even years after the aggression (Komar et al., 2021). Data with evidentiary value was collected, but medical and psychological care was also provided to the victims, in a safe and respectful environment. This practice moves away from the instrumentalist forensic vision, focused exclusively on evidence, and aligns with a broader paradigm, where forensic science serves human dignity.

The examination of verifiable medical physical evidence gathered from the victims and their aftermath was combined with qualitative research (Komar et al., 2021), which is typical of forensic anthropology in cases of serious human rights violations (Parra et al., 2024). This type of research is based on in-depth interviews and is supplemented by documentation of prior information (Komar et al., 2021). Using the framework of the International Protocol on the Documentation and Investigation of Sexual Violence in Conflict, this procedure made it possible to process the data in a comprehensive and logical manner that was tailored to the particulars of the case and the amount of time that had passed since the incidents. The combination of thorough testimonies, historical documentation, and verifiable medical forensic findings enhanced the evidentiary solidity and aided in both the judicial investigation and the validation of the international protocol's practicality (Komar et al., 2021). According to Rubini et al. (2024), sexual violence during armed conflicts is a serious human rights violation that also goes unnoticed by forensic investigators. Forensic examinations are typically conducted at a late stage, frequently in the context of migration, asylum, or armed conflict, when there is little chance of obtaining biological evidence (Rubini et al., 2024; Komar et al., 2021). Survivors are denied reliable documentation that could aid in legal or international accountability procedures because of this delay. Additionally, the propensity to concentrate on broad psychological or physical effects rather than findings unique to sexual violence adds to the crime's invisibility (Rubini et al., 2024). Given this, forensic science in humanitarian actions becomes a crucial area to develop: skilled multidisciplinary teams could meticulously record the aftermath of violence at an early stage, guaranteeing clinical care as well as the generation of trustworthy evidence with legal and protective value. Incorporating forensic procedures into humanitarian contexts would acknowledge sexual assault as a public health and legal matter, offering survivors not only medical assistance but also resources to pursue justice, restitution, and safety. It is critically necessary to invest in resources, procedures, and training to improve this humanitarian-forensic component (Rubini et al., 2024; Komar et al., 2021; Wells 2017; Tidball-Binz, 2020; Cordner and Tidball-Binz, 2017).

Contemporary approaches to sexual violence in conflict are moving from a punitive and fragmented perspective to a comprehensive and victim-centered understanding (UN, 2025). This shift involves not only new tools and protocols but also an ethical transformation of forensic practice. Sexual violence in war cannot be addressed exclusively from the perspective of law or medicine: it requires a critical articulation of knowledge, a sensitivity to the social and political conditions in which it occurs, and a clear will to preserve the truth for the victims, even in the most adverse contexts.[5] In this context, forensic assistance takes on a new dimension: it is no longer just an investigative technique, but a form of care, memory, and humanitarian action (Mugisho et al., 2022; Mukwege and Berg, 2016).

6.3 Structural and Operational Challenges in Conflict Contexts

In addressing sexual and gender-based violence in contexts of armed conflict, the existence of international protocols, ethical standards, and methodological tools such as the International Protocol on the Documentation and Investigation of Sexual Violence in Conflict represents undeniable advances. However, the

[5] According to the UN, effective and victim-sensitive criminal proceedings in cases of conflict-related sexual violence will be made possible by strong political will, improved technical and operational capacity of national rule of law institutions and actors, and increased cooperation, coordination, coherence, and awareness among actors. This will lead to greater accountability for such crimes and ultimately contribute to long-term peace, security, and development. See https://www.un.org/sexualviolenceinconflict/our-work/team-of-experts/?utm_source=chatgpt.com

gap between normative design and practical application is deep and persistent, especially in environments marked by structural violence, institutional weakness, and technical precariousness. In countries such as the DRC, these tensions are manifested at all levels of the forensic process, from the initial complaint to the preservation of evidence, including the protection of victims and the training of the personnel involved (Médecins Sans Frontières, 2021; Physicians for Human Rights, 2024; OHCHR, 2014; UN, 2025). This reflection is essential not to idealize forensic intervention in the abstract but to adapt it to complex, fragile, and, often, hostile realities.

6.3.1 Scenarios of Protracted Conflict and Institutional Weakening

The first major obstacle faced by forensic documentation processes in conflict contexts is the very nature of the environment. In places like the DRC, where armed conflicts span decades, state institutions are often weakened, fragmented, or co-opted by armed actors (Kiakuvue et al., 2024; Médecins Sans Frontières, 2021; Naimer et al., 2017; Physicians for Human Rights, 2024). This situation generates a rupture in the institutional fabric that makes it impossible to guarantee the continuity of investigative actions, the safeguarding of evidence or the effective protection of victims (UN, 2025).

Systematic violence does not occur in a vacuum: it is inserted in a context where the state is often perceived as absent, complicit, or ineffective (UN, 2025). Victims, aware of this reality, tend to distrust judicial and health institutions (Arrief, 2011; Kiakuvue et al., 2024; Mukwege and Nangini, 2009). This reduces the chances of formal reporting, limits access to forensic medical services, and makes it difficult to build strong court cases. Moreover, in many rural or remote areas, institutional presence is simply nonexistent, and any documentation effort requires costly travel, security risks, and complex logistics (Médecins Sans Frontières, 2021; UN, 2025).

6.3.2 Systemic Impunity and Obstacles to Access to Justice

Even when victims manage to overcome initial barriers and access a medical or judicial institution, they face a system saturated with impunity. The ineffectiveness of criminal justice systems in many countries in conflict is exacerbated by corruption, political interference, and a lack of judicial independence (Arrief, 2011; OHCHR, 2014; UN, 2025). In contexts where the perpetrators are members of the state or non-state armed group or actors with local power, victims fear reprisals, social isolation, or criminalization, which reinforces their silence (UN, 2025).

Impunity generates a deterrent and revictimizing effect. Many persons who have been subjected to sexual violence in areas in conflict do not report because they have seen how other victims were ignored or unprotected (UN, 2025). In the absence of institutional guarantees, testimonies are lost, evidence is not collected in time, and the possibilities of a judicial process are diluted (Médecins Sans Frontières, 2021; Physicians for Human Rights, 2024; OHCHR, 2014). This reality stresses the function of forensic science, which, without a receptive and competent judicial structure, loses its transformative capacity and becomes an archive without a voice; however, first responders who provide health support, if well trained in documenting forensic evidence, can alleviate this problem.

6.3.3 Forensic Limitations: Lack of Protocols, Training and Resources

One of the main operational challenges in conflict contexts is the absence of installed forensic capabilities (Arrief, 2011; Obenson and Enow Orock, 2017). In many countries with protracted conflicts, public health systems lack specialized personnel in forensic medicine, obstetrics, and gynecology, or forensic clinical psychology. In the DRC, for example, there is no uniform national policy for the forensic examination of survivors of sexual violence, but it is not consistently applied across the country, and the tools used vary widely among institutions, NGOs, and international agencies (Physicians for Human Rights, 2024).

In addition, most of the clinical forms used until a few years ago, such as those of NGOs, were designed for humanitarian, not judicial, purposes. This means that they do not collect key information that can be used as evidence in criminal cases, whether at the local or international trials. As observed in the pilot process of the International Protocol in DRC, previous medical records were incomplete, subjective, and in many cases poorly transcribed, which made them useless from an expert point of view (Komar et al., 2021). This finding underscores the need to train medical personnel in forensic interviewing procedures, structured symptom recording, and careful collection of physical evidence, including photographs, documentation of injuries, and preservation of biological samples (Médecins Sans Frontières, 2021; Naimer et al., 2017). Infrastructure also represents a critical constraint. Many health centers do not have basic equipment such as examination lamps, sample collection kits, refrigerators to preserve evidence, or secure software to store clinical data.

6.3.4 Time as a Forensic Enemy: Delay, Disappearance and Deterioration

In cases of sexual violence, time is a determining factor. Physical evidence, such as bruises, genital injuries, DNA, semen, and biological remains, has a limited time frame for documentation. After a few days, many of these indicators disappear or degrade, making it impossible to use them in judicial processes. However, in armed conflict contexts, immediate access to forensic medical services is the exception, not the norm. Although first responders to stabilize health, they can provide substantial added value, with constant training.

It often takes days, weeks, or even months for victims to seek care, whether due to fear, geographic isolation, stigmatization, or lack of available services (Arrief, 2011). When a victim of sexual assault does make it to a medical facility, they frequently do so without understanding how crucial it is to save their clothes, refrain from washing them right away, or protect other types of documentation. It might even be less important at that terrible time than protecting their health and self-respect. It is important to realize that the victim may not always react by refusing to take a bath because they may feel dirty and experience severe emotional distress, which may cause them to desperately seek hygiene in an attempt to regain control over their body. Since other factors can be documented, this circumstance, along with inadequate information and guidance brought on by weak and poorly coordinated health systems, contributes to the loss of immediate evidence. But before these incidents happen, forensic scientists and medical teams need to collaborate. Even if a lot of time has gone by, they still need to look for ways to spot traces, marks, and physical and psychological aftereffects. The professionals who have the challenging task of recording the traces are the ones affected, not the victim. In order to provide the victim with comprehensive care, it is also necessary to acknowledge the subjective effects of trauma, lessen revictimization, and improve access to justice and compensation.

6.3.5 Inequality in the Capacities of Medical and Judicial Personnel

Another important structural challenge is the profound inequality in the training and awareness of health, police, and judicial personnel. In many contexts, health personnel lack specific training in cases of sexual violence, are unaware of or insensitive to the importance of recording their findings in medical records that could potentially be used in future legal proceedings, and even reproduce stereotypes or practices that revictimize victims. Some professionals minimize symptoms, doubt the victim's story, or impose bureaucratic barriers that prevent adequate care (Médecins Sans Frontières 2021).

On the other hand, police officers and prosecutors often do not understand the probative value of forensic examinations, do not know how to safeguard the chain of custody, or dismiss evidence due to a lack of technical knowledge. In this training vacuum, the information collected is lost, misinterpreted, or not presented in a useful way in legal proceedings (Kidenda et al., 2022; Naimer et al., 2017).

The experience of the UNJHRO team in Kasai shows that, with adequate training and technical support, it is possible to transform and strengthen these dynamics. In one region of the DRC, the use of the International Protocol was accompanied by training sessions for local health personnel, who learned how to conduct sensitive interviews, record clinical information in a structured manner, and refer victims to specialized services. This type of intervention, although limited in scale, shows the potential of forensic science in humanitarian assistance to empower local teams and improve the quality of interventions (Komar et al., 2021).

6.3.6 Risks for Victims and Intervening Personnel

Finally, any forensic documentation process in armed conflict contexts carries significant risks for both victims and those who assist them (Ferro Ribeiro and van der Straten Ponthoz, 2017). Survivors may be subject to reprisals, stigmatization, or exclusion from the community if they are identified as having participated in a judicial process (Arrief, 2011; Médecins Sans Frontières, 2021). Forensic interviews, if not conducted with a sensitive approach focused on trauma and informed consent, can reopen psychological wounds, cause retraumatization, and erode the person's emotional well-being. It is never an interrogation, but rather an interview, a respectful conversation that always takes into account the sensitivity of the situation.

Similarly, medical, judicial, or humanitarian personnel who document these cases may face threats, institutional pressure, or direct violence from perpetrators or their allies. In some cases, documenting sexual crimes is considered a subversive act, and professionals who do so are singled out or persecuted (Physicians for Human Rights, 2024).

For this reason, the International Protocol and other guidelines insist that documentation must be voluntary, safe, victim-centered, and appropriate to the context. Any intervention must be based on a risk assessment, guarantee the confidentiality of data, protect the identity of victims, and establish secure channels for safeguarding the information collected. Documentation cannot become a second form of violence: it must be an opportunity for redress and empowerment (Ferro Ribeiro and van der Straten Ponthoz, 2017).

6.4 Case Study: DRC Post-conflict and the Implementation of the International Protocol

This section aims to highlight the application of the International Protocol on the Documentation and Investigation of Sexual Violence in Conflict based on a case study of the forensic process carried out in the DRC. We present very general information not only to demonstrate the technical advantages of implementing a standardized forensic protocol but also to reveal the real challenges of its application in an environment marked by suffering.

The intervention, carried out between 2020 and 2021 by a forensic team from the United Nations Joint Human Rights Office (UNJHRO) in collaboration with the Military Prosecutor's Office and local medical professionals, aimed to recover clinical and testimonial evidence of cases of sexual violence committed during an armed conflict in the DRC between 2016 and 2017. The experience constituted a regional pilot test for the application of the International Protocol, allowing for a comparison of two different realities: on the one hand, the use of humanitarian forms of medical care in affected village X, which were developed shortly after the conflict through a well-known international organization (during 2018); on the other hand, the direct application of the forensic protocol in a scenario of mass sexual violence in village Y, very close to X.

6.4.1 X Case: Clinical Documentation with Humanitarian Approach

Case X is a clear example of how the lack of a uniform forensic framework for preliminary documentation or initial response to health stabilization can reduce the evidentiary value of the case in trials related to sexual violence in armed conflict. It is well known publicly that, in the Greater Kasai region, between 2016 and 2017, various armed groups violently subjugated the civilian population. Among the devastating consequences are the systematic rape of women and girls as part of war tactics and ritual initiation ceremonies, and the killing of civilians, including men, women, and children (Komar et al., 2021).

In this context, victims who survived the attacks were treated by a non-governmental organization that provides humanitarian medical support internationally. Between May 2017 and March 2020, health professionals from this NGO conducted examinations and recorded their findings on forms for medical certificates of sexual violence against women (Certificat Médical Violence Sexuelles Adulte/Mineur(e)). These forms, designed for medical rather than forensic purposes, were subsequently analyzed by the UNJHRO forensic team.

The evaluation of these records revealed critical limitations in the protection of forensic information:

1. *Incomplete or inaccurate records:* Of 481 forms, only 341 (71%) could be used. The loss of material was due to missing narratives, illegible photocopies, and faulty transcripts.
2. *Delays in reporting and loss of physical evidence:* The average time between the assault and the medical evaluation was 312 days, with a median of 459 days. Only 13% of the victims had relevant genital findings, and in only five cases could the injuries be directly linked to the assault, thanks to examinations performed within 48 hours.
3. *Variability and bias in medical examinations:* Twenty different physicians participated, with heterogeneous documentation practices. The collection of biological samples was inconsistent, and a small group of physicians accounted for the majority of genital findings.
4. *Transcription errors and terminology issues:* The forms were completed by third parties (nurses or translators), which led to linguistic inconsistencies and variations in critical legal terms such as "rape," "sexual abuse," or "sexual assault."

While these records provided valuable information on the extent of the violence, their evidentiary value was limited. Analysis of this dataset served as a baseline for assessing the potential of the International Protocol, highlighting areas where a standardized instrument could improve the quality and comprehensiveness of the information.

6.4.2 Y Case: Direct Application of the International Forensic Protocol

Unlike case X, where the clinical evaluation was not forensic in nature, case Y provided an opportunity to directly apply the International Protocol for the Documentation and Investigation of Sexual Violence in Conflict, adapted to local conditions and with forensic assistance from the United Nations Joint Human Rights Office (UNJHRO). In November 2019, local authorities ordered the intervention of medical professionals from the Technical and Scientific Police, who had been previously trained by UNJHRO forensic specialists, to examine 20 victims between 20 and 45 years old. The forensic operation was carried out months later, between June and July 2020, when the forensic team assessed that local professionals were now trained to carry out the evaluations, always accompanied by the UNJHRO forensic team.

Although more than 1,200 days had passed since the attacks, the protocol was adapted to include additional variables that would allow for differentiation between injuries resulting from the attack and those associated with the victims' subsequent sexual or medical history. Questions were added about the age at which they first had sexual relations, pregnancies, surgical procedures, and history of violence, thereby broadening the interpretive context of the results.

The process combined in-depth community interviews, typical of qualitative research in forensic anthropology, with previously available documentation and medical analyses of verifiable physical and psychological sequelae. This integration reinforced the probative validity of the findings and allowed for the comparison of testimonies with medical, physical, and psychological evidence. The International Protocol guided data collection with a logical and comprehensive flow, covering details of the assault (time, place, number and description of assailants, threats, use of weapons) and the physical and psychological impact on victims.

The results demonstrated substantial improvements compared to non-forensic clinical documentation from X case:

- 100% capture of variables compared to a range of 0–82% in NGO forms.
- Inclusion of critical forensic information missing from humanitarian documentation, such as the perpetrator's language, drug or alcohol use, and detailed descriptions of each sexual act.
- Consistency and uniform quality of assessments thanks to technical oversight and training of local staff.
- Although the proportion of relevant genital findings remained low (0.5%), in line with studies questioning the validity of examinations performed after

96 hours, the overall evidentiary value was reinforced by the richness of context and the accuracy of the documented narrative.

6.4.3 Comparative Analysis and Lessons Learned

The comparison between X case and Y case highlights a key aspect: the difference lies not only in the professionalism of those documenting, but in the tool used to do so. The use of a protocol designed for non-forensic humanitarian clinical care, although essential for the health of victims, does not guarantee the collection of data with full forensic value. In contrast, the application of the International Protocol, even in contexts of late reporting and material limitations, allows for the generation of a more robust case file for future legal proceedings.

In X case, the available information was fragmented, subject to interpretation, and vulnerable to distortion. In Y case, the standardized structure of the protocol and its rigorous application produced more complete and comparable data, increasing the possibility of linking testimonies with patterns of perpetration and contextual elements of the conflict.

This learning has practical implications: in conflict environments where institutional re-victimization and lack of resources are the norm, the first and perhaps only documentation of a case should aim to be comprehensive and forensically valid. Failure to do so may mean irreparable loss of evidence.

To ensure the scientific validity of the findings and empirically strengthen the procedures in this DRC region, the International Protocol was applied to two specific cases (Case Z and Case B).

Although the forensic medical examination of Case Z was conducted between 1,277 and 1,289 days after the assault, the application of the protocol identified persistent clinical and psychological signs. When examining 188 women between the ages 20 and 78, the results showed physical abnormalities, old scars on the genitals and other parts of the body, and serious psychological effects such as fear, profound sadness, and reliving trauma. The protocol's scientific ability to organize and validate data was demonstrated through the use of complementary questionnaires, which made it possible to distinguish injuries directly related to sexual assault from those caused by other life events. The experiences of 59 survivors (50 women and 9 men), ranging in age from 16 to 76, were documented in Case B, which occurred in Kasaï province during attacks by an armed group between 2016 and 2017. Through the direct application of the protocol, the team discovered physical scarring, functional disabilities, gait problems, and genital prolapses, all frequently linked to assaults by multiple assailants. The protocol's scope was expanded by involving psychologists in the assessment process, who addressed the survivors' emotional and social impacts, in addition to their physical ones.

Collectively, these cases demonstrate that the International Protocol is a modified scientific instrument that ensures the methodical and reliable collection of data, going beyond medical documentation. This method contributes to the comprehensive care of survivors while providing crucial evidence for justice. This adaptation of the International Protocol underwent a thorough review process before being published in a prestigious international journal in order to ensure the tool's validation and to meet international standards regarding the rigor of medico-legal practice (Komar et al., 2021).

6.4.4 Role of Forensic Team UNJHRO and the Implementation of the International Protocol

In the DRC, the UNJHRO has been instrumental in recording and examining grave human rights abuses during armed conflicts.[6] The forensic team is a crucial part of its structure because it gives the gathering and preservation of evidence scientific and methodological rigor, which is necessary to support legal proceedings pertaining to war crimes, crimes against humanity and, in general, the fight against impunity.

The Human Rights Council voiced its alarm in March 2017 about the humanitarian situation in the Greater Kasai region, where mass graves were frequently used after massacres and summary executions.[7] In response, a Technical Assistance Team was sent to Kananga, Kasai Central, in June of that year. Its task was to support and counsel the military prosecutor in the investigation of abuses that had occurred in the impacted provinces.[8]

The International Protocol on the Documentation and Investigation of Sexual Violence in Conflict has emerged as a crucial tool in this regard. This tool, which was created to standardize documentation procedures and guarantee victim protection, has been examined, tested, and adapted by UNJHRO's forensic team to address the unique circumstances of the Congo. Its implementation made it possible to create precise protocols for gathering testimonies, handling medico-legal evidence, and supporting survivors during court proceedings in Greater Kasai, an area severely impacted by high rates of sexual violence during the armed conflict.

In addition to its technical aspect, the Protocol's implementation aided in an institutional strengthening process. In order to support the sustainability of practices and the preservation of victims' dignity, the forensic team has provided training in trauma-sensitive documentation techniques to local physicians, judges, prosecutors, and security personnel. This strategy guarantees that cases of sexual violence can be brought to court with credible and admissible evidence, which helps to increase public confidence in the legal system.

The experience that was initially created in Greater Kasai has now spread throughout the DRC's entire territory.[9] Significant progress has been made in bringing together a thorough response to grave human rights abuses, where forensic practice serves as a link between the nation's truth, justice, and

[6] See further information in https://www.ohchr.org/en/hr-bodies/hrc/kasai-region/index
[7] See further information in https://www.ohchr.org/en/hr-bodies/hrc/ite-kasai-drc/index
[8] See further information in https://docs.un.org/en/A/HRC/RES/38/20
[9] See further information in https://docs.un.org/en/A/HRC/RES/48/20

reconciliation processes and the memories of the victims. In 2021, a forensic intervention plan was defined, with a dual objective: on the one hand, to adequately document cases of sexual violence committed years earlier and, on the other, to test the feasibility of applying the International Protocol in post-conflict contexts with structural limitations (Komar et al., 2021)

A version in French of the original protocol was provided to the team by the *Physicians for Human Rights* (PHR), including the following sections (Komar et al., 2021):

1. General data, sociodemographic and circumstances of the event.
2. General medical information and gynecological-obstetric history.
3. A structured and pressure-free account of the event.
4. Documentation of physical and psychological symptoms consistent with sexual violence.
5. Forensic medical evaluation and clinical signs of violence.
6. Expert conclusion and clinical judgment of the professional.

In addition, procedures were incorporated to obtain informed consent, guarantee confidentiality, provide psychosocial assistance, and ensure that the examination did not imply additional harm to the victims.

6.4.5 Local Adaptation: Inclusion of Sociocultural and Clinical Variables

One of the key achievements of the process was the forensic cultural contextualization of the protocol. The interviews were conducted by forensic anthropologist in the local Tshiluba language, with interpreters previously trained in ethical principles, a focus on trauma and narrative neutrality. The victims were accompanied by women leaders of the community, which generated an environment of greater trust.

In addition, the form included variables relevant to the local context, such as:

- Traditional marital status (not formally registered).
- Community perception of the fact (stigma, acceptance or exclusion).
- Economic impact of the event (loss of home, livelihood, mobility).
- Obstetric consequences (unwanted pregnancies, miscarriage, infertility).

These variables enriched the understanding of the multidimensional impact of violence, beyond the medical level, and contributed to strengthening expert conclusions with a comprehensive approach.

In total, 267 women and girls who survived sexual violence in cases Y, Z, and B were examined. Approximately 85% were adult women, mostly between 15 and 60 years old, engaged in subsistence farming or informal trade, and who had remained silent for years for fear of reprisals or social exclusion. For many, this was the first time they recounted their experiences in a safe and respectful environment. The implementation of the International Protocol allowed for the systematic documentation of the physical and psychological after-effects, transforming the survivors' accounts into scientifically valid forensic evidence for justice.

6.4.6 Adaptation Results: Quality, Completeness and Forensic Utility

The results of the process were highly positive. Compared to previous clinical forms used by humanitarian NGOs, reports produced with the International Protocol showed greater completeness, narrative coherence, and legal utility. While previous forms contained vague phrases ("presumed gang rape," "generalized abdominal pain"), the new reports made it possible to:

- Record the exact circumstances of the event.
- Describe symptoms and lesions with precise clinical language.
- Identify signs of psychological trauma consistent with sexual violence.
- To make well-supported clinical judgments with possible probative value.

The process also validated the hypothesis that late documentation can be equally useful, provided it is done with technical rigour, a sensitive approach and community support. In all cases, the women reported that the examination represented a moment of symbolic reparation, even if the judicial result is still pending. This reinforces the idea that the act of documenting is not only a technical procedure but also a process of resignifying trauma.

6.5 Lessons Learned and Replicability

The X, Y, Z, and B cases offer multiple relevant lessons to replicate in other contexts:

International standards can be applied in adverse contexts, if they are properly adapted, and local staff are trained, and the adapted tool published internationally.

Forensic documentation can be carried out years after the fact, without losing value, as long as good clinical practice is respected and a structured record is made.

The victim-centered approach is essential. The active participation of women and girls, informed consent, choice of language, and community accompaniment were key to success.

Interdisciplinary work is essential. Forensic doctors, forensic anthropologists, psychologists, lawyers, translators, and local leaders worked together to ensure a safe, useful, and ethical intervention.

The use of standardized forms improves the quality of evidence, allows comparison between cases, and strengthens the clinical chain of custody in judicial processes.

Forensic assistance is also an act of restorative justice and humanitarian action. Although criminal prosecution is desirable, institutional recognition of the harm suffered has a value in itself.

6.6 Methodological Comparison: International Protocol vs. Clinical Form

In efforts to adequately document cases of sexual violence in contexts of armed conflict, the quality, accuracy, and usefulness of the data collection tool is critical. The methodologies applied in the field and, in particular, the clinical forms used have a direct impact on the possibility of using the information collected as evidence in judicial processes or accountability mechanisms. In this context, this section offers a methodological comparison between two widely used instruments: the International Protocol on the Documentation and Investigation of Sexual Violence in Conflict (hereinafter referred to as the International Protocol) and the standard clinical form.

Both instruments have been applied in emergency contexts and reflect different approaches in terms of objectives, structure, depth, required training, and legal applicability. Based on the forensic experience of the UNJHRO team in DRC (Kasai), this comparison allows us to understand not only the technical differences but also the practical implications in terms of victim protection, possibility of justice, and documentary value.

6.6.1 Differences in Objectives: Medical Assistance vs. Forensic Evidence Collection

The main difference between the Clinic no forensic form and the International Protocol lies in their institutional objectives:

ONGs is a medical-humanitarian organization whose priority is to provide immediate care, safeguard the victim's health, and avoid secondary harm. Its clinical form has as its central purpose to document physical and psychologic symptoms for the purpose of guiding medical treatment, without explicit guidance toward the legal use of the information.

The International Protocol, on the other hand, is designed with a clear evidentiary vocation. Its purpose is to turn the act of documentation into a tool for accountability. This does not imply neglecting the medical well-being of the victim but places the collection of evidence within a forensic and judicial logic, with a multidisciplinary and inter-institutional approach.

This fundamental difference explains many of the methodological decisions observed in both formats.

6.6.2 Form Structure: Level of Detail and Organization of Information

In terms of structure, the Clinic form tends to be shorter and more clinical, generally composed of:

- Basic personal data.
- Overview of physical symptoms.
- Gynecological observations.
- Presumptive diagnosis.
- Medical prescription and clinical follow-up.

This instrument, although agile and focused on health, does not include a complete narrative of the event, omits contextual variables of the crime environment, and rarely integrates an analysis of consistency between the story, clinical findings, and expert conclusion.

The International Protocol form, in contrast, presents:

- An informed consent and identity protection section.
- Expanded sociodemographic information.
- Structured narrative of the event according to the victim's account.
- Variables on the context of the crime (location, armed actors, victim-aggressor relationship).
- Detailed forensic clinical examination (injuries, physical signs, psychological state).
- Forensic conclusion with professional judgment of the evaluator.
- Registration of complementary evidence (clothing, photographs, biological samples).

This structure responds to an evidentiary and articulated logic, allowing the construction of a forensic medical history that can be used as evidence before a national or international court.

6.6.3 Technical Language vs. Clinical Accessibility

Another substantial difference relates to the use of language and the training required to use each instrument.

The clinic form uses a more accessible language, compatible with general medical personnel, often without specialized training in forensic medicine or forensic gynecology-obstetrics. This allows for wide application in emergency contexts and also implies greater variability in the quality of the data collected and low standardization in clinical descriptions.

For its part, the International Protocol requires a higher technical level. Clinical observations must follow a logical structure, and the intervening professional must be trained in forensic principles, chain of custody, trauma documentation, and victim-centered approach. This requirement limits its spontaneous use but allows the legal value of the final report to be significantly raised.

It became clear from the Y, Z, and B cases that local medical staff needed special training to fully comprehend and apply the International Protocol's terminology and procedures, even though they were clinically trained. Without this kind of instruction, the standardized form frequently came across as overly complicated or frightening, which limited its practical application. This disparity emphasizes importance forensic science in humanitarian work, especially when it comes to documenting sexual violence, which is acknowledged as a serious human rights violation and a war crime under international law.

In times of peace, forensic science in humanitarian actions helps by creating training, coaching, and simulation exercises in addition to making these tools available. Before encountering hostile or crisis situations, practitioners can familiarize themselves with the methodology thanks to these preparatory efforts. Strengthening technical capacity through hands-on coaching gives local teams the competence and confidence to rigorously document sexual violence using international standards.

In the end, this procedure closes the gap between forensic accountability and clinical practice. It guarantees that professionals have the necessary abilities to convert survivors' testimonies into trustworthy forensic evidence when called upon to document war crimes, thereby promoting justice and upholding human dignity.

6.6.4 Consent, Confidentiality, and Data Protection

Both instruments recognize the importance of informed consent, but address it with different levels of formality and traceability. The Clinic form includes a general statement of consent for health care but does not delve into the secondary use of the information (e.g., for legal processes or public reporting). It also does not usually include a specific section to protect the identity or assess risks of retaliation for the victim.

The International Protocol, on the other hand, contains a detailed section on informed consent, which specifies:

- The medical and judicial use of data.
- The ability to withdraw consent at any time.
- Mechanisms for protecting the identity of the victim.
- Risk assessment and referral to protective services.

This ethical approach ensures not only greater safety for the victim but also the future validity of the evidence, by reducing the risk of legal challenge for procedural rights violations.

6.6.5 Judicial Value and Use in Litigation

In terms of legal utility, the difference between the two instruments is substantive. Clinic forms, designed for clinical purposes, do not cover the chain of custody, expert validation of findings, or the narrative consistency required to be presented as forensic evidence. This implies that, in general, their evidentiary weight is minimal.

On the contrary, the forms of the International Protocol are explicitly designed to be integrated into judicial proceedings, whether in national or international courts. They are designed as expert documents, and their authors act as forensic experts before the judicial authorities. Its structure facilitates the logical analysis between facts, findings, and conclusion, complying with the standards of admissibility of evidence in adversarial and inquisitorial systems.

The significance of Case X goes beyond the medical findings, even though it clinically documents instances of sexual violence. Professionals in forensic medical clinic can better understand the extent and trends of abuse by reading and analyzing the documentation. Forensic anthropologists' contributions are especially pertinent in this regard. Their specific proficiency in conducting in-depth interviews makes it possible to systematically record qualitative data, which enhances and supplements the clinical data.

Under the direction of anthropological procedures that place a high value on establishing trust and cultural sensitivity, survivors in community X were able to recount their experiences in a controlled and courteous setting. In addition to documenting the actual traumatic event, these interviews also covered more general topics like social repercussions, perpetration patterns, and effects at the local level. The qualitative accounts gave a more complete picture of the violence, its effects, and its systemic nature when paired with the clinical data.

The significance of interdisciplinary approaches in the documentation of sexual violence is thus demonstrated by Case X. Recognizing sexual violence as a grave violation of human rights and a war crime that can be prosecuted requires the scientific rigor of the evidence as well as the preservation of survivors' voices, which are ensured by the integration of clinical, medico-legal, and anthropological perspectives.

6.6.6 Adaptability to Adverse Contexts

One of the most relevant aspects when comparing instruments for documenting sexual violence in armed conflict is their ability to adapt to adverse contexts. These scenarios, marked by insecurity, institutional weakness, scarcity of human and material resources, and structural mistrust of the victims toward the state, constitute particularly challenging environments for the application of any standardized protocol. In this framework, it is essential to assess whether an instrument is operationalizable without compromising its fundamental principles.

Clinical form stands out for its simplicity and adaptability. It was designed to be implemented quickly by general medical personnel, even in conditions of extreme urgency, such as camps for displaced people, field hospitals, or primary health care centers. It does not require complex technological equipment or advanced knowledge in forensic medicine. This versatility has been key to its use in multiple humanitarian crises. However, this same accessibility entails a methodological limitation: by prioritizing immediate medical care, it reduces its potential to generate useful evidence in criminal justice processes or international accountability mechanisms.

In contrast, the International Protocol may seem, at first glance, more difficult to implement in fragile contexts. Its comprehensive design, technical language, and forensic orientation could be interpreted as barriers to field use. However, Y, Z and B cases experience shows that, with contextual adaptations and appropriate pedagogical strategies, the protocol can be perfectly implemented even in rural communities affected by conflict. In this case, the protocol was translated into the local language, its content was synthesized into more manageable forms, and practical training was provided to health professionals with little forensic experience. This customization process made it possible to maintain the methodological integrity of the protocol without sacrificing its applicability.

In addition, the protocol promotes a flexible logic: it is not a question of imposing a rigid standard, but of offering adaptable guidance based on ethical, scientific, and legal principles. Its implementation in adverse contexts does not depend so much on technology or infrastructure, but on political will, adequate training, and ethical commitment. Thus, more than an exclusive instrument, the protocol is positioned as a scalable tool that can articulate forensic assistance with human rights and humanitarian actions.

6.7 Forensic Protection as a Humanitarian Act

Sexual violence in contexts of armed conflict is not only a crime; it is an act of domination, collective punishment and dehumanization. Its purpose goes beyond physical harm: it seeks to break the community fabric, sow fear, stigmatize victims, and consolidate structures of impunity (Karvatska et al., 2024). In this context, forensic intervention, when carried out with an ethical, scientific, and victim-centered approach, transcends its technical dimension to become a profoundly humanitarian act, a tool for symbolic restitution, historical truth, and access to justice.

This section proposes a reinterpretation of forensic assistance as a humanitarian act, especially when addressing sexual violence in armed conflict. It argues that forensic practice, far from being a cold or instrumental discipline serving a prosecutor's request or investigating judge within the parameters of the request, constitutes a form of care, a humanitarian response focused on preserving what is invaluable: the dignity of individuals and the possibility that their stories will not be silenced. This perspective implies breaking with standardized and bureaucratic views of forensic science to recover its transformative potential in contexts where pain has been systematically ignored.

6.7.1 Beyond Evidence: Forensic Science in Humanitarian Contexts

In the context of armed conflict, many victims of sexual violence do not have access to formal justice or guarantees that their cases will be prosecuted (OHCHR, 2014). In these contexts, forensic intervention cannot be limited to the production of expert evidence, but must be understood as an act of recognition of the damage suffered. When a person narrates their experience in a safe environment, when their body is examined with respect and their testimony is rigorously documented, a form of institutional and social validation is generated that had often been denied (Mukwege and Nangini, 2009).

This recognition, even if it does not lead to a criminal conviction, has enormous symbolic, psychosocial, and humanitarian values. The victims express that they feel listened to, respected, believed. The forensic interview, when conducted with a focus on trauma and informed consent, can become a milestone in the reparation process, a way of resignifying suffering and recovering one's own narrative (Ferro Ribeiro and van der Straten Ponthoz, 2017). In the words of a survivor interviewed in Mulombodji: *"It's the first time that someone has asked me about what I went through without judging me."* The human forensic action begins here.

6.7.2 The Ethics of Care in Forensic Contexts

Forensic assistance in situations of sexual violence requires an ethic of care that recognizes the fragility, pain, and asymmetry inherent in the process (Ferro Ribeiro and van der Straten Ponthoz, 2017; WHO, 2003, 2016). Victims have experienced a radical breakdown in their bodies, relationships, and environments, and any technical intervention can reactivate that trauma if not handled sensitively. Forensic documentation, in this sense, is not neutral: it can be healing or it can be revictimizing (Ferro Ribeiro and van der Straten Ponthoz, 2017).

Adopting an ethics of care involves:

- Guarantee the voluntary nature of the process: documentation should never be forced.
- Adapt the pace to the emotional state of the person, allowing pauses, omissions, or even the suspension of the exam.
- Create safe, intimate, and culturally appropriate environments for interview and physical examination.

- Avoid unnecessary questions, moral judgments, or suspicious attitudes.
- Always offer psychosocial support and referral options.

When these principles are respected, forensic intervention ceases to be just a procedure and becomes an act of dignified accompaniment. Thus, forensic science is aligned with the humanitarian principles of humanity, impartiality, and respect for the dignity of the person (Ferro Ribeiro and van der Straten Ponthoz, 2017).

6.7.3 The Role of Informed Consent as a Pillar of Dignity

Informed consent is not an administrative requirement; it is the ethical foundation that transforms a medical examination into a respectful and non-invasive act (Ferro Ribeiro and van der Straten Ponthoz, 2017; Kurner and Marelli, 2020). In the case of sexual violence, where the body has been turned into a field of aggression, regaining control over decisions is a profoundly restorative act.

Therefore, in forensic science in humanitarian contexts, consent must be:

- *Specific:* general acceptance is not enough, but each stage of the process (interview, physical examination, sampling, use of information, etc.) must be clearly explained.
- *Reversible:* the person can withdraw their consent at any time, without negative consequences.
- *Understandable:* it must be provided in the victim's language, with accessible explanations, avoiding technical terms.
- *Voluntary:* without coercion, implicit blackmail or institutional pressures.

Respect for this principle is a way of restoring agency to victims, of reaffirming their ability to decide about their bodies, their history, and their future. In this sense, forensic science in humanitarian assistance is not only based on scientific principles but also on ethical and deontological foundations that prioritize autonomy and protection against new forms of institutional violence (Ferro Ribeiro and van der Straten Ponthoz, 2017; Kurner and Marelli, 2020).

6.7.4 Documenting to Protect: Prevention as a Humanitarian Dimension

Another central aspect of forensic science in humanitarian assistance is its preventive and protective potential. Properly documenting cases of sexual violence, even years later, makes it possible to build patterns, identify structural dynamics of violence, and demand collective responsibility. Through rigorous documentation, affected communities can make visible what was intended to be hidden, question the perpetrators, and pressure states to adopt measures of non-repetition (Ferro Ribeiro and van der Straten Ponthoz, 2017; ICRC, 2016; Kurner and Marelli, 2020).

In this sense, forensic work is not only reactive; it is also proactive, insofar as it generates conditions for a stronger institutional response, more informed public policies, and mechanisms for collective reparation. In contexts such as the DRC, where sexual violence has been used as a strategy of war, the existence of well-documented forensic archives can be a key input for truth commissions, hybrid tribunals, or international transitional justice mechanisms.

6.7.5 The Role of the Community and Local Knowledge

Forensic science in humanitarian assistance also requires incorporating a community-based and participatory perspective. Forensic interventions are often perceived as external impositions, disconnected from local knowledge, values, and social dynamics. This can generate rejection, resistance, or misunderstanding, even when the intention is positive.

Therefore, any forensic humanitarian assistance process must include community leaders, women's organizations, religious actors, or traditional authorities, not as ornamental elements, but as active agents in the process. Their participation in awareness-raising, accompaniment, cultural validation of the process, and subsequent referral is key to ensuring legitimacy, sustainability, and effectiveness.

In DRC, for example, forensic interviews were only possible because the victims were accompanied by women from their own community whom they trusted. These social mediators not only facilitated understanding of the process but also helped mitigate stigma, provide emotional support, and ensure that the experience was perceived as restorative rather than a new form of exposure.

6.7.6 Forensic Science and Humanitarian Action: A Necessary Link

Historically, there has been a tendency to separate forensic practice from the humanitarian field, under the premise that the former pursues judicial objectives while the latter responds to immediate needs for protection and care. This dichotomy, however, has been challenged in recent decades, particularly in contexts of mass violence, enforced disappearances, and war crimes.

The experience of organizations such as the International Committee of the Red Cross (ICRC), Physicians for Human Rights (PHR) or the Office of the United Nations High Commissioner for Human Rights (OHCHR) shows that forensics can be integrated into humanitarian missions without losing its technical rigor or its evidentiary vocation. On the contrary, when a logic centered on dignity is adopted, forensic assistance contributes to humanitarian ends: alleviating suffering, restoring rights, and preserving the truth.

The International Protocol embodies this integration by conceiving forensic documentation not as an end in itself, but as a means to ensure justice, prevent repetition, and empower victims. This ethical and strategic vision places forensic assistance at the very heart of contemporary humanitarian action.

6.8 Ethical Considerations and Protection of Information

In the forensic approach to sexual violence in contexts of armed conflict, ethical considerations cannot be understood as mere secondary guidelines. They constitute the guiding core that determines the validity, legitimacy, and, above all, the humanity of the intervention (Wells, 2017). Unlike other areas of specialization, here the handling of information involves not only issues of scientific veracity, but also the life, safety, dignity, and recovery of people in situations of profound vulnerability (Wells, 2017). Documenting these types of crimes requires a delicate balance between the imperative of justice and the obligation not to cause harm (Ferro Ribeiro and van der Straten Ponthoz, 2017; Wells, 2017).

This section develops four key subthemes that comprise a comprehensive ethical architecture: confidentiality in risk scenarios; the dangers of re-victimization, coercion, and misuse of information; the integration of the principles of the International Protocol and ICRC standards; and finally, the opportunities and risks that emerging technologies present in the documentation of these types of crimes.

6.8.1 Confidentiality in Contexts of Risk

Confidentiality is a cardinal principle in forensic assistance to victims of sexual violence. However, its actual implementation in contexts of armed conflict faces significant obstacles. Areas affected by mass violence often lack secure storage infrastructure, data protection protocols, and reliable institutional mechanisms (Kiakuvue et al., 2024; Médecins Sans Frontières, 2021; Physicians for Human Rights, 2024). In some cases, even judicial or health authorities may be in collusion with armed actors, making state systems themselves potential threats.

Therefore, the guarantee of confidentiality cannot be limited to the verbal promise. It requires concrete technical and policy decisions: the use of codes instead of names, the secure physical custody of forms, the encryption of electronic data, strict access restriction, and the training of staff in information security practices. But beyond technological measures, confidentiality must be understood as an ethical attitude: not sharing any detail without express authorization, not assuming the good faith of the default institutions, and always prioritizing the safety of the victim over judicial or statistical purposes.

In X, Y, Z, and B cases, for example, the International Protocol forms were encoded with alphanumeric systems not directly linked to real names. Cross-referencing was only possible in the presence of two independent operators with separate keys. This strategy made it possible to document 267 cases without compromising the safety of the victims, even in an environment with the presence of high armed groups.

6.8.2 Risks of Revictimization, Coercion, or Misuse of Data

One of the biggest ethical dilemmas in documenting sexual violence is the risk of revictimization. The forensic process, when not carried out carefully, can replicate the logic of abuse: a body exposed, interrogated, dissected, often without control over what is said, shown, or archived. Poorly formulated questions, overly technical interviews, invasive examinations, or the subsequent non-consensual use of information can cause profound retraumatization (Ferro Ribeiro and van der Straten Ponthoz, 2017; WHO, 2003, 2016).

Added to this are risks of institutional coercion. In certain contexts, access to medical services, shelter, or humanitarian aid is implicitly conditional on the provision of information or the agreement to participate in legal proceedings. This practice, although not always explicit, constitutes a form of instrumentalization of the victims, which erodes their autonomy and violates their dignity. Even more troubling is the misuse of data by government actors, media outlets or even humanitarian agencies, which sometimes display accounts or statistics without prior consent, transforming a story of suffering into a commodity for reports, campaigns or institutional justifications.

Forensic ethics requires, in the face of these risks, a policy of "minimum exposure." Do not collect more data than necessary. Do not store information that will not be used securely. Do not show testimonials or photos without written authorization. And always verify that people's participation is free, informed and reversible.

6.8.3 Principles of the International Protocol and ICRC Standards

The International Protocol on the Documentation and Investigation of Sexual Violence in Conflict offers a solid ethical architecture that articulates the rights of victims with the technical-legal requirements of forensic documentation. At its core, the Protocol sets out six guiding principles: security, confidentiality, informed consent, nondiscrimination, respect, and professional competence (Ferro Ribeiro and van der Straten Ponthoz, 2017).

These principles are largely in line with the standards developed by the ICRC, particularly in its guidelines for the treatment of detainees, the protection of vulnerable people and the preservation of sensitive medical records (ICRC,

2016; ICRC, 2019). Both sources agree that information about sexual violence is "hyper-sensitive" and should be treated as such, even beyond conventional frameworks of medical or judicial ethics.[10]

The convergence between the Protocol and ICRC standards can be summed up in the following essential practices:

- Never collect information if it cannot be adequately protected.
- Prioritize the well-being of the victim over the institutional or investigative interest.
- Document only if there is a reasonable expectation that the information will be used with respect, security, and consent.
- Develop procedures for destroying, archiving, or declassifying information, based on victims' future decisions.

Both frameworks recognize that silence can be a valid and ethical option. Documentation is not always better than not documenting. In certain contexts, protecting a person may entail temporarily forgoing the collection of evidence. This stance requires institutional maturity, a people-centered ethic, and forensic practice that is not governed solely by the logic of punishment. However, when cases are opened, whether at the individual or group level, they must be addressed holistically and integral, as in the case of Mulombodji.

6.8.4 Emerging Technologies: Advantages and Risks in Forensic Documentation (MediCapt, GBVIMS)

Emerging technologies have opened up new possibilities for the safe, standardized, and efficient documentation of cases of sexual violence in conflict contexts. Tools such as MediCapt, https://phr.org/issues/sexual-violence/medicapt/ (developed by Physicians for Human Rights) and the Gender-Based Violence Information Management System (GBVIMS, https://www.gbvims.com/) (used by humanitarian agencies[11] such as UNFPA, IRC or UNICEF[12]) represent a

---

[10] María Carolina Aissa de Figueredo (ICRC Advisor for Humanitarian and Political Diplomacy) offers a number of suggestions for striking a balance between the duty to report and the safety and dignity of victims in the July 4, 2024, ICRC blog post, "Forced to report: mandatory reporting of sexual violence in armed conflict" (blogs.icrc.org). She recommends that states examine their legal frameworks to make sure that mandatory reporting does not impede victims' access to psychosocial support and medical care, always putting the survivor's autonomy and informed consent first. In accordance with international humanitarian law, she suggests that humanitarian actors create transparent, culturally aware procedures that include exceptions for situations in which reporting would jeopardize the victim's safety. In order to achieve protection and justice without jeopardizing the trust and well-being of those who have been victims of these crimes, she also suggests bolstering professional training in the treatment of victims of sexual violence, guaranteed information confidentiality, and encouraging inter-institutional coordination.

[11] See further information in https://www.gbvims.com/?utm_source=chatgpt.com

[12] See further information in https://www.unicef.org/documents/guidance-implementing-gbvims-government-actors?utm_source=chatgpt.com

paradigm shift in the way sensitive information is collected, stored, and analyzed round the world.[13]

MediCapt, for example, is a mobile application that allows forensic findings to be digitally recorded, clinical photographs to be attached, information to be automatically encoded and sent to secure servers.[14] The system integrates standardized forms with digital consent and restricted access, reducing human error, preventing physical document tampering, and improving evidence traceability. In pilot trials in DRC and Kenya (Kidenda et al., 2022; Naimer et al., 2017), MediCapt has proven to be effective even in rural areas, provided that it is accompanied by local training and cultural adaptations.

For its part, the GBVIMS works as a platform to collect anonymous data on cases attended by different agencies, allowing the analysis of patterns, types of aggressors, risk areas, and service needs (*The Gender-Based Violence Information Management System (GBVIMS)*[15]). Its added value lies in the fact that it avoids double counting, protects the identity of individuals, and facilitates inter-institutional coordination without sharing identification data.

Confidentiality, consent, responsible use, protection against harm, critical technological integration, and coordination with international regulatory frameworks are all pieces of the same puzzle: ensuring that forensic practice draws on this information is a fruitful path that can strengthen evidence in the future, as well as the protection of information.

In war zones, where the bodies of women and victims in general have become territory of conquest, protecting information is protecting life. Ethical documentation means resisting oblivion, without turning pain into spectacle or truth into a commodity. Ultimately, it is about returning science to its most noble function: serving humanity. Critical thinking on the need to protect evidence and victims' data, avoiding unnecessary exposure, even in judicial settings.

6.9 Towards a Resilient Forensic System in Adverse Contexts

Traditional forensic systems, designed in peace contexts and supported by stable infrastructure, often collapse or become ineffective in armed conflict settings. In these environments, characterized by institutional fragmentation, persistent insecurity, citizen mistrust, and scarce resources, there is an urgent need to rethink the role of forensic science and transform it into a resilient tool able to operate in humanitarian settings.

---

[13] See further information https://www.gbvims.com/what-is-gbvims/where-gbvims-is/?utm_source=chatgpt.com

[14] See further information https://phr.org/issues/sexual-violence/medicapt/?utm_source=chatgpt.com

[15] See further information https://www.gbvims.com/

This section explores the keys to designing a forensic system that not only meets international standards but is also adaptive, contextual, participatory, and victim-centered. The aim is to reconstruct forensic practice based on a logic that combines justice, care, and memory, integrating technical knowledge with a deep understanding of local social realities.

6.9.1 Training of Local Personnel with International Standards

The cornerstone of a forensic science in humanitarian action is the training of local staff with strong technical skills and an ethical understanding of the context in which they work. Rather than relying exclusively on foreign experts or one-off external interventions, it aims to strengthen the internal capacities of local communities and structures, training professionals who remain in the territory, speak the language of the population and understand cultural, social, and political dynamics.

This training must go beyond traditional technical content. It should include:

- Principles of humanitarian ethics and human rights.
- Trauma management and empathic communication with victims.
- Forensic documentation of sexual and gender-based violence.
- Protection of information and responsible use of technologies.
- Contextual adaptation of international protocols.

The experience of organizations such as the ICRC, UNJHRO, or Physicians for Human Rights shows that on-site training programs, when articulated with universities, professional associations, and local communities, can generate networks of experts, technicians, doctors, and psychologists capable of sustaining forensic assistance even in fragile contexts. This strategy empowers local actors, breaks with the logic of the "imported expert" and fosters a social appropriation of the truth.

6.9.2 Flexible Yet Robust Protocols, Adaptable to Multiple Scenarios

One of the main challenges of forensic assistance in conflict zones is the application of protocols designed for ideal contexts, with sophisticated equipment, specialized personnel, and safe environments. Faced with this reality, there is a need to have protocols that maintain methodological rigor but can be adapted to adverse conditions.

The key is to conceive of protocols not as rigid forms, but as ethical-operational frameworks that guide decision-making even in conditions of uncertainty. An adapted protocol should:

Allow partial documentation when it is not possible to complete all steps.
Prioritize victim safety over obtaining evidence.

Offer alternatives in the collection of evidence according to the resources available.

Be understandable to non-forensic users, such as medical personnel or community agents.

The International Protocol on Sexual Violence in Conflict has proven to be adaptable, especially when broken down into modules and translated into local languages. For example, simplified forms were developed in DRC, based on the principles of the protocol, which could be applied by rural health personnel without formal forensic training (Komar et al., 2021). The key was training, accompaniment, and continuous review of procedures.

Flexibility does not mean giving up rigor. It means prioritizing the ultimate ends of the process: protecting, documenting, repairing. An adapted protocol is, in essence, an instrument of equity, which allows the truth to be recorded even when conditions are not optimal.

6.9.3 Articulation Between Health, Justice and Humanitarian Action

Forensic humanitarian action cannot be sustained in isolation. It requires an intersectoral articulation between the health system, the justice system and historical memory initiatives. In conflict contexts, this articulation is even more critical, as each sector faces its own institutional and ethical boundaries.

The health system is often the first point of contact with victims. Therefore, they must be trained not only to provide medical care, but also to recognize signs of sexual violence, activate forensic documentation routes, and ensure informed consent. The justice system, for its part, must ensure that forensic reports are received with respect, that they do not become instruments of secondary criminalization or stigmatization, and that the procedural rights of victims are preserved.

Finally, memory is the third axis. Many times, the forensic truth does not reach a court. But it can feed truth commissions, historical reports, symbolic reparation processes, or mechanisms of public recognition. Forensic science, when integrated into these narratives, ceases to be just a technical tool and becomes a source of collective legitimation.

A Forensic humanitarian action is built not only with good intervention of mobilization or assistance, but with ethical and strategic alliances between sectors that understand that documenting is also protecting, and that justice, health, and memory are not separate paths, but parts of the same human response to barbarism.

6.9.4 The Integrated Forensic Approach in Transitional Justice

In post-conflict periods, transitional justice processes represent a crucial way to respond to the harm suffered by victims. In this scenario, a forensic approach must take center stage, not only as a source of evidence but also as a mechanism for the institutional validation of suffering, the reconstruction of truth, and the prevention of impunity.

Transitional justice, comprising judicial and extrajudicial mechanisms such as special tribunals, truth commissions, collective reparations, and institutional reforms, is enriched when it incorporates a forensic humanitarian assistance dimension that:

- Rigorously documents the violence and the consequences suffered by victims and communities.
- Provides independent evidence in contexts of narrative dispute.
- Allows for the recognition of systematic patterns of violence.
- Contributes to the symbolic reparation of victims by recognizing their testimony as true and worthy of memory. In many countries, the integration of forensic work into transitional justice processes has proven to be a tool for institutional legitimacy and trust (UN, 2025). Not only has evidence been provided to the courts, but an official narrative about the conflict has been constructed that incorporates the victims' experiences as a central axis of the process.

To achieve this, it is essential that forensic work be integrated from the very design of transitional justice mechanisms, with the active participation of victims and a rationale that prioritizes reparation over punishment. Forensic science can and should be a bridge between individual suffering and collective responsibility.

6.10 Conclusion

In contexts of armed conflict, sexual- and gender-based violence has ceased to be a marginal consequence and has become one of the most brutal and effective strategies of collective subjugation. Beyond physical destruction, this violence seeks to disintegrate the social fabric, instill fear and reaffirm power relations through the bodies of women, girls, boys, adolescents, and, to a lesser extent, men. As highlighted by Dr. Denis Mukwege, witness to this reality in the Democratic Republic of Congo, the violence exerted on bodies not only hurts people: it fractures entire communities, devastates generations, and perpetuates trauma in silence. His famous statement, *"women's bodies have become a true battlefield and rape is being used as a weapon of war,"*[16] is not a rhetorical metaphor, but a crude diagnosis of a systematic practice that requires equally structural and committed responses.

[16] These words were spoken when Dr. Denis Mukwege accepted the Sakharov Prize for Freedom of Thought awarded by the European Parliament. This occurred during his acceptance speech on November 26, 2014, in Strasbourg. See https://www.europarl.europa.eu/topics/en/article/20141125STO80503/sakharov-laureate-denis-mukwege-women-s-bodies-have-become-a-true-battlefield?utm_source=chatgpt.com

Faced with this reality, forensic science plays a crucial role, provided it manages to embrace its ethical and humanitarian dimension with the same force as its technical dimension. Forensic protection, far from being limited to the identification of injuries or the collection of evidence, must be a tool that preserves dignity, a bridge between the trauma experienced and the often distant, but essential, possibility of reparation. In this sense, documentation is not just about recording: it is about preserving, about protecting information. It is about preserving the truth of what happened. It is about preserving the history of communities that have been systematically violated. It is also about preserving the possibility of a different future that can be rebuilt and assessing its aftermath so that it never happens again.

However, for this potential to be realized, it is imperative to rethink the foundations upon which traditional forensic practice has been built, including decisively activating the humanitarian component of forensic science in this regard. In emergency contexts or precarious institutional frameworks, such as those that characterize many zones of armed conflict, forensic systems designed according to Western standards are ineffective. Robust protocols and technically competent professionals are insufficient if they cannot adapt to changing realities, where the protection of the victim must prevail over the search for evidence, and where silence is sometimes a legitimate form of resistance. It is in this silence that forensic science in humanitarian actions contributes to freezing these episodes.

Therefore, forensic sciences in humanitarian action can no longer be understood as the mere ability to manage death in armed conflicts and the lives of those who are related to it, a task that has fulfilled and continues to fulfill. Its scope is enormous; it must also be understood as a humanitarian commitment to the most vulnerable people, those who have suffered sexual violence, as a practice that adapts to the environment, but without losing its roots in the fight against impunity and the defense of human rights, while always preserving confidentiality. This approach requires ongoing training, investment in local capacities, and a deep connection between the health system, the justice system, and humanitarian action mechanisms. It also requires concrete actions from the institutional framework: knowing when to intervene and when not to, knowing how to listen without invading, and knowing how to recognize that the damaged body deserves care, protection, and not judgment.

Sexual violence as a weapon of war is not a new phenomenon, but it remains one of the most silenced. Testimonies collected in areas like DRC, forensic analyses conducted by local and international teams in post-conflict, and reports prepared by organizations such as the International Committee of the Red Cross and the United Nations all agree on the urgency of a comprehensive, ethical, and sustainable approach. Forensic science in humanitarian assistances can contribute enormously to this task, through training for health workers, instilling sensitivity, and building capacity where these people seek care, or where they are evacuated for care. There, in the first response to stabilize health, the possibility of protecting forensic information arises. In this framework, forensic assistance becomes a form of protection. Every piece of evidence documented with respect and every piece of evidence protected with integrity are acts that challenge the project of erasure that sexual violence seeks to impose.

As Dr. Mukwege warned (2020), the silence imposed by shame, fear, or lack of resources must be replaced by a policy of care, recognition, and justice. *"We believe that survivors are entitled not only to holistic care, but also to holistic justice: prosecution of perpetrators and instigators, reparations for victims and affected communities, truth-seeking mechanisms, and guarantees that these crimes will not be repeated for survivors and society. It is only by using all these transitional justice approaches that the impunity gap can be closed"*.[17]

In this task, forensic science has an inalienable responsibility. It is not about intervening only when the case reaches a national or international court. It is about being present from the beginning, on the ground, alongside the victims, constructing an alternative narrative to the history of barbarism: a narrative where truth is not an instrument of pain, but a promise of reparation.

To preserve, then, is to protect… this means precisely that Forensic science must mobilize health actors to contribute to ethical identification and documentation, to accompany with humanity, and to build systems that, even in the midst of conflict, keep alive the possibility of justice, transforming sexual violence into proof not only of the horror suffered but also of the hope that can still be rebuilt.

References

Ali Bitenga, A. and Mutondo, K.M. (2022) Behind the weapon of war: sexual violence in wartime as a reflection of social attitudes towards women in peacetime. *Journal of Sexual Aggression*, **28**(2), 149–163.

Ali Bitenga, A., Mukwege, A., Mutondo, K.M., Apasa, R.B., Mugisho, G., Amisi, C., *et al.* (2025) Bridging theory and praxis in the comprehensive treatment of conflict-related sexual violence in the Great Lakes Region of Africa. *Global Public Health*, **20**, 1.

Anstett, E. (2023) Destruction, mass violence, and human remains. In: *Anthropology of Violent Death: Theoretical Foundations for Forensic Humanitarian Action* (eds. R.C. Parra and D.H. Uberlaker). Wiley, pp. 91–104.

Arrief, A. (2011, November 30) Sexual Violence in African Conflicts. (CRS Report No. R40956). Congressional Research Service, Library of Congress. https://crsreports.congress.gov.

Bitenga Alexandre, A., Moke Mutondo, K., Bazilashe Balegamire, J., Emile, A., and Mukwege, D. (2021) Motivations for sexual violence in armed conflicts: Voices from combatants in eastern Democratic Republic of Congo. *Medicine, Conflict and Survival*, **37**(1), 15–33. https://doi.org/10.1080/13623699.2021.1882365.

[17] Bukavu June 19, 2020, *Statement by Dr. Denis Mukwege on the International Day for the Elimination of Sexual Violence in Conflict*. See https://panzifoundation.org/statement-by-dr-denis-mukwege-on-the-international-day-for-the-elimination-of-sexual-violence-in-conflict/?utm_source=chatgpt.com

Cordner, S. and Tidball-Binz, M. (2017) Humanitarian forensic action: Its origins and future. *Forensic Science International*, **279**, 65–71.

Ferro Ribeiro, S., and van der Straten Ponthoz, D. (2017) *International Protocol on the Documentation and Investigation of Sexual Violence in Conflict.*

Garrido, R. (2021) Mapping the invisible rape: Men and boys as victims of sexual violence in armed conflict. *Nação e Defesa*, **159**, 151–168.

International Committee of the Red Cross (ICRC). (2016, September 22) Q&A: Sexual violence in armed conflict.

International Committee of the Red Cross (ICRC) (2019). Policy on the Processing of Biometric Data by the ICRC. https://www.icrc.org/en/publication/4261-icrc-rules-on-personal-data-protection.

International Criminal Court (ICC). (2013) Elements-of-Crimes. www.icc-cpi.int.

International Criminal Court (ICC). (2021) Rome Statute of The International Criminal Court. www.icc-cpi.int.

Karvatska, S., Gnatuyk, T., and Labyk, A. (2024) Sexual and gender-based violence in Armed Conflicts: Problems of defining and creating a prevention mechanism. *Baltic Journal of Legal and Social Sciences*, **2**, 5–12. https://doi.org/10.30525/2592-8813-2024-2-1.

Kiakuvue, Y.N., Kanyere, F.S., Mukubu, D.M., Ruhindiza, B.M., and Mukuku, O. (2024) Sexual violence among female survivors in Goma, in the Democratic Republic of the Congo: epidemiology, clinical features, and circumstances of occurrence. *Scientific Reports*, **14**(1). https://doi.org/10.1038/s41598-024-65412-7.

Kidenda, S., Muchai, R., Green, L., McHale, T., Mishori, R., and Nelson, B.D. (2022) Evaluating the effectiveness of a mobile application to improve the quality, collection, and usability of forensic documentation of sexual violence. *PLOS ONE*, **17**(12), e0278312. https://doi.org/10.1371/journal.pone.0278312.

Komar, D., El Jundi, S., Parra, R.C., and Perich, P. (2021) A comparison of the international protocols for the forensic assessment of conflict-related sexual violence victims. *Journal of Forensic Sciences*, **66**(4), 1520–1523. https://doi.org/10.1111/1556-4029.14691.

Kurner, C., and Marelli, M. (2020) *Handbook on Data Protection in Humanitarian Actions.* https://www.icrc.org/en/publication/430501-handbook-data-protection-humanitarian-action-second-edition (accessed December 8, 2025).

Latek, M. (2014) *Sexual violence in the Democratic Republic of Congo (At a Glace).* European Parliamentary Research Service. . https://www.europarl.europa.eu/thinktank/en/document/EPRS_ATA%282014%29542155?utm_source=chatgpt.com (accessed December 8, 2025).

Leatherman, J.L. (2011) *Sexual Violence and Armed Conflict.* Polity Press, Cambridge.

Médecins Sans Frontières. (2021) Sexual violence in the Democratic Republic of Congo: The critical need for a comprehensive response to address the needs of survivors. https://www.msf.org/sexual-violence-democratic-republic-congo (accessed December 8, 2025).

Médecins Sans Frontières (2021) Sexual violence in the Democratic Republic of Congo: MSF report 2021 [Report]. MSF. https://www.msf.org/sites/default/files/2021-07/MSF%20DRC_SEXUAL%20VIOLENCE%20REPORT.pdf (accessed December 8, 2025).

Mugisho, G.M., Maroyi, R., Nabami, S., Kasherwa, A.C., Bitenga, A., and Mukwege, D. (2022) Sexual and gender-based violence victims' satisfaction of the support services through the holistic model of care in the Democratic Republic of Congo. *Discover Social Science and Health*, **2**(1). https://doi.org/10.1007/s44155-022-00025-x.

Mukwege, D. (2024) healing the survivors of sexual violence. *Bulletin of the World Health Organization*, **102**(3), 157–158. https://doi.org/10.2471/BLT.24.030324. PMID: 38434185; PMCID: PMC10898282.

Mukwege, D. and Berg, M. (2016) A Holistic, Person-Centred Care Model for Victims of Sexual Violence in Democratic Republic of Congo: *The Panzi Hospital One-Stop Centre Model of Care. PLOS Medicine*, **13**(10), e1002156. https://doi.org/10.1371/journal.pmed.1002156.

Mukwege, D.M. and Nangini, C. (2009) Rape with extreme violence: The new pathology in South Kivu, Democratic Republic of Congo. *PLOS Medicine*, **6**(12), e1000204. https://doi.org/10.1371/journal.pmed.1000204.

Naimer, K., Brown, W., and Mishori, R. (2017) MediCapt in the Democratic Republic of the Congo: The design, development, and deployment of mobile technology to document forensic evidence of sexual violence. *Genocide Studies and Prevention*, **11**(1), 25–35. https://doi.org/10.5038/1911-9933.11.1.1455.

Obenson, K. and Enow Orock, G. (2017) An overview of the challenges facing death investigation systems in certain resource limited countries. *Journal of Forensic and Legal Medicine*, **50**, 58–62. https://doi.org/10.1016/j.jflm.2017.05.011.

Office of the High Commissioner for Human Rights (2024) *OHCHR report 2023*. United Nations. https://www.ohchr.org/sites/default/files/documents/publications/ohchr-reports/ohchr-report-2023.pdf (accessed December 8, 2025).

Office of the United Nations High Commissioner for Human Rights (2022). Istanbul Protocol: Manual on the Effective Investigation and Documentation of Torture and Other Cruel, Inhuman or Degrading Treatment or Punishment (Professional Training Series No. 8/Rev. 2). United Nations. https://www.ohchr.org/sites/default/files/documents/publications/2022-06-29/Istanbul-Protocol_Rev2_EN.pdf.

Office of the United Nations High Commissioner for Human Rights (2023, 12 de diciembre) Report on the human rights situation in Ukraine, 1 August to 30 November 2023. https://www.ohchr.org/sites/default/files/2023-12/23-12-12-OHCHR-37th-periodic-report-ukraine-en.pdf (accessed December 8, 2025).

Office of the United Nations Hight Commissioner for Human Rights (OHCHR). (2014) Progress and Obstacles in the fight against impunity for sexual violence in The Democratic Republic of The Congo.

Parra, R.C., Anstett, E., Perich, P., and Buikstra, J.E. (2020) Unidentified deceased persons: Social life, social death, and humanitarian action. In Roberto C. Parra, Sara C. Zapico, and Douglas H. Ubelaker (Eds.), *Forensic Science and Humanitarian Action: Interacting with the Dead and the Living*. Vol. 1, pp. 79–99. John Wiley & Sons.

Parra, R.C., Condori, L.A., and Ubelaker, D.H. (2024) Forensic anthropology and the mitigation of cognitive biases in the investigation of human rights violations: Operationalization of a comprehensive theoretical model. *Forensic Anthropology*, **7**(1). https://doi.org/10.5744/fa.2023.0024.

Parra, R.C., Vigo-Corea, D.M., and Perich, P. (2023) Kill, kill again and destroy: When death is not enough. In: *Anthropology of Violent Death: Theoretical Foundations for Forensic Humanitarian Action* (eds. R.C. Parra and D.H. Ubelaker). Wiley, pp. 109–132.

Physicians for Human Rights. (2024) "Massive Influx of Cases": Health Worker Perspectives on Conflict-Related Sexual Violence in Eastern Democratic Republic of the Congo. https://phr.org/our-work/resources/massive-influx-of-cases-sexual-violence-drc/ (accessed December 8, 2025).

Rubini, E., Valente, M., Sguazzi, G., Trentin, M., Ragazzoni, L., and Gino, S. (2024) Forensic medical examination after conflict-related sexual violence: A scoping review of the literature. *Journal of Forensic and Legal Medicine*, **106**, 102736. https://doi.org/10.1016/j.jflm.2024.102736.

Sivakumaran, S. (2007) *Sexual violence against men in armed conflict. European Journal of International Law*, **18**(2), 253–276.

Tidball-Binz, M. (2020) Using forensic science to care for the dead and search for the missing. In: *Forensic Science and Humanitarian Action: Interacting with the Dead and the Living* (eds. R.C. Parra, S.C. Zapico, and D.H. Ubelaker), Vol. 1. John Wiley & Sons, pp. 3–23.

Ubelaker, D.H., Zapico, S.C., and Parra, R.C. (2020) Humanitarian action: New approaches from forensic science. In: *Forensic Science and Humanitarian Action: Interacting with the Dead and the Living* (eds. R.C. Parra, S.C. Zapico, and D.H. Ubelaker), Vol. 1. John Wiley & Sons, pp. 717–723.

United Nations (UN). (2025, July 15) *Conflict-related sexual violence: Report of the Secretary General* (Report No. S/2025/389). United Nations Security Council. https://documents.un.org/doc/undoc/gen/n25/108/72/pdf/n2510872.pdf.

United Nations Office on Drugs and Crime (UNODC). (2024) *Forensic Evidence* Processing in Gender-Based Violence Cases.

Weishut, D.J.N. (2015) Sexual torture of Palestinian men by Israeli authorities. *Reproductive Health Matters*, **23**(46), 71–84. https://doi.org/10.1016/j.rhm.2015.11.019.

Wells, D. (2017) Sexual violence interventions: Considerations for humanitarian settings. *Forensic Science International*, **276**, 1–4. https://doi.org/10.1016/j.forsciint.2017.04.004.

World Health Organization (WHO). (2003) Guidelines for medico-legal care for victims of sexual violence.

World Health Organization (WHO). (2016) Strengthening the Medico-Legal Response to Sexual Violence. https://www.who.int/publications/i/item/WHO-RHR-15.24 (accessed December 8, 2025).

CHAPTER 7

Quality Management in Forensic Science in Panama: Advances, Challenges, and Perspectives

José Vicente Pachar Lucio
Institute of Legal Medicine and Forensic Sciences of Panama, Panama

7.1 Introduction

Forensic science is an essential component of investigations and the administration of justice, as it provides key scientific evidence to resolve primarily civil and criminal litigation.

The implementation of quality management systems in forensic sections and laboratories ensures technical competence, traceability of procedures, and reliable results (Houck and Siegel, 2015).

In Panama, the IMELCF (National Institute of Forensic Medicine and Forensic Sciences) is the only government institution responsible for providing expert services in Legal and Forensic Medicine, Criminalistics, and Forensic Laboratories throughout the country.

The Institute of Legal Medicine and Forensic Sciences (IMELCF) originated in what was formerly known as the "Forensic Medicine Office," a department of the Ministry of Government and Justice until 1973, when Law No. 34 of May 8 was enacted, assigning it to the Public Prosecutor's Office as an auxiliary body in judicial investigations. Subsequently, Law No. 29 of October 25, 1984, which adopted the Judicial Code of Panama, created the Institute of Forensic Medicine and attached it to the Office of the Attorney General.

In 2006, with the approval of Law 50 of December 13, the institute, which at that time only offered forensic medicine expert services and some laboratories, was reorganized and attached to the Public Prosecutor's Office to provide scientific and technical advice to the administration of justice regarding investigations

Forensic Science and Quality Management: Addressing the Era of Standardization in Challenging Environments, First Edition. Edited by Roberto C. Parra and Allan G. Alvarez-Godoy.

and the scientific and medical-scientific description of forensic findings and evidence. This law also stipulated that management positions should be filled through a competitive examination based on professional merit, established labor guarantees for officials, and guaranteed autonomy in administrative and human resources management.

The following year, in 2007, the National Assembly approved Law 69 on December 27, and the Criminalistics, Forensic Services, and Forensic Laboratories Departments of the defunct Technical Judicial Police were transferred to the IMELCF. In this way, all scientific forensic services related to forensic sciences were integrated into a single civil institution. It is an institution with operational, administrative, and human resource management autonomy, which provides technical and scientific forensic services impartially, at the request of the competent authority, on a permanent basis, nationwide.

Starting in 2019, the IMELCF launched an ambitious accreditation project aligned with international standards and aimed at unifying and strengthening the practice of its experts.

7.2 Regulatory Framework and International Context

ISO/IEC standards are international standards designed to ensure the quality, safety, efficiency, and compatibility of products, services, and systems. They are often applied to information technology, quality, laboratory management, and security systems (See table 7.1).

ISO/IEC 17025 – General requirements for the competence of testing and calibration laboratories – is fundamental to forensic laboratories. It establishes requirements for the quality management system and technical competence and ensures that results are valid and reproducible.

ISO/IEC 17020, on the other hand, establishes operating requirements for various types of inspection bodies, such as Field Criminalistics Sections, ensuring that procedures comply with standardized criteria.

In the context of forensic science, these standards provide structured frameworks to ensure that processes, analyses, and results are reliable, reproducible, and internationally valid. Forensic science requires high precision, traceability, and objectivity, as its results have legal implications. Therefore, its application translates into greater credibility in the courts, a reduction in errors and biases, and recognition, both within the country (International Organization for Standardization [ISO], 2017, ISO, 2012). Several Latin American countries have undertaken similar efforts, albeit at different levels of development, making Panama's progress especially relevant in the regional context (UNODC, 2021).

Table 7.1 IMELCF accredited laboratories and sections.

ENTE	Laboratorio/Sección	NORMA ISO/IEC
ANAB	Field Criminalistics – Ancón	17020
ANAB	Field Criminalistics – West Panama	17020
ANAB	Field Criminalistics – San Miguelito	17020
ANAB	Forensic Ballistics	17025
ANAB	Forensic Documentology	17025
ANAB	Forensic Fingerprinting	17025
ANAB	Forensic Planimetry	17025
ANAB	Controlled Substances – Ancón	17025
ANAB	Controlled Substances – Veraguas	17025
ANAB	Biomolecular Analysis (DNA)	17025
CNA	Forensic Toxicology	17025
CNA	Forensic Chemistry	17025
CNA	Forensic Biology	17025

ANAB: ANSI *National Accreditation Board*.
CNA: National Accreditation Council of Panama (In English languaje: Consejo Nacional de Acreditación de Panamá).

7.3 Accreditation Progress in Panama

With the financial and logistical support from the United States Embassy in Panama, the IMELCF applied for accreditation of its laboratories and sections with the American accreditation body ANAB (ANSI National Accreditation Board) in 2019, starting with the Documentation laboratories and the Biomolecular Analysis Unit (ADN). Both achieved ISO/IEC 17025 accreditation after a rigorous process of method validation, internal quality control, and staff training. The accreditation process has continued and has been extended not only to laboratories and sections in the capital but also to other cities in Panama.

The following table presents a summary of the sections and laboratories accredited through April 2025.

In this way, we have consolidated a robust institutional system aligned with international best practices. It is worth noting that the Ancón Field Criminalistics Section was one of the first to obtain ISO/IEC 17020 accreditation, making Panama one of the first Latin American countries to achieve this milestone.

Furthermore, our experts have collaborated as facilitators in Central American and Asian countries.

The accreditations have positively influenced public and judicial confidence in forensic reports (ANSI National Accreditation Board [ANAB], 2022).

7.4 Challenges Faced During the Process

7.4.1 Technical and Operational Challenges

At the IMELCF, we did not have facilities specifically designed for the operation of forensic sections and laboratories, and we were not prepared to meet the necessary technical, environmental, and traceability requirements. In the first stage, adjustments were made to the DNA and Documentation laboratories.

Since the accreditation process requires specialized knowledge, time, and rigorous documentation to demonstrate technical competence, experts received training both domestically and internationally.

Another element to consider was metrological traceability, with the aim of ensuring that all instruments are calibrated and traceable to national and international standards, a complex and costly process.

Furthermore, an internal quality control plan was implemented, necessary to implement robust procedures to ensure the continued validity of the results.

7.4.2 Staff Training and Competence

Recognizing that it is essential for staff to be competent not only technically but also in their understanding of the management system and regulatory requirements, ongoing training programs were developed, both within and outside the country, with the support of the United States Embassy.

During the process, we observed that some experts viewed the system as an additional bureaucratic burden to their expert duties, so administrative and educational measures were taken to reinforce effective change management. Likewise, a system was established to periodically assess competencies, although it was not institutionalized.

7.4.3 Documentation and Information Management

Another challenge faced was managing the document overload. The standards require a large amount of procedures, records, and objective evidence that must be kept up-to-date.

Furthermore, we had to consider that the ISO/IEC 17025 standard (2017 version) introduced a risk-based approach that was novel and difficult to implement.

In addition, countless efforts have been made to ensure that all documentation is controlled and easily accessible to authorized users.

7.4.4 Financial and Economic Resources

For the first accreditations, the IMELCF was responsible for the adaptations of the laboratories and sections. The United States Embassy supported us with donations of equipment, calibrations, expert training, and consulting services. They also made payments to the accrediting body ANAB. Currently, IMELCF finances its new accreditations and maintenance audits with its own resources, through its association with the ANAB accreditation body and with the accrediting body Consejo Nacional de Acreditación (CNA) of Panama.

7.4.5 Quality Management and Organizational Culture

Beginning in 2018, with the change in the general management of IMELCF, the commitment of senior management was notable, not only in rhetoric, which allowed for the sustainability and continuity of the system.

One of the most difficult challenges to face was the lack of a culture of continuous improvement, which hindered the internalization of quality principles.

Internal and external audits were and are stressful and require specific preparation and training.

7.4.6 Integration with Other Systems and Their Users

The coexistence with other regulatory frameworks, such as the Panamanian legal provisions on the practice of expert reports, established in the Code of Criminal Procedure, caused friction and conflicts with service users who, accustomed to the previous system, were stuck in a culture of paper expert reports, without control over the results, but within the timeframes established in national regulations.

Clients did not understand that compliance with quality standards guarantees the technical and legal validity of the results. Judges and prosecutors lack understanding of the foundations and importance of quality standards, which translates into a lack of interest in the quality management system, difficulties in justifying institutional resources before the corresponding authorities, and the risk of judicial decisions that ignore key differences between accredited and nonaccredited results. This weakens the defensibility of expert reports and exposes the IMELCF laboratory or section to unnecessary questioning, even when working with high standards.

We addressed this challenge by holding workshops for prosecutors, judges, and public defenders on the importance of traceability, chain of custody, method validation, and more. We also showed them how the system reduces errors, ensures the traceability of analyzed samples, and improves the defense of cases against challenges. It was particularly significant that, in a hearing involving a high-profile corruption case, poor quality management, specifically in the chain of custody of digital evidence, affected the outcome expected by the Public Prosecutor's Office and the community at large.

Along the same lines, lawyers failed to see the relationship between technical quality and procedural guarantees, so we emphasized that accreditation guarantees impartiality, traceability, and competence – fundamental pillars of due process.

The implementation of quality systems requires a profound cultural transformation that affects known and established procedures, operational hierarchies, and organizational dynamics (Ponce and Leyva, 2019). Furthermore, it is difficult to guarantee the financial sustainability of the system, especially once the initial phase of international support has ended.

7.5 Institutional and Social Impact

The standardization of procedures, the use of validated methods, and systematic documentation have increased the Panamanian judicial system's confidence in IMELCF expert reports. Furthermore, accreditation has strengthened international cooperation and positioned Panama as a regional example in forensic quality management. This has direct implications for the protection of human rights, due process, and the effectiveness of the justice system (National Institute of Justice [NIJ], 2013).

7.6 Conclusions

The implementation of quality management systems at the IMELCF in Panama has proven to be a fundamental process for ensuring the reliability and validity of forensic analyses. This effort has allowed IMELCF to obtain national and international accreditation, positioning Panama as a benchmark in the Central American region. Despite technical, operational, financial, and staff training challenges, institutional commitment and international cooperation have been key to overcoming these obstacles. The standardization of procedures and continuous improvement have strengthened the judicial system's confidence in expert reports, contributing to the protection of human rights and due process.

References

ANSI National Accreditation Board (ANAB). (2022) *Accreditation of Forensic Laboratories.*

Houck, M.M. and Siegel, J.A. (2015) *Fundamentals of Forensic Science. Academic Press.* https://www.imelcf.gob.pa/.

National Institute of Justice (NIJ). (2013) Strengthening Forensic Science in the United States: A Path Forward.

Organización Internacional de Normalización (ISO). (2012) ISO/IEC 17020:2012 Conformity assessment – Requirements for the operation of various types of bodies performing inspection.
Organización Internacional de Normalización (ISO). (2017) ISO/IEC 17025:2017 General requirements for the competence of testing and calibration laboratories.
Ponce, J. and Leyva, R. (2019) *Gestión de la calidad en laboratorios forenses. Editorial Forense.*
United Nations Office on Drugs and Crime (UNODC). (2021) Forensic Science and Criminal Justice: An International Perspective.

CHAPTER 8

Peruvian Efforts to Strengthen the Quality of Forensic Practice: Limitations and Advances in Standardization

Gian Carlo Iannacone[1], Marleny Huerta-Valdivia[1], Jorge Vasquez-Guerrero[1], and Roberto C. Parra[2,*]

[1] *Institute of Legal Medicine and Forensic Sciences of Peru, LIma, Peru*

[2] *The Specialized Forensic Team of the United Nations Joint Human Rights Office (UNJHRO) in the Democratic Republic of the Congo*

8.1 Introduction

In Latin America, the progress of forensic sciences in terms of quality management has been quite differentiated. In some countries of the region, quality management processes have advanced significantly, and their sustainability has strengthened their capacities, mainly in more accessible sectors. Colombia continues to be the regional leader in this area, although deficiencies persist, mainly in forensic branch in the interior of the country. Nevertheless, the progress made is undeniable and has become a reference point for other countries. Nations such as Chile, Guatemala, and Honduras have followed this Colombian leadership with varying degrees of efficiency and continuity. In contrast, several countries have attempted to advance, but their efforts have often amounted to good intentions rather than concrete, sustainable achievements. Peru is among these countries, continuously struggling to strengthen its quality management systems, particularly in the management of forensic and analytical laboratories, where international accreditation and highly standardized processes are increasingly required.Forensic science in Peru also has not been able to take off due to innumerable factors that have blocked its concrete development. Deficient administrations, precarious infrastructures, and an uncontrolled

*The views expressed herein are those authors and do not necessarily reflect the views of the United Nations.

Forensic Science and Quality Management: Addressing the Era of Standardization in Challenging Environments, First Edition. Edited by Roberto C. Parra and Allan G. Alvarez-Godoy.

deficit of budgetary and logistical shortcomings have been the main sources of underdevelopment of a forensic system that requires greater attention. Nevertheless, the system is functioning, with enormous difficulties, but it is trying to maintain sustainability in a scenario of enormous needs for the practice of forensic sciences and the proper administration of justice. To address this issue, this paper navigates in such a system, where the challenges become evident to cope with an absolutely challenging context. The Peruvian forensic system includes two important organizations; firstly the Institute of Legal Medicine and Forensic Sciences of Peru (IMLCF-Peru) and then the Peruvian National Police Criminalistics Directorate; however, we will focus only on IMLCF-Peru, since it has the greatest organizational and operational development and scope for the approach to cases. The Peruvian forensic system can be a Latin American sample, which can serve as a way of diagnosing the current situation of forensic sciences in Latin America and the complexities that other Latin American countries experience for their real development.

8.2 Brief Review of the IMLFC-Perú

February 15, 1918, marked an important milestone in the history of Peruvian forensic sciences, the inauguration of the central morgue of Lima as well as the first academic publication entitled "Legal Medicine in Peru" (Avendaño, 1918). Avendaño's publication highlights the importance of strengthening forensic medicine and the need to create an institute of forensic medicine for Peru as had been happening in other areas in the world (Ubelaker, 2015), and in the Latin American context in particular where Colombia (Giraldo, 2014; Rodriguez-Zorro and Constantin, 2015), Chile (Bustos-Streeter and Intriago-Leiva, 2015), and Uruguay (Rodriguez-Almada, 2015) stand out. Avendaño's publication (1918) was at the forefront of the knowledge of the time, where in addition to narrating the history of the gestation and development of forensic sciences, he visualizes the future of the discipline within the framework of an institutional organization of a scientific nature. Certainly, during the inaugural speech of the morgue, Leonidas Avendaño Ureta also emphasized that this place had to become a true Institute of legal Medicine (Fernández, 1955; Avendaño 1960; Avendaño, 1918). He also emphasized that "without the aid of science, the law is deficient and justice is blind" (Avendaño, 1960). Leonidad Avendaño Ureta had managed the construction of an adequate space to develop forensic autopsies for the city of Lima and also to incorporate a chief of autopsies, Guillermo Fernandez Dávila, who wrote his doctoral thesis entitled "Autopsia medico-legal" that same year. This document is the first forensic standard in the history of forensic science in Peru, which sought to achieve the quality of the practice; it also represents one of the first antecedents of its kind in Latin America. Since the inauguration of the Lima morgue, Avendaño and Fernandez worked together for nine years seeking the constant improvement of forensic practice through research and publication of their results. However, while everything seemed to be in place to consolidate the institute of legal medicine at that time, several external events of lack of political decision-making, ignorance about the importance of scientific evidence, and limited budget prevented its takeoff and further development. The institute of legal medicine had to wait about 70 years for someone to create it, although always in precarious conditions, while other countries in the region were already creating and consolidating modern forensic systems. Peru was also at the forefront of the subject at that time, but as is the case even today, Peru was not able to overcome the challenges and make them a reality.

Established in 1985, IMLFC-Peru was initially under the jurisdiction of the Ministry of Justice. However, in 1992, it was reassigned to the Public Prosecutor's Office, an autonomous constitutional entity, responsible for prosecutorial investigations within judicial processes in Peru. In this new framework, the IMLFC-Perú assumed the role of a scientific-technical advisory body for prosecutors, offering specialized services that aid in the investigation of crimes, thereby supporting the administration of justice.

By 2002, the IMLFC-Perú underwent a significant reorganization, transforming into a nationally representative institute within the Public Prosecutor's Office. This reorganization process coincided favorably with the 2004 amendments to the Peruvian Criminal Procedure Code, which underscored the importance of expert evidence in an accusatory system (Salas, 2011). Today, the IMLFC-Perú's forensic services are primarily centralized in Lima (capital of Peru), providing national headquarters reference services (in orange). Also, there are three high-resolution medical legal units (Level-III) aimed at segmenting forensic services nationally into three regions: north (red), center (gray), and south (green) (Figure 8.1). This segmentation is intended to allow dedicated forensic service in Lima. However, despite efforts, centralization of forensic services and this situation often face challenges, such as delays in acquiring materials and supplies for laboratory services and less implementation of specialized equipment in the three Level-III sites.

Additionally, the IMLFC-Perú has 27 Level-II medical legal units across the nation. These medical legal units were established over the years without a strategic plan, leading to a level of implementation often akin to that of Level-III medical legal unit in some cases. This has consequently escalated the cost of operating services due to the lack of strategic prioritization in the organization for network attention.

Both Level-III and Level-II services are supported by Level-I medical legal units (164 sites), which offer basic forensic services as the forensic clinical area (medical and psychological forensic services) and thanatological service. In the

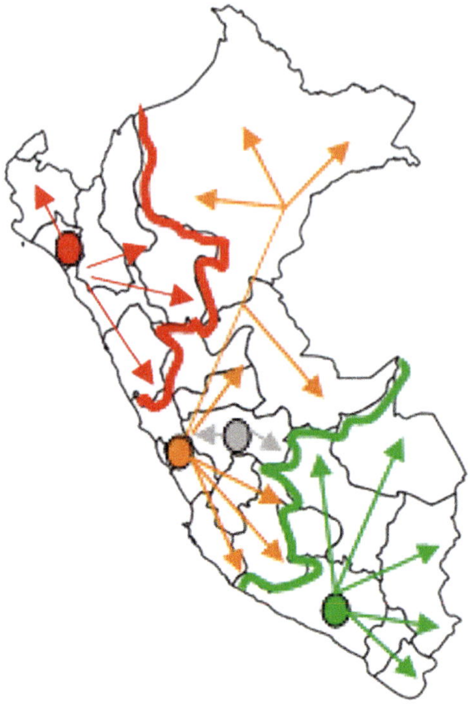

Figure 8.1 The map of Peru illustrates the division of its territory into 24 departments and a constitutional province. The coverage of Level-III forensic services is represented for the northern region as red, the southern region as green, and the central area is primarily attended to by the national reference headquarters (Lima) as orange. Also, the central area has a Level-III medical legal unit as gray, which exclusively covers the departmental area.

case of thanatological service with a morgue are only present in 26 of the 164 Level-I medical legal units out of a total of 55 morgues nationwide, then 29 medical legal units of Level-II and Level-III have a morgue. For facilities that do not have a morgue, there are often agreements with local hospitals to provide space for autopsies. However, these agreements have administrative problems, often resulting in delays in payments for services due to scarce resources. This deficit makes it difficult to improve infrastructure, which often does not meet the minimum standards required to perform necropsies.

In this context, the attention of the IMLFC-Perú partially covers the demand of the 34 districts of the prosecutor's office that are distributed nationwide (https://cfe.mpfn.gob.pe/gis_mp/gis_mpfn/map_default.phtml). The service coverage at the level of psychological forensic service has been implemented in 100% of the Level-II and Level-III medical legal units, followed by biology forensic services in 90% at the national level and in the case of the other forensic services they are present in less than 50% of the medical legal units (Table 8.1). These coverage limitations are due to high operating costs, as is the case of DNA and toxicology

Table 8.1 Distribution of the national presence of the forensic services of the IMLFC-Perú. Services with less than 50% national in gray.

Forensic service	National facilities
Legal medicine	100%
Psychology	100%
Biology	90%
Toxicology	45%
Pathology	21%
DNA	12%
Radiology	21%
Psychiatry	12%
Anthropology	66%
Odontology	87%

laboratories. In other cases, it is due to the lack of availability at the national level of forensic professionals.

According to the difficulties described above, there are international recommendations for forensic institutes in relation to ensuring the quality of forensic services, which is even more necessary in conditions of deficiencies in infrastructure, equipment and personnel (De Francisco Enciso et al. 2016 and Martin-Fumadó et al. 2016). Thus, it will be able to address the three critical macro-problems of the IMLFC-Peru for the optimal management of forensic processes that will positively impact the timeliness of services:

a. Deficiency of a system for control, distribution and use of stocks, which has generated over the years requests for materials, supplies and equipment without support that impact the programming of the annual budget.
b. Poor scheduling of work in forensic services, generating, in many cases, the false notion that there is a shortage of forensic professionals.
c. Deficiency of a system for monitoring forensic processes through indicators that allow measuring the opportunity to deliver results. This problem has been generated by the lack of integration of existing forensic systems (client-server versions) that are not interconnected.

Finally, although these problems have been known by several senior managers of the IMLFC-Peru, it has not been possible to address them adequately due to the budget gaps that have dragged on over the years, which is a common problem in several forensic institutions of Latin America, Asia, and Africa.

8.3 Macro-level Process Flow of the IMLFC-Perú Forensic Services

The IMLFC-Perú, in accordance with the basic international criteria for forensic investigation (Lee & Pagliario 2013), provides information to answer prosecutor questions as When? How? and What? with the contribution of thanatological and clinical forensic services. In this sense the degree of precision and accuracy in their conclusions will depend on the support of the auxiliary examination laboratories, aiming to adequate support to the prosecutorial hypothesis. Also it is important in order to clarify the causes of a criminal case, identify those persons involved in the case through the answer the prosecutor question Who? through the homologation of an individual with the trace of a criminal case or in other contexts looking of biological connections (genealogical affiliations) applied to human rights or humanitarian law or in a criminalistic case that involves an unidentified body.

Therefore, the IMLFC-Peru currently has a forensic processes that contribute to the prosecutor work in order to finally be able to provide results that finally answer the prosecutor question Why? and thus the prosecutor can frame it within the national legal norm in force and contribute to the proper administration of justice (Figure 8.2):

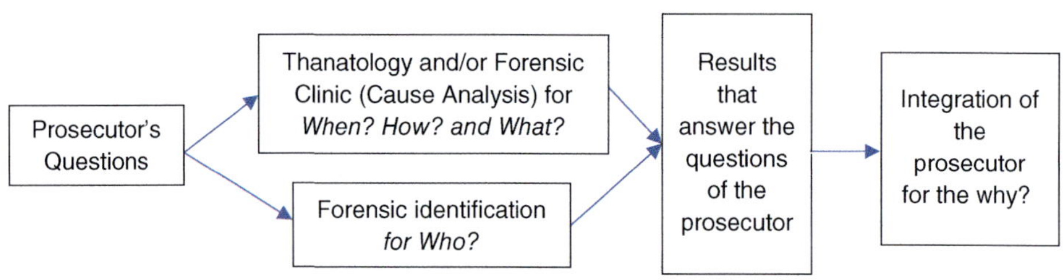

Figure 8.2 Process flow that supports the forensic work at the Institute of Legal Medicine and Forensic Sciences of Peru (IMLFC-Perú).

However, although at a macro level there is a comprehensive expertise approach, even each IMLFC-Peru process by type of forensic service still does not have adequate integration, and this is mainly due to:

a. Obsolete organizational structure of the IMLFC-Peru, which has remained the same for more than 20 years, not allowing the development of networks by forensic services for an adequate integration of multidisciplinary forensic analysis.
b. Insufficient integration between the prosecutor and forensic, which allows using only those traces that are informative for evaluation of the forensic case, leaving aside what is redundant or not relevant for the forensic analysis.

c. Insufficient integration of processes and procedures between forensic services: which currently respond to a need within each service, without considering what will serve or should be integrated into the next forensic service.
d. Priority of deadlines over comprehensive work, common for forensic services to avoid greater complexities of analysis that could provide in many cases a comprehensive evaluation of the trace, in order to provide solid answers to the investigative questions that the prosecutor has.
e. Cultural aspects of forensic professionals, related to the fact that the most appropriate forensic analysis is generated in the best way by the qualities and experience of a person than by the trained person who performs the analysis with the appropriate procedures, thus favoring the paradigm; it does not matter much what happened in later stages of the forensic services, if the expert opinion was carried out by a certain person with experience, it is an unquestionable truth.
f. Insufficient weighting of forensic examinations, each result in this context has a weight according to its potential to provide information and in this context, it forces both the forensic and prosecutor to be able to reach a level of acceptance, thus generating the need for greater integration of forensic analysis, which the aim of a are solid and objective support.
g. Insufficient opportunity, solidity, and quality of the forensic results, when the forensic results do not obtain the expected results to solve the case in court, then the goals programmed at the institutional level are not met, bringing with them two consequences; on the one hand, at the budgetary level, not being able to have a larger budget for the following year due to not being able to meet the programmed annual goals; and on the other hand, deficient state policies are generated as a consequence of the lack of effectiveness of the forensic system, since the results are biased due to poor management for the integration of processes (intra-forensic and prosecution system), insufficient process optimization, and misuse of resources.

8.4 Integration of Processes Within the Framework of the Sydney Declaration

In forensics, there are two main approaches to ensuring the quality of results:

a. *Formal accreditation and certification:* which consider the implementation of ISO systems as a nonmandatory measure but highly recommended to be able to obtain to guarantee the quality of the forensic report in court (Koehler, 2013; Zhai et al. 2020, Doyle 2019). These systems, such as ISO 17025, set rigorous standards for technical competence and quality management in forensic laboratories, ensuring that procedures and results are consistent and reliable to increase the credibility of forensic laboratories and facilitate the acceptance of their results in court.

b. *Quality assurance culture:* which is supported by the quality assurance through integrated processes, without necessarily resorting to ISO certification. This approach is based on the creation of a culture of quality within forensic organizations, where continuous quality control practices are implemented and continuous improvement is encouraged (ASCLD Train the Director, 2020; Gough, 2000; Levy et al., 2005). For example, the Sydney Declaration (Roux et al. 2022) emphasizes the importance of quality assurance through integrated processes and the active participation of all members of the organization as the basis for providing quality expertise to the justice system.

In this context, the second approach presents a significant opportunity for international associations in the forensic field to assume a more proactive role in contributing to the quality assurance of forensic institutions. In this sense, organizations such as the International Association for Forensic Science (IAFS), the Ibero-American Academy of Criminalistics and Forensic Studies (AICEF), the International Society for Forensic Genetics (ISFG), the Latin American Association of Forensic Anthropology (ALAF), among others, can lead initiatives to promote quality standards and provide resources and training to forensic professionals. In this context, these partnerships could facilitate international collaboration and the exchange of best practices, thus contributing to the continuous improvement of quality in the forensic field at a global level.

In the case of IMLFC-Peru, a few years ago the need to have ISO in some services became evident. For example, during the period from 2005 to 2007, the IMLFC-Perú made preparations to obtain ISO 9001 certification for the DNA Laboratory in Lima. Subsequently, in the years 2015 to 2016, this certification was extended to the toxicology service, specifically in relation to alcohol tests by gas chromatography. As a result, the certification was achieved in the years 2007 and 2016, respectively. However, in 2018 it was decided not to continue with this certification, because the senior management of the IMLFC-Perú considered that it was more convenient to have an accreditation of the quality of the product for both DNA and alcohol tests with ISO 17025, which specifically in the case of DNA tests should include the recommendations of the International Society for Forensic Genetics (ISFG) (Morling et al. 2002 and Gjertson et al. 2007), but despite the efforts made to date, ISO 17025 has not been achieved.

It is worth mentioning, in the context of lessons learned, what have been the main reasons that have prevented reaching the objective of ISO 17025 at the IMLFC-Perú:

a. Budgetary problems to hire an external organization to help with the accreditation project and also limited resources to maintain and calibrate the equipment. In addition, the delay in the delivery of forensic results due to budgetary reasons and poor procurement.

b. Discontinuity of the ISO system, the interruption of an already established ISO quality system to begin the implementation of a new ISO system caused this practice to be abandoned over time.
c. Insufficient training, in the context of ISO, it prevented adequate quality awareness among those involved in the process, which hindered the continuity of the ISO system, even if there was no formal certification, which as of 2018 was no longer available.

In the last years, based on the lessons learned from 2020 onward, it was considered appropriate as an alternative option for the IMLFC-Peru to implement ISO 17024 (International Accreditation Forum, 2003; Anastasopoulos, 2021; ISO, 2016), which is a process of certifying people in relation to their competencies. In this sense, with the implementation of this system, it will ensure the quality of the competencies to be an expert in accordance with international standards. However, in this context of certification, it must be considered that it cannot be assured that the components that make up that forensic report are of quality, that is, the forensic can be doing things well as a forensic professional, but in the case of the procedures that the forensic use as an input for his forensic analysis could be deficient, since that is not necessarily being controlled. On the other hand, continuity in this type of certification is an important factor because if at any time the certifying body does not have the certifying capacity due to problems of availability of resources such as budgetary resources, it puts at risk the certifications carried out and those pending recertification.

In the context of successes and failures in the implementation of ISO systems and despite the fact that the levels of process integration are still incipient, it is advisable, within the framework of the ISO 17024 implementation process in the IMLFC-Peru, to include the criteria mentioned in the Sydney Declaration to achieve the objective of greater forensic analysis integration. These criteria are detailed in Figure 8.3:

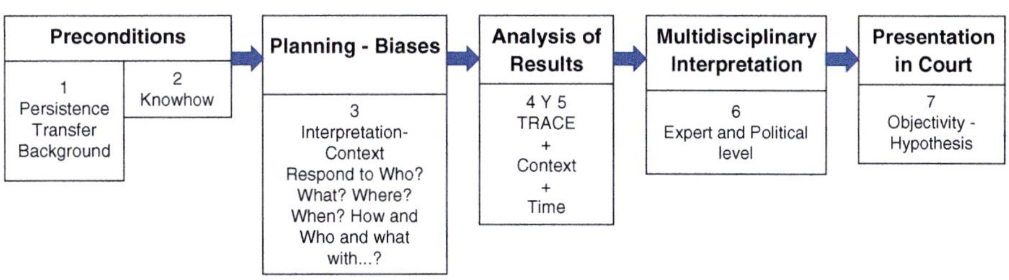

Figure 8.3 Sydney declaration steps.

8.5 Strategies from IMLFC-Peru for Quality Assurance: Applying the Declaration of Sydney as an Efficient Alternative

An example of process improvement and quality assurance in forensic institutions to achieve integrated forensic results is the experience accumulated by IMLCF-Peru in the last 20 years, in relation to each of the stages contemplated in the Sydney Declaration.

8.5.1 Preconditions in the Framework of Forensic Process

One of the essential stages of the forensic analysis process is the chain of custody, which is a transversal process that in recent years at the IMLFC-Peru has been gaining progressive importance in accordance with the current regulations in Peru. In this sense, it is necessary to point out that the chain of custody, as stated Saks and Koehler (2005) and Dawnay and Sheppard (2023), offers the following advantages:

a. Preserve the integrity of the evidence, so that it is handled carefully and safely from its origin to its presentation in court, thus guaranteeing its legal admission.
b. Provide confidence to all actors within the judicial process.
c. Provide protection of individual rights, which are fundamental in any legal system, thus ensuring a fair and equitable legal process.
d. Contribute to the prevention of impunity.
e. Contribute to international collaboration for an adequate exchange of information and collaboration between jurisdictions, especially in transnational cases.

In this sense, the correct application of the chain of custody minimizes the probability of its breakdown (Meintjies-van Del Walt 2001, 2010; Olaborede and Meintjies-van Del Walt, 2020), thus mitigating the risks of:

a. Loss of integrity of the evidence.
b. Diminished capacity for judicial admissibility.
c. Reduced ability to establish responsibility.
d. Test contamination.
e. Distrust in the judicial process.
f. Impunity.

Therefore, considering the reasons stated above, the IMLFC-Peru has implemented a specific Chain of Custody regulation in 2024. Prior to this formalization of the chain of custody, standards applicable to the chain of custody of the assets seized by the Prosecutor's Office were used, which were not the most appropriate for the proper management of the traces necessary for forensic analysis. This new IMLFC-Peru regulation establishes procedures that include:

a. Protection, perennialization, collection of samples in case of segmentation or separation, packaging, labeling, transfer, review, and reception.
b. The guidelines for assigning the forensic professional to carry out the analysis and the criteria for sending the evidence to other areas of the IMLFC-Peru for the corresponding analysis.
c. The criteria of preservation over time.
d. The criteria for temporary and definitive storage, which are defined by each of the areas of the IMLFC-Peru and in accordance with current regulations.

It should be noted that, with regard to the last two criteria (preservation over time and storage criteria), the IMLFC-Peru still faces overcrowded conditions in the sample custody areas, especially in pathology and DNA services, which are the most critical. This situation entails a risk of deterioration and, therefore, of loss of the evidentiary capacity of these samples.

On the other hand, although this Chain of Custody regulation has been developed by the IMLFC-Peru considering what is necessary to ensure the quality and integrity of the evidence, it has not considered three relevant aspects for an adequate interpretation of traces according to Kokshoorn (2023):

a. Persistence – Evidentiary capacity over time of a sample.
b. Transfer – Ability of a sample to maintain the same information in different places and media than where it was initially found.
c. Background – Magnitude of pre-existing information (contaminants) that may interfere with the collection and interpretation of a sample.

In this context, for example, the IMLFC-Peru in relation to sexual assault cases takes samples from victims in order to evaluate the presence of sperm and prostate cells at the forensic biology and DNA services. However, it is crucial to assess the transfer capacity factor, which is affected by the choice of sample collection material. For example, when cotton swabs are used for sampling, they retain the biological material with greater capacity, but in the processing stage they release this material with greater difficulty. For this reason, one mitigation measure is to opt for nylon fiber swabs, which retain a little less biological material, but release it more easily (Buchan & Ledeboer, 2014). In addition, technology has advanced, and there are improvements in cotton swabs that make them comparable to nylon swabs in their ability to yield cells (Seiberle et al., 2022). It is also necessary to consider the transfer factor in the way the evidence is packaged and transported. For example, the risk of cross-contamination is significantly increased if swabs are placed in the same packaging, especially if this packaging is susceptible to breakage.

On the other hand, with regard to the persistence capacity factor, the use of cotton swabs negatively affects these cases, since they do not have preservatives that prevent biological degradation. This generates a decrease in the suitability of the biological material and, therefore, a reduction in its evidentiary capacity. In contrast, nylon swabs, which contain suitable buffer solutions, allow for greater persistence of biological material over time (Smith et al. 2021).

Finally, in relation to the "Background" factor, the chain of custody regulations recently approved by the IMLFC-Peru does not include criteria determining the magnitude of pre-existing background information. A relevant mitigation measure would be the collection of a blank sample from the area where the evidence is collected. In the case of sexual assault cases, this could involve taking a sample of clothes from the victim and/or suspect in a part where there is no biological fluid.

In addition, it is important to consider other factors that are not included in the technical process of the IMLFC-Peru chain of custody regulations. These factors include, for example, logistical and administrative aspects of the user area, which impact the execution of these procedures. In the case of the IMLFC-Peru, from the logistical point of view, there is a lack of adequate identification of the ideal collection material for each type of sample collection, and the acquisition processes are often difficult to acquire the best quality, since the lowest price is valued more in the government regulatory system.

In relation to the transport of samples, the user area of IMLFC-Peru sends them to the place of analysis using public mail systems, which are designed for the sending of documents, not for the transport of samples. This is due to the absence of a supplier or system of its own for transporting forensic samples in the country. Due to these difficulties, in some circumstances the forensic professionals are responsible for personally bringing the samples to the place of analysis. However, in all cases, the chain of custody of such transport is not signed, especially in shipments made by public mail, which clearly affects the evidentiary capacity of the samples in court.

At this point, based on what has been mentioned in the previous paragraphs, the possibility of IMLFC-Peru obtaining ISO 21043-1:2018 certification (International Organization for Standardization, 2018) can be considered in the medium to long term. This standard is compatible with the current chain of custody regulations, with the proposed improvements, in terms of the improvement, reliability, transparency and reliability of forensic trace, as well as the requirements for the examination of crime scenes, the activities carried out within the facilities and the quality requirements in the forensic process. However, their implementation and, even more, their maintenance over time are critical factors in government organizations, as is the case in Peru.

In summary, if the limitation to quality assurance lies in the need to have an ISO certification, and considering that in Latin American, African, and Asian countries this formal certification represents a budgetary barrier, it would be advisable to:

a. Organizations count and demonstrate through records, included in an appropriate chain of custody regulation, that the handling of samples ensures quality.
b. The development of the chain of custody procedure is supported by adequate training of forensic professionals.
c. The recognition by a third party such as the case of national and/or international forensic inter-organization networks in order to ensure the best preconditions that forensic organizations must have for the analysis of samples.

8.5.2 Planning and Evaluation of Biases for a Correct Forensic Analysis

In the scope of the accusatory process implemented in the judicial system of Peru, the prosecutor is in charge of accusing and to do so he must answer questions related to Who? What? Where? When? How? as well as Who and with what? and which can be achieved through the scientific-technical evaluation of the forensic areas of the IMLFC-Peru.

It is in this context, the IMLFC-Peru receives in a decentralized manner the requests from prosecutors to be able to answer the questions they have about the traces, so that they can be transformed into evidence and thus support their accusation hypotheses. However, it is currently common for the Prosecutor's Office not to formulate investigative hypotheses or to do so inadequately, which affects the forensic work of the IMLFC-Peru. For example, the prosecutor in charge usually opts for a type of scanning of the crime scene so that the forensic scientists obtain relevant samples and that way of working, as the investigation progresses, the prosecutors build their hypotheses based on the results of the forensic analyses, which compromises the objectivity of the process and leaves the forensic scientist responsible for adopting the hypotheses that must be contrasted in their analyses.

However, it is important to note that there are tests that do not require the explicit generation of a prior hypothesis. However, a hypothesis analysis by the prosecution would be necessary to avoid unnecessary testing that does not contribute significantly to the investigation. For example, in the case of a robbery suspect caught in a bar during the early hours of the morning, an alcoholic test would not be relevant, given the context of the case.

At this point, in the framework of adequate planning in order to avoid bias in the forensic analyses, it is advisable to use the Bayesian method, which emerges as a versatile tool that can be applied to a wide range of forensic analysis, especially in contexts where different forensic areas are integrated, thus guaranteeing maximum reliability (Aitken et al., 2024). In an integrated forensic reporting process, each forensic professional evaluates their results by contrasting hypotheses proposed by the prosecutor through the analysis of the probability of the Prosecutor's Hypothesis (Hp) and evaluated with the clues (I), in contrast with the alternative hypothesis, commonly the position of the defense (Hd) with respect the clues (I), which is known as a priori probability (AP).

Thus, whether in each individual forensic analysis or in an integrated analysis of forensic analyzes (application of Bayesian networks), the trace (E) is evaluated by a likelihood ratio (LR) conditional on the a priori hypothesis (PHs). Both ratios translate into a posterior probability (PP), to be assessed at trial, which is represented as follows.

In this scenario, the IMLFC-Peru, in close collaboration with the Attorney General's Office, has carried out training for both forensic professionals and prosecutors in recent years, with the aim to the prosecutors to be able to formulate their investigative hypotheses appropriately, addressing the questions of What? How? and When? while forensic professionals understand the need to integrate their analyses with the prosecutorial investigation. That is, forensic analysis must not only provide results on the traces but also provide the answers that prosecutors need for their investigative hypotheses.

Likewise, to contribute to the objective of greater use of the Bayesian method and integrated forensic analysis, a specific catalog of services has been identified and approved for each forensic area of the IMLFC-Peru. This catalog details the requirements and information necessary for each forensic analysis. However, to date, it has not been possible for a significant number of forensic analyzes at the IMLFC-Peru to adopt Bayesian methodology, much less achieve greater integration of forensic analysis processes through its application.

Despite the difficulties mentioned in the previous paragraph, they can still be corrected by reflecting in the procedures of the forensic areas the hierarchical level of the hypotheses that the forensic professionals are going to examine, since this facilitates the degree of integration between the different forensic areas. This hierarchical determination allows for better coordination and collaboration, ensuring that the analyzes carried out by each area effectively contribute to the general objectives of the research and thus where the Bayesian method can be used, it will be valued. These hierarchical levels according to Schaapveld et al. (2019) include the following:

a. *Accusation level:* Answers whether a person is the perpetrator of the crime and answers the questions of the reasons or motives for the facts (Why?) and that will be evaluated in court.
b. *Activity level:* Answers the questions of how the evidence arrived in relation to the actors involved in the case, that is, if the aggressor actor committed the acts on the victims within the period of time (When?), the authenticity and integrity of the trace is verified.

c. *Source Level:* The nature of the source of the trace is determined in order to make sense of its origin (How? and What?).
d. *Sub-Source Level:* It is determined if the source belongs to any of the actors (victim and/or aggressor), that is, if at a qualitative and quantitative level the source belongs to the victim and/or aggressor (Who?).
e. *Sub-Sub-source level:* It is determined whether one of the actors contributes or is a source of the evidence (who?).

For example, you can have a complaint of sexual assault case without penetration, where it involves a suspect (S) and a victim (V). The events occurred in the bathroom of a house, where there was a meeting of friends. The hierarchical levels of analysis would be (Figure 8.4):

a. *Activity:* The prosecutorial investigation is essential at this point with the support of forensic crime scene professionals, with the following propositions:
   i. (S) and (V) have been at the party and in the bathroom of the party.
   ii. (S) put the finger into (V's) vagina.
   iii. A random person may have put their finger into (V's) vagina.
b. *Source Level I – Transfer, Persistence and Recovery:* The contribution of auxiliary exams such as forensic biology laboratories are relevant to this level, with the following propositions:
   i. (S) indirectly transfers the epithelial cells to the vagina of (V) by transferring biological material left at the scene.

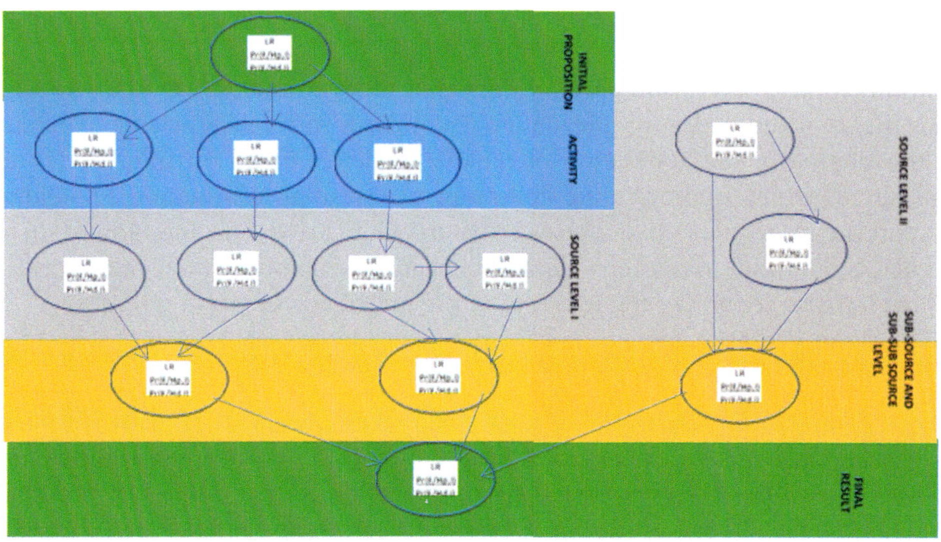

Figure 8.4 Analysis model by hierarchical levels and Bayesian networks (see description text) that corresponds to the analysis based on an initial proposition with the analyses by activity levels, source, sub-source, and sub-sub-source.

    ii. The cells of the finger of (S) are transferred to the vagina of the (V).
    iii. A chance that cells from a random person's finger are transferred to the vagina of the (V).
    iv. The cells from a random person's finger are transferred to the vagina of the (V) and it is compatible with (S).
c. *Source Level II – Other factors:* The contribution of auxiliary exams such as forensic biology laboratories are relevant to this level, with the following propositions:
    i. The (V) Vagina has a Background
    ii. The (V) Vagina Background is compatible with (S)
d. *Sub-source and sub-sub-source level:* The contribution of DNA laboratories are relevant to this level, with the following propositions:
    i. The DNA result of the suspect is a component of the mixture of the genetic profiles of the vagina (V).
    ii. The DNA result of a random person is a component of the mixture of the genetic profiles of the vagina (V).
    iii. The DNA result of the Vagina Background of the (V) is component of the genetic profile of the vagina (V).

8.5.3 Analysis of Forensic Results

In the field of forensic work, it is essential that the forensic report has the greatest possible forensic information, so that the prosecutor can place the facts in the appropriate context and thus, when formulating the accusation during the trial, can base his hypotheses on a solid way. The strength of the accusation depends largely on the quality and quantity of information presented, thus guaranteeing the integrity and veracity of the judicial process.

In this context, the Sydney Declaration is of utmost importance, as it encourages the implementation of international standards in forensic science. Thanks to this approach, the generation of reliable evidence based on solid evidence is ensured, which optimizes the collection of essential information to solidly support the prosecutor's hypotheses (Wilson-Wilde 2018). The adoption of such standards not only strengthens the accuracy and credibility of the evidence presented but also reinforces the integrity of the judicial process as a whole.

To achieve this objective, it is necessary to consider several aspects that ensure the quality and objectivity of forensic analysis:

a. *Biases in the analysis:* Identify and minimize biases in the techniques used, as well as cognitive biases or prejudices that may affect the interpretation of the results by the forensic professional. Here the professional competencies of each forensic scientist become important to address each analysis, where the widest range of criteria must be maintained so that both forensic professionals who strictly follow the procedures and those who challenge them to go further

(Neuteboom & Ross 2024) can provide the greatest amount of information to be reported with the least possible bias.

b. *Analysis models:* Establish standardized models and protocols for analysis, which may include statistical methods, machine learning algorithms, or techniques specific to each forensic discipline (DNA, ballistics, etc.). Artificial intelligence is a key tool for automating and standardizing analysis criteria that will be widely used in the next 5–10 years.
c. *Best practices and protocols:* Ensure quality through validation and accreditation, allowing forensic laboratories in the future to obtain accreditation according to the ISO/IEC 17025 standard, which is a benchmark for technical competence and quality in forensic analysis. However, it does not necessarily imply obtaining formal accreditation but rather implementing it as a quality system model to achieve quality assurance.

Additionally, these three points are significantly affected if context and time are not taken into consideration when interpreting the results (Weber & Lednev 2020):

a. *Context:* Interpret the results by answering questions such as Where was the evidence found? Under what circumstances? and also include the place where the traces were found and testimonies.
b. *Time:* Consider how long the trace has been in the place, as well as when it was collected and the time elapsed until its forensic analysis, because this period of time can generate degradation, contamination, or alteration, which can affect the results by reducing the potential of information contained in the trace.

To address the needs described in the previous paragraphs, IMLFC-Peru has formulated three projects that are currently in the process of implementation and which are financed by the Inter American Development Bank (IDB).

These projects seek to improve thanatological and clinical forensic analysis, ensuring that the trace on the bodies of victims, aggressors, and crime scenes do not disappear or diminish their potential to provide relevant information. In addition, in the field of identification, it seeks to provide timely attention to cases analyzed with DNA using an automated network of laboratories interconnected with a genetic profiling center (DNA Bank) through the development of a computer system for the management of genetic information to improve the capacity and opportunity to identify people involved in criminal acts.

In this sense, the three projects will be described, highlighting their scope, progress, and problems in the last years:

8.5.3.1 Necropsy Attention in Remote Areas of Peru

The IMLFC-Peru has a network of 55 morgues distributed nationwide, whose infrastructure and equipment conditions vary from good to regular. Approximately 50% of these morgues are located in the capitals of Peru's departments

(24 departments and 1 constitutional province). This distribution focuses mainly on the areas of greater population density, which presents a problem for the timely performance of necropsies, taking into consideration that this affects the ability to retrieve relevant information for forensic cases.

This problem is not exclusive to Peru. Other countries also face resource limitations, inadequate infrastructure, and the need to improve training and protocols. These deficiencies impact the adequate evaluation of the causes of death and also the timely responses to emergency cases for the management of corpses and their respective identification. In that sense, collaboration between different state agencies and the implementation of effective state policies are crucial to better manage criminal forensic cases, as well as mass casualty situations (Komolafe et al., 2020).

In several countries such as Colombia, Guatemala, El Salvador, Honduras, Mexico, among others, mobile forensic units have been an alternative solution with the aim to improve the efficiency and accuracy of forensic investigations in cases of crime scenes or mass disasters. These units are equipped with advanced technology that allows for comprehensive post-mortem examinations to be performed on-site. This technology is also useful, especially in rural areas where access to forensic facilities may be limited, and thus becoming a valuable tool to improve the timeliness and accuracy of forensic analysis, especially in emergency situations or in areas with limited resources.

Under these conditions, in the case of Peru, autopsies in vehicles are an innovative alternative in the field of forensic medicine. These mobile units allow for on-site autopsies, which can be crucial in situations where time is a critical factor or in remote areas where access to suitable facilities is limited.

The project identified the places with the greatest need for timely necropsies in Peru. These regions include the northeastern high forest, the Inter-Andean Valley (central and southern zone), and the Altiplano (southeast zone). To address geographic diversity, the implementation of mobile morgues that can be adapted to these remote areas was proposed, allowing the autopsy service to be brought to remote places, overcoming the difficulties of existing communication routes. Therefore, the objective of this project is to ensure that forensic information about corpses remains relevant to support forensic analysis.

However, the development of this project faces several challenges:

a. *Geography and size of mobile morgues:* Peru's diverse geography presents significant challenges. In the north-eastern high jungle and part of the central Inter-Andean Valley, heavy rains and narrow, unpaved roads make it difficult to travel. In the southern Inter-Andean Valley, roads are narrow, unpaved, and steep. In the southern Altiplano, low temperatures and high altitude further complicate the situation. This requires the design of three types of mobile morgues or one versatile type that can operate in all of these conditions, which increases the costs.

b. *Mobile morgue implementation:* Mobile morgues can range from a basic level with a necropsy table and a conservation chamber to more advanced units with spaces to perform basic biological and toxicological analysis. Geography limits the size of mobile morgues, which can affect their operational capacity.
c. *Operating cost:* Include refueling, maintenance of both the vehicle and equipment, and other operating expenses. These costs can be significant, especially in remote areas.
d. *Management decisions:* The frequent changes in the management of the high authorities of IMLFC-Peru have generated uncertainty about the viability of the project. The lack of continuity in management decisions and the constant evaluation of the proposed solution have affected the progress of the project.

Currently, the project is being re-evaluated with options including implementing cold rooms or upgrading existing morgue units. However, the scope of the project approved by the IDB is a mobile solution that brings thanatology (necropsy) services closer to the most remote communities. One of the alternatives evaluated is the use of vans that deploy a tent for necropsies, with a folding necropsy table.

At this point, the critical part lies in the management decisions of senior management at the IMLFC-Peru, where the initial conceptions of the solutions have not been maintained. This translates into a project whose requirements in the plan were not completely solid or shared within a good stakeholder analysis of the project.

8.5.3.2 Opportunity for Auxiliary Services in Thanatology and Forensic Clinic

The project aims to improve the timeliness of auxiliary exams. This includes the decentralization of alcohol analysis test and toxicological analyses in toxicology laboratories, as well as the increase of processing capacity in two pathology laboratories that geographically divides Peru into northern and southern regions. In the case of the central part of Peru, it would be covered by Lima. In addition, in the case of biology laboratories, not only the decentralization of services is sought but also the methodological innovation to address cases of sexual violence, especially in the context of violence to the women and their families.

In the specific case of the biology laboratories project, molecular analyses using real-time PCR equipment will be implemented to determine the presence of male DNA in sexual assault cases (Lin et al. 2018; Ginart et al. 2024) as a screening prior to DNA laboratory analysis. Then the project seeks to unite the molecular biology methodology with the routine work of forensic biology laboratories that includes microscopy analysis to detect sperm by using acid phosphatase tests and rapid tests for the detection of prostate antigens.

Likewise, this initiative in forensic biology laboratories is, thanks to the current improvement of commercial kits, for the quantification of human DNA by PCR in real time, where it is expected to solve between 30% and 35% of cases in which male biological fluids are not found in the swabs of rape cases. This would avoid the need to send these samples for genetic profiling analysis, reducing processing time and allowing prosecutors to have timely information to support their investigative hypotheses with other evidences.

In relation to the coverage of this project, it considers five IMLFC-Peru medical legal units that will work in a network to attend this type of forensic analysis in the north region (2 laboratories), center region (1 laboratory) and south region (2 laboratories).

In terms of processing time, forensic biology laboratories currently take about a day in the classic microscopic analysis to determine the presence of sperm and/or prostate cells. Regardless of the result, the samples are sent to the DNA lab, where analysis can take up to 30 days. In most cases, only samples that test positive are sent to the DNA lab, which can affect the sensitivity of the test for detecting male cells. With the new molecular flow, a fraction of the swab is destined for microscopic evaluation and another for real-time PCR analysis, with an analysis duration of approximately three days and referring to DNA laboratories only those that tested positive for the presence of male DNA, with a processing time of 30 days. Although this flow can add up to two more days in the area of forensic biology, the benefit is that 30–35% of cases could be supported in a timely manner with other evidence by the tax authority. In addition, the time in the DNA laboratory would be compensated by reducing the time to send reports to the authority.

Despite this innovative approach, currently the forensic biology laboratories of IMLFC-Peru have been affected in their execution due to deficiencies in the infrastructure for their implementation that were not fully considered in the formulation of the project, as well as the competence for these new technologies by the professionals of these laboratories.

These same problems have also been seen in the case of the other part of the project in the case of the pathology and toxicology laboratories where at first the management raised the need to acquire equipment in order to expand the services of these laboratories. However, in a new management they raised the need to improve the infrastructure of the entire process in these laboratories, which was not contemplated in the scope of the project and has generated a delay in its execution.

8.5.3.3 DNA Databank in Cases of Sexual and Criminal Violence

Throughout the world, DNA databases have proven to be an invaluable tool in solving crimes, allowing both the identification of suspects and the exoneration of innocent. These databases have greatly enhanced the capacity of forensic institutions to solve cases, whether recent cases or cold cases. However, this progress is not without its challenges, as the privacy and ethics concerns, as well as the urgent need to establish clear policies for the management and use of genetic information, even today continue to be issues of utmost importance (Amankwaa & McCartney 2019).

The successful implementation of DNA databanks requires the consideration of several key factors, as noted by Iannacone & Parra (2020). One of these factors is the availability of reference samples, which must be compared with the evidence database. To achieve this aim, it is necessary to consider the scope of the DNA databank. For example, in the case of the bank that is about to be implemented in the IMLFC-Peru may initially be established within the scope of the organization's function and expanded through legislation of the country where it is defined as the inclusion criteria for the DNA databank. Additionally, a key factor is to guarantee the quality of genetic profiles in the laboratory, which is essential for the reliability of the tests, and another key factor is the adequate knowledge of the population structure. Then the ideal context is created for successful comparisons within the database.

In this context, the project pursues two fundamental objectives. First, the automation of processes in the three DNA laboratories located in the northern, central, and southern regions in Peru, in charge of dealing with cases of rape and criminalistics. Second, the implementation of a genetic profiling center, within the framework of the agreement signed with the FBI for the use of the CODIS (Combined DNA Index System).

Regarding the second component of the project, it is crucial to highlight that the implementation of a genetic profiling center can follow three work schemes:

a. *Independent server in each DNA laboratory:* Each laboratory would have its own DNA database. However, this scheme presents problems such as the impossibility of ensuring the uniform quality of genetic profiles and the dispersion of genetic profiles related to the same case due to being probably in different DNA databases.
b. *Centralized server in a DNA laboratory:* In this scheme, a laboratory centralizes the server with the DNA database, receiving information from the contributing laboratories. Although the quality of genetic profiles is ensured, the central laboratory is overloaded, which must fulfill two roles: contributing laboratory and DNA databank. This could call into question information security and make it difficult to establish uniform organizational standards.
c. *Centralized genetic profiling center:* This scheme proposes a dedicated center where the server with the DNA databank is hosted, receiving profiles from the contributing DNA laboratories. This model ensures the quality of genetic profiles and facilitates the establishment of quality standards to be followed by contributing laboratories. In addition, it allows the implementation of international standards such as ISO/IEC 27001 on information security and ISO/IEC 27701 on data protection.

The project is adapted to the scheme described in point C. To this end, a computer system will be developed for the management of genetic profiles, which includes both reference and trace samples. This system is designed to ensure the integrity, security, and quality of genetic data, aligning with international best practices and complying with established ISO standards. In this way, an efficient and reliable management of genetic information is guaranteed.

In addition, this computer system for the management of genetic profiles will allow the collection and connection of the contributing laboratories with the genetic profiling center (Figure 8.5). In this same system, the analysis of the quality of the genetic profiles will be carried out in a pre-bank phase and their uniqueness will be verified in the bank phase, comparing them with the profiles stored on the server. This will ensure that genetic profiles meet the standards needed to be used in the genetic profile search systems such as the CODIS system. Likewise, the results of the matches will be stored on the server.

In addition, a communication module will be included between the center and the contributing DNA laboratories, aimed at attending to and resolving

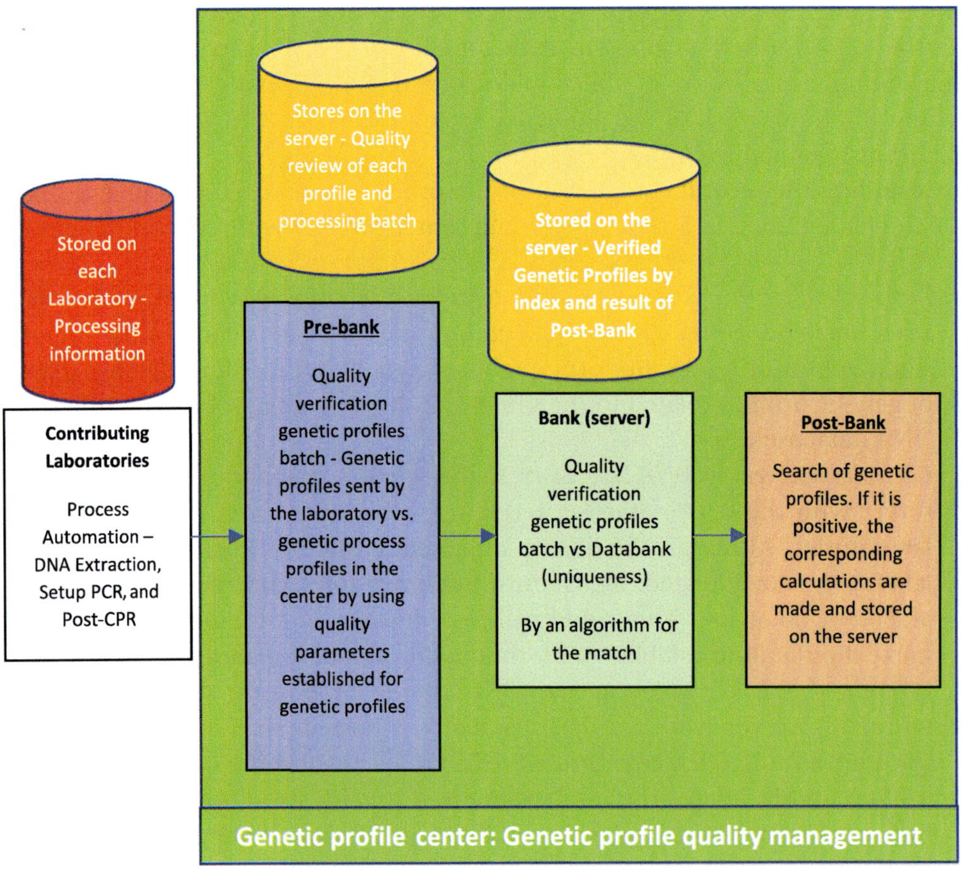

Figure 8.5 System of genetic profile center.

observations that may arise in the pre-bank, bank, and post-bank stages. A communication module will also be implemented to manage profile search requests and the sending of matching results to applicants. Thus, this comprehensive approach will ensure efficiency and accuracy in the handling of genetic data.

However, this project has been affected by changes in the management of IMLFC-Peru, which has changed the prospects for implementation, both in the equipment for the automation of the laboratories, associated with the needs of existing infrastructure, and in the implementation of the genetic profile quality management system in the genetic profiling center. These factors have delayed the execution of the project and, consequently, the implementation of the agreement signed with the FBI to implement the CODIS system in Peru.

8.5.4 Multidisciplinary Interpretation of Forensic Results

The multidisciplinary approach in the forensic field is essential to improve precision and efficiency in the identification and analysis of bodies within the framework of a forensic report. According to international experience as mentioned by Baldino et al. (2023), a detailed protocol for the management of bodies is vital, which allows collaboration and effective communication between different disciplines. This protocol also should include recommendations for sample collection, flow of sample analysis, and parameters for search documentation to optimize forensic results and facilitate case resolution.

In Peru, there are relevant experiences of multidisciplinary work, such as the national program for the prevention and eradication of violence against women and members of the family group, established under Law No. 30364. In the case of IMLFC-Peru, this program aims to optimize the work of the forensic areas as forensic medicine, forensic psychology (Gesell chambers), forensic biology laboratories, and forensic toxicology; based on existing demand at the IMLCF-Peru, where in the forensic clinical examinations, 60% of the attention corresponds to medico-legal examinations of injuries, while the other 40% is divided between psychological examinations (55%), sexual integrity examinations (15%), and post-facto examinations (20%).

In recent years, inter-institutional support based on national policies has been strengthened, evidenced in the repowering and implementation of new Gesell chambers at the national level, in addition to the 129 Gesell chambers and 62 interview rooms available in the IMLFC-Peru because currently only 80% of the chambers and 65% of the interview rooms are in operation. The main causes of these problems are the availability of personnel and deterioration of computer equipment, audio and video equipment, as well as infrastructure problems and difficulties in managing the process; for example, in the case of psychological forensic evaluations, about 50% of appointments in Gesell chambers are not made due to the management of the prosecutors. One option to solve this problem is to have a computer system for appointments, which allows recording and alerting of appointment cancellations so that the prosecutor's office can take the corresponding actions to optimize them.

Another example of multidisciplinary work at IMLFC-Peru is the search for missing persons in Peru and the fight against impunity between 1980 and 2000. In 2003, the Truth Commission presented a report that generated actions and policies in state institutions. That same year, the Specialized Forensic Team (EFE) was created at the IMLFC-Peru. Subsequently, in 2016, the law of missing persons (Law 30470) was approved, and in 2018, the Peruvian government published legislative Decree No. 1398, creating the DNA database bank for missing persons and the missing persons office.

Over the years, these management actions have been taken as a result of better integration of the areas involved in identification in the IMLFC-Peru, with the aim of increasing success in identification and avoiding errors. Likewise, these relationships have been strengthened through inter-institutional agreements but with some administrative difficulties. For example, sending genetic profiles of bone remains to the DNA database of the Ministry of Justice of Peru required existing legislation and the signing of inter-institutional agreements to specify technical aspects of collaboration; that is, the existence of the law was no enough, and additionally the institutions agreed on how they should carry out the collaboration without violating their functions.

Furthermore, the implementation of these actions in relation to the forensic process has improved coordination and efficiency in the identification of missing persons, ensuring more rigorous and precise procedures, in accordance with international recommendations (Parra et al. 2020). On the other hand, collaboration between international agencies has also facilitated access to advanced resources and technologies, which contributes significantly to the quality and speed of identification processes.

However, there is still much to be done since only approximately 30%–35% of the estimated total of missing persons has been identified and more than 20 years have passed since the attention to this humanitarian problem, which it has been affected over time by limited budgetary, internal management, and political problems.

8.5.5 Presentation in Court by the Forensic Professionals

ISO/IEC 17024:2012 is an international standard that specifies requirements for bodies that certify people. This standard ensures that certifications are unbiased and that evaluation processes are consistent and reliable. Certification under this standard is crucial to ensuring that forensic professionals possess the competencies necessary to perform their work effectively and ethically. Its key components are:

a. *Impartiality and Transparency:* The standard establishes that certification bodies must operate in an impartial and transparent manner. This includes managing conflicts of interest and implementing policies that ensure objectivity in the certification process.

b. *Technical Competence:* Certification bodies must demonstrate technical competence in the areas they certify. This includes having qualified staff and appropriate procedures for assessing candidates competencies.
c. *Evaluation Process:* The standard details the requirements for the evaluation process, including the planning, execution, and review of exams. This ensures that the evaluations are fair, valid, and reliable.
d. *Maintenance of Certification:* ISO/IEC 17024:2012 also sets out requirements for the maintenance of certification, including periodic recertification and handling of complaints and appeals.

Within the framework of Peruvian legislation, which follows an accusatory model, the relevance of adequate training for the assurance of the quality of expert processes is a factor of great importance. IMLFC-Peru has identified this need as one of its main goals in recent years.

In this context, the IMLFC-Peru, through international collaboration, has taken steps to initiate the accreditation process of the institute through the National Institute of Quality (INACAL) with the ISO/IEC 17024:2012 standard. This accreditation will allow IMLFC-Peru to certify its forensic professionals, ensuring that they meet international standards of competence and quality.

For these certifications of forensic professionals, schemes of processes to be certified with their respective standards have been established. In the first stage, it will focus on the medical forensic clinical area, specifically on the medico-legal evaluation of injuries and sexual integrity examinations (rape cases). In the second stage, the area of forensic psychology will be addressed.

These certifications ensure the quality of forensic processes and support the skills, competencies, and knowledge of experts in court. This not only improves the quality of forensic investigations but also strengthens the confidence of the public and the judicial system in the results presented.

The implementation of the ISO/IEC 17024:2012 standard in the IMLFC-Peru represents a significant step toward the professionalization and standardization of forensic processes in the country. This standard not only ensures that forensic professionals are properly qualified but also ensures that certification processes are fair, transparent, and trustworthy. The adoption of these standards will contribute to a more robust and reliable judicial system, benefiting both forensic professionals and society at large.

8.6 Conclusion

This document briefly describes three relevant aspects of INMLFC-Peru in the field of quality assurance: (1) the most relevant limitations which remain constant over time, (2) the efforts to achieve optimum quality and sustainable efficiency of its processes, and (3) the resilience of a forensic system that constantly adapts to the adversity of its own reality.

The first aspect has been historically dragged along, even since its gestation as the Peruvian forensic science system, including, but not limited to, the political will and decision-making to concretize the impulse of an organization such as IMLFC-Peru, which is necessary for the social balance and the correct administration of justice in the fight against impunity. This situation leads to precarious organizational systems, nebulous strategic development plans, and therefore action plans without a specific direction, without necessary infrastructure, serious technological deficiencies, and operating budget, and of course, inadequate leadership and senior management components without management experience or vision of development. These factors make IMLFC-Peru navigate constantly in a turbulent scenario, becoming a highly challenging administrative context.

The second aspect is linked to the strength and experience of its members, who try to carry out various improvements for their development in this turbulent navigation we talked about before. However, all these efforts are always minimized when faced with sustainability, which includes, but is not limited to, lack of budget and inadequate decision-making by the administrators on duty, who on several occasions, as has happened in the history of IMLFC-Peru, do not have sufficient vision or limitations to help steer the organization. These episodes cause IMLFC-Peru to continue navigating in turbulence but in circles, without being able to get out of the storm.

The third and final aspect is the fuel reserve of the organization, which has managed to learn from its shortcomings and adapt to complex and challenging scenarios. The application of an alternative and contemporary way of looking at forensic sciences is boosting the possibility of getting out of the storm and navigating without turbulence, although the dilemmas continue, as political decisions and the lack of budget and infrastructure have made them a difficult challenge to face. Finally, we must emphasize that the words expressed at the beginning of the last century "without the help of science, the law is deficient, and justice is blind" (Avendaño, 1960) are still valid. If these words are heard and understood in their real magnitude, the IMLFC-Peru can change its history, from a mediocre way of observing, conceiving, organizing, and practicing forensic sciences to start to really compete as modern contemporary forensic sciences demand.

References

Aitken, C., Taroni, F., and Bozza, S. (2024) The role of the bayes factor in the evaluation of evidence. *Annual Review of Statistics and its Application*, **11**, 203–226. https://doi.org/10.1146/annurev-statistics-040522-101020.

Amankwaa, A.O. and McCartney, C. (2019) The effectiveness of the UK national DNA database. *Forensic Sci Int Synerg*, **21**(1), 45–55. http://doi.org/10.1016/j.fsisyn.2019.03.004.

Anastasopoulos, G. (2021) Workshop on persons certification (ISO/IEC 17024) cl.4 & cl.5. *International Accreditation Forum*. Recuperado de https://iaf.nu/wp-content/uploads/2021/05/02_GA_ISO_17024_IAFILAC_presentation.pdf.

ASCLD Train the Director – Quality Assurance: Beyond Accreditation. (2020) *Forensic Technology Center of Excellence*. Recuperado de https://forensiccoe.org/quality-assurance-beyond-accreditation/.

Avendano, J. (1960) Pasado y presente de la Medicina legal en el Perú. *Anales de la facultad de. Medicina.*, **43 N2**, 392–408.

Avendano, L. (1918) La Medicina Legal en el Perú. *Anales de la facultad de Medicina*, **N1**, 210–233.

Baldino, G., Mondello, C., Sapienza, D., Stassi, C., Asmundo, A., Gualniera, P., *et al*. (2023) Multidisciplinary forensic approach in "complex" bodies: Systematic review and procedural proposal. *Diagnostics*, **13**(2), 310. https://doi.org/10.3390/diagnostics13020310.

Buchan, B.W. and Ledeboer, N.A. (2014) Emerging technologies for the clinical microbiology laboratory. *Clinical Microbiology Reviews*, **27**(4), 783–822. https://doi.org/10.1128/cmr.00003-14.

Bustos-Streeter P., Intriago-Leiva M. (2015). The Chilean Forensic Medical Service. . En Ubelaker, DH. *The Global Practice of Forensic Science. Wiley Blackwell*. 29–38 pp.

Dawnay, N. and Sheppard, K. (2023) From crime scene to courtroom: A review of the current bioanalytical evidence workflows used in rape and sexual assault investigations in the United Kingdom. *Science and Justice*, **63**(2), 206–228. https://doi.org/10.1016/j.scijus.2022.12.006.

De Francisco Enciso, E., Errejón García, A.M., and Vicente Mendoza, M. (2016) El nuevo modelo de organización de la medicina forense en España. El servicio de organización y calidad: una propuesta de mejora. *Revista Española de Medicina Legal*, **42**(2), 81–85. https://doi.org/10.1016/j.reml.2015.11.001.

Doyle, S. (2019) A review of the current quality standards framework supporting forensic science: Risks and opportunities. *Wiley Interdisciplinary Reviews: Forensic Science*, **2**(1), e1365. https://doi.org/10.1002/wfs2.1365.

Fernandez – Davila, G. (1955) Centenario de la catedra de Medicina Legal. *Anales de la facultad de. Medicina*, **38 N4**, 1069–1079.

Ginart, S., Garrigos Calivares, L., Caputo, M., Corach, D., and Sala, A. (2024) Improving the efficiency of Y-chromosome detection and the quality of STR typing in forensic casework with an in-house made qPCR and HRM system based on SYTO™ 9 chemistry. *Forensic Sci Int.*, **354**, 111893. https://doi.org/10.1016/j.forsciint.2023.111893.

Giraldo-Giraldo CA. (2014) Medicina legal en Colombia. Crónica de un centenario y de sus antecedentes *CES Medicina*, vol. **28**, núm. 2. 325–335.

Gjertson, D.W., Brenner, C.H., Baur, M.P., Carracedo, A., Guidet, F., Luque, J.A., *et al.* (2007) ISFG: Recommendations on biostatistics in paternity testing. *Forensic Science International: Genetics*, **1**(3), 223–231. https://doi.org/10.1016/j.fsigen.2007.06.006.

Gough, T. (2000) Quality assurance in forensic science: the UK situation. *Accreditation and Quality Assurance*, **5**(9), 389–393. https://doi.org/10.1007/s007690050137.

Iannacone, G.C. and Parra, R.C. (2020) Genetic structure and kinship analysis from the Peruvian Andean area. In: *Forensic Science and Humanitarian Action* (eds. R.C. Parra, S.C. Zapico, and D.H. Ubelaker). https://doi.org/10.1002/9781119482062.ch30.

International Accreditation Forum. (2003) Guidance on the application of ISO/IEC 17024. *International Accreditation Forum.* by https://iaf.nu/resolutions/guidance-on-the-application-of-iso-iec-17024/ (accessed December 8, 2025).

International Organization for Standardization. (2018) ISO 21043-2:2018 *Forensic sciences* — Part 2: Recognition, recording, collecting, transport and storage of items. https://www.iso.org/obp/ui/en/#iso:std:iso:21043:-2:ed-1:v1:en (accessed December 8, 2025).

ISO. (2016) How to develop schemes for the certification of persons: Guidance of ISO/IEC 17024. *International Organization for Standardization.* Recuperado de https://www.iso.org/es/contents/data/publication/10/03/PUB100384.html.

Koehler, J.J. (2013) Proficiency tests to estimate error rates in the forensic sciences. *Law, Probability and Risk,* **12**(1), 89–98. https://doi.org/10.1093/lpr/mgs028.

Kokshoorn, B. (2023). Transfer, persistence, prevalence and recovery of biological traces. *En* D. Taylor & B. Kokshoorn *(Eds.), Forensic DNA trace evidence interpretation* (pp. 26–45). CRC Press. https://doi.org/10.4324/9781003273189-3.

Komolafe, A.O., Adefidipe, A.A., Olorunsola, I.S., Akinyemi, H.A.M., Ogunrinde, O.V., Alade, O.T., *et al.* (2020) Medicolegal autopsies and causes of death in mass casualties in a developing country and challenges encountered. *Nigerian Journal of Health Sciences,* **20**(1), 17. https://doi.org/10.4103/njhs.njhs_25_20.

Lee, H.C. and Pagliaro, E.M. (2013) Forensic evidence and crime scene investigation. *Journal of Forensic Investigation,* **1**(2), 5. https://doi.org/10.13188/2330-0396.1000004.

Levy, S., Bergman, P., and Frank, A. (2005) Quality assurance in forensic science. *Accreditation and Quality Assurance,* **10**(6), 361–367. https://doi.org/10.1007/s007690050361.

Lin, S.W., Li, C., and Ip, S.C.Y. (2018) Performance study on three qPCR quantification kits and their compatibilities with the 6-dye DNA profiling systems. *Forensic Sci Int Genet.,* **33**, 72–83. https://doi.org/10.1016/j.fsigen.2017.11.016.

Martin-Fumadó, C., Cuatrecasas Castellsagués, O., and Fontcuberta Adalid, C. (2016) Gestión por procesos en medicina forense: Lean. *Revista Española de Medicina Legal,* **42**(3), 126–127. https://doi.org/10.1016/j.reml.2016.02.001.

Meintjes-van der Walt, L. (2001) *Expert evidence and the right to a fair trial: A comparative perspective. South African Journal on Human Rights,* **17**(3), 301–319. https://doi.org/10.1080/02587203.2001.11827628.

Meintjies-Van Der Walt, L. (2010) The chain of custody and formal admissions. *South African Journal of Criminal Justice,* **23**(3), 371–384. https://hdl.handle.net/10520/EJC53048.

Morling, N., Allen, R.W., Carracedo, A., Geada, H., Guidet, F., Hallenberg, C., *et al.* (2002) Paternity Testing Commission of the International Society of Forensic Genetics: Recommendations on genetic investigations in paternity cases. *Forensic Science International,* **129**(3), 148–157. https://doi.org/10.1016/S0379-0738(02)00289-X.

Neuteboom, W. and Ross, A. (2024) Shall the twain ever meet? *Australian Journal of Forensic Sciences,* **1–7**. https://doi.org/10.1080/00450618.2024.2363823.

Olaborede, A. and Meintjes-van der Walt, L. (2020) *The dangers of convictions based on a single piece of forensic evidence. Potchefstroom Electronic Law Journal,* **23**, 1–38. https://doi.org/10.17159/1727-3781/2020/v23i0a6169.

Parra, R.C., Palma, M.R., Calcina, O., Tejada, J., Condori, L.A., and Baraybar, J.P. (2020) Peruvian forensic experience in the search for missing persons and the identification of human remains. In: *Forensic Science and Humanitarian Action* (eds. R.C. Parra, S.C. Zapico, and D.H. Ubelaker). https://doi.org/10.1002/9781119482062.ch41.

Rodriguez-Almada H. (2015). Legal Medicine and Forensic Science in Uruguay. En Ubelaker, DH. *The Global Practice of Forensic Science. Wiley Blackwell.* 335–350 pp.

Rodriguez-Zorro A. Constantin AE. (2015) Forensic Science in Colombia. En Ubelaker, DH. *The Global Practice of Forensic Science. Wiley Blackwell.* 49–66 pp.

Roux, C., Bucht, R., Crispino, F., De Forest, P., Lennard, C., Margot, P., *et al.* (2022) *The Sydney declaration – Revisiting the essence of forensic science through its fundamental principles. Forensic Science International,* **332**, Article 111182. https://doi.org/10.1016/j.forsciint.2022.111182.

Saks, M.J. and Koehler, J.J. (2005) The coming paradigm shift in forensic identification science. *Science,* **309**(5736), 892–895. https://doi.org/10.1126/science.1111565.

Salas Beteta, C. (2011) La eficacia del proceso penal acusatorio en el Perú. *Prolegómenos. Derechos y Valores,* **14**(28), 263–275.

Schaapveld, T.E.M., Opperman, S.L., and Harbison, S. (2019) Bayesian networks for the interpretation of biological evidence. *WIREs Forensic Sci.,* **1**, e1325. https://doi.org/10.1002/wfs2.1325.

Seiberle, I., Währer, J., Kron, S., Flury, K., Girardin, M., Schocker, A., *et al.* (2022) Collaborative swab performance comparison and the impact of sampling solution volumes on DNA recovery. *Forensic Science International: Genetics,* **59**, 102716. https://doi.org/10.1016/j.fsigen.2022.102716.

Smith, C., Cox, J.O., Rhodes, C., Lewis, C., Koroma, M., Hudson, B.C., *et al.* (2021, 2021) Comparison of DNA typing success in compromised blood and touch samples based on sampling swab composition. *J Forensic Sci.,* **66**(4), 1427–1434. https://doi.org/10.1111/1556-4029.14694.

Ubelaker, D.H. (2015) *The Global Practice of Forensic Science. Wiley Blackwell.* 1–360.

Weber, A. and Lednev, I.K. (2020) *Crime clock* – Analytical studies for approximating time since deposition of bloodstains. *Forensic Chemistry,* **19**, 100248. https://doi.org/10.1016/j.forc.2020.100248.

Wilson-Wilde, L. (2018) The international development of forensic science standards – A review. *Forensic Science International,* **288**, 1–9. https://doi.org/10.1016/j.forsciint.2018.04.009.

Zhai, W., Zhang, N., and Hua, F. (2020) The development of forensic science standards in China. *Forensic Science International: Synergy.* https://doi.org/10.1016/j.fsisyn.2020.06.001.

CHAPTER 9

Guatemalan's Efforts to Strengthen the Quality of Forensic Practice: Limitations and Advances

Ruth Garcia-Marroquin[1] and Allan G. Alvarez-Godoy[2]
[1] *Forensic Science Laboratories, INACIF-Guatemala, Guatemala City, Guatemala*
[2] *International Forensic Consultant, The Hague, Netherlands*

9.1 Introduction

9.1.1 Generalities About Guatemala

Guatemala (from the Nahuatl word Cuauhtemallan meaning "place of many trees") is one of the five countries located in the central part of the American continent. According to its constitution, it is a democratic republic, with 22 departments. Its capital and most populous city is Guatemala City. It is also the most populous country in Central America with 18, 607, 184 inhabitants according to the latest official census carried out in 2022. It is bordered to the north and west by Mexico; to the east by Belize, the Atlantic Ocean, Honduras, and El Salvador; and to the south by the Pacific Ocean. It was the cradle of the great Mayan civilisation whose vestiges are maintained mainly in the north of the country, where the Mayan pyramids of El Gran Jaguar in the sacred city of Tikal and La Gran Danta considered the largest ancestral pyramid in the world, located in the archaeological site of El Mirador, both places are located in the northern department of El Peten and remind us of the pre-Columbian history of this beautiful country.

The official language of Guatemala is Spanish; however, as part of its ancestral legacy, 23 Mayan languages are recognised as being spoken in different regions, making it a multicultural country.

Guatemala gained independence from Spain on September 15, 1821, and since then, it has experienced a series of significant events that have shaped the most

Forensic Science and Quality Management: Addressing the Era of Standardization in Challenging Environments, First Edition. Edited by Roberto C. Parra and Allan G. Alvarez-Godoy.

relevant being the proclamation of the Republic of Guatemala in 1847 and the Triumph of the Liberal Reform in 1871. In 1898, the presidential term of Manuel Estrada Cabrera began, which was the beginning of one of the dark periods in the history of Guatemala; during his government—in 1901—the company of the United States of America—the United Fruit Company (UFCO)—began commercial operations in the country, and with this, there was a clear North American interference in the commercial and political affairs of the Central American nation. In 1944, the Guatemalan people, tired of the military regimes, began a revolt that gave way to the October 20 revolution, initiating on this date 10 years of a true democracy that brought with it important changes for the benefit of the population; this only lasted 10 years, since in the face of the possible communist threat, the United Fruit Company (UFCO) intervened again and in 1954 President Juan Jacobo Arbenz y Guzmán, elected by popular vote, was removed from office through a coup d'état. In the following years, the country plunged into a civil war, also called "the internal armed conflict," which lasted approximately 36 years. On February 4, 1976, a devastating earthquake affected the central area of the Republic, leaving more than 22,000 dead; in 1980 there was another coup overthrowing the government of the day, leaving General José Efrain Ríos Mont as head of state. Due to the authoritarian policies presided over by Ríos Mont and in the face of a series of violations of human rights, especially of life, another coup d'état took place in 1983, leaving General Oscar Humberto Mejía Victores in power. When Mejía Victores came to power, despite the fact that the internal armed conflict continued, general elections were called whose objective was to create a new national constituent assembly and thus consider reforms to the political constitution of the republic; this is how in 1985 the first democratic elections took place after several decades of military regimes and in January 1986 the first nonmilitary president took office, elected by popular vote, Mr. Marco Vinicio Cerezo Arévalo; in 1996, when Mr. Álvaro Arzú Irigoyen was president, the peace accords were signed between the representatives of the Guatemalan guerrillas and the military, putting an end to the civil war that left more than 200,000 victims and 45,000 disappeared, who are still being sought today; this event is of special relevance because it was General Otto Pérez Molina who at that time represented the military commanders of the Government of Guatemala; 16 years later he would be popularly elected president of Guatemala, but before the end of his constitutional term as President of the Republic in the period 2012–2016, government corruption in 2015 forced him to leave his mandate, returning our country to be an international focus in the face of the excesses of corruption generated by the rulers of the day. President Otto Pérez Molina and Vice President Ingrid Roxana Baldetti were imprisoned and tried for acts of corruption and are still serving sentences.

The reforms to the political constitution of the Republic of Guatemala gave way for a series of events that also mark a before and after in matters of justice. On May 31, 1929, government decree 1-618 was published, which gave the green light to the creation of the Public Ministry of the Republic of Guatemala, defining it as the entity in charge of criminal prosecution and with this, marking a before and after in the investigation and clarification of crimes and modernizing the justice sector by implementing the oral and public trial, leaving aside judicial practices behind closed doors and sentences based on testimonial evidence, among others.

However, as the new reforms were being implemented, there was still a long way to go for the consolidation of an independent forensic system. Under the hierarchy of the Judicial Branch in each department, including the capital city, until December 2007, the forensic services of thanatology (morgues) continued to operate. Other hospital institutions also continued to provide medico-legal autopsy services, these being the Guatemalan Institute of Social Security (IGSS) and the Military Medical Hospital at the service of the military institution.

9.1.2 Dispersion of Guatemalan Forensic Science and the Need to Harmonize Management

Similarly, the expert services that had the capacity to process evidence and analyze it continued to be dispersed in two different institutions. One of these was the National Civil Police through the Directorate of Criminal Investigations. Until November 2007, the ballistics, documentoscopy, biology, and dactyloscopy laboratories operated, the latter being particularly important due to its maintenance of the criminal file of fingerprints. Today, by legal mandate, the fingerprint archive continues to operate, since the National Civil Police is the institution in charge of administering the criminal registry of persons who are arrested for any crime.

From its creation until November 2007, the Public Prosecutor's Office operated its crime laboratory, which integrated services based on the needs of investigations, starting with the incorporation of forensic medical services. These services included evaluating living victims of crimes and assisting prosecutors at crime scenes to preliminarily establish possible causes of death. Various locations within the central zone gradually welcomed the addition of laboratories for fingerprinting, documentoscopy, biology, physicochemistry, vehicle identification, controlled substances, and toxicology.. Faced with the need to integrate the services provided by the crime laboratories in a single environment, the high authorities of the Directorate of Criminal Investigations of the Public Ministry in July 1999 created the Technical and Scientific Department, an entity that until November 2007 was in charge of eight crime laboratories, such as ballistics, biology, dactyloscopy, copy documents, physical chemistry, vehicle identification, controlled substances, and toxicology. This new department in the General Prosecutor's Office from July 1999 to November 2007 was consolidated as a forensic laboratory with national and even international recognition. Prior to this, an event that marked the urgent need to have specialised units for managing crime scenes was the attack and murder of a high-ranking hierarch of the Catholic Church, Monsignor Juan Gerardi, an event that was framed as a political assassination, which occurred on April 26, 1998, and whose crime scene was not properly managed. Contamination prevailed, especially by people outside the investigation—firefighters, the press, high authorities of the government faith, etc.—resulting in little or almost no scientific proof. In response to this new act of violence, the General Prosecutor's Office accelerated the implementation of crime scene groups, which had operated since July 1999.

9.2 National Institute of Forensic Sciences of Guatemala (INACIF)

Faced with the uncertainty generated by considering that the prosecuting entity had under its administration the scientific evidence through the crime laboratories that operated under its direction, as well as in the same way, the institution in charge of issuing sentences – the judicial body – had under its administration the different headquarters of forensic thanatology and in the face of the uncertainty faced by the Prosecutor's Office as it was not clear from whom to request an expert's report: yes to their own laboratories of the technical scientific department or to the National Civil Police, the same institutions at the service of the justice sector and different civil society organizations evidenced the need to create an independent forensic institution that would house both the forensic laboratories as well as everything related to medico-legal evaluations.

After the publication of governmental agreement 32-2006, the Congress of the Republic of Guatemala, in 2006, enacted the law that established the National Institute of Forensic Sciences of Guatemala (INACIF).

With the law already approved, a new challenge was presented for the different instances of the justice sector: that the newly created INACIF would not only remain in a publication of the official gazette; in this way, 18 months after its creation, finally on July 18, 2007, the first director of this new forensic institution, Dr. Míriam Dolores Ovalle de Monroy, officially began her work. From the time she took office, she tirelessly worked to form administrative teams that would facilitate a smooth transition of the responsibilities that had previously belonged to various institutions providing forensic services.

Among the relevant events following the inauguration of the new INACIF authorities, we find two important events:

- *November 8, 2007:* The crime laboratories are incorporated into INACIF.
- *December 4, 2007:* The transfer of the forensic medical services of the Judicial Branch and the Public Prosecutor's Office to INACIF is carried out.

The organizational structure of the National Institute of Forensic Sciences was established as follows:

1. Board of Directors represented by the highest authorities of seven institutions as follows:
   - President of the Judicial Branch
   - Attorney General and Head of the Public Prosecutor's Office
   - Minister of the Interior
   - Director of the Public Defender
   - Resident of the College of Chemists and Pharmacists of Guatemala
   - President of the College of Physicians and Surgeons of Guatemala
   - President of the Association of Lawyers and Notaries of Guatemala
   - Director of the Victim's Institute (adhered, according to the government agreement of 2022)
2. General Directorate represented by a professional – the general director who after a public selection process is elected and appointed by the board of directors; his administration lasts five years and he has the option of being reelected once.
3. Three different departments:
   - Scientific Technical Department
   - Financial Administrative Department
   - Training Department
4. Units among these are those of our interest:
   - Metropolitan Forensic Medicine Unit of Thanatology
   - Crime Laboratories Unit
   - Regional Forensic Medicine Unit of Thanatology and Forensic Clinic
   - Metropolitan Forensic Medicine Unit–Clinical Area
   - Forensic Psychology Unit
   - Expert Management Unit

After this date, a new era began in the technical-scientific investigation of the Guatemalan justice system; the opinions to be issued by the INACIF experts become autonomous, meaning this is a great challenge for the same institution that from this date onwards will have to ensure all the quality of the expert reports.

On November 8, 2007, INACIF began its forensic activities with the incorporation of nine crime laboratories, the vision at all times being to strengthen new forensic services, which have always been considered essential for the investigation. In 2008, the Fire Trajectory Laboratory was implemented. The Genetics Laboratory was established in 2009, and the Computer Ballistics Laboratory, the first fundamental forensic database for criminal investigation, followed in December 2010.

In 2014, the Forensic Acoustics Laboratory formally began activities; in 2017, the incorporation of the Forensic Computer Laboratory was achieved and in

2022, the Forensic Entomology and Environmental Analysis laboratories were established.

Finally, in September 2024, the Archaeology service was incorporated, forming a new laboratory together with Forensic Anthropology.

As of October 31, when this writing is completed, INACIF has 14 crime laboratories, which are summarized below.

9.2.1 Acoustics Laboratory

INACIF's Forensic Acoustics Laboratory is active and officially recognized as a specialized area that performs voice analysis expertise for criminal investigations, with rigorous procedures that include sampling in a soundproof booth and internationally validated technical-scientific analysis (Instituto Nacional de Ciencias Forenses de Guatemala, n.d.-a).

It is made up of five expert analysts, including professionals in sound engineering, telecommunications, and criminalistics. Voice appraisals are carried out through comparisons using NUANCE software, as well as the BATVOX system. The laboratory has a soundproof booth where voice samples are taken that will be useful for comparison analyses.

Acoustics Laboratory

AÑO	Total Cases Admitted
2017	251
2018	293
2019	355
2020	261
2021	727
2022	591
2023	790
2024	748

Source: INACIF statistical tables 2017–2024.

9.2.2 Environmental Analysis Laboratory

INACIF's Environmental Analysis Laboratory was inaugurated on November 16, 2021, at the institute's headquarters in zone 1 of Guatemala City. This laboratory is the first at the national level specialized in carrying out forensic expert reports on environmental matters, especially to detect contaminants in water and soil.

The investment for its creation was approximately 6.5 million quetzales, with contributions from the central government's own funds and international donations from the United States Agency for International Development (USAID).

Its functions include forensic analysis of pesticides, herbicides, heavy metals, harmful organic and inorganic substances, hydrocarbons, and other pollutants, using internationally validated methods to ensure the quality and scientific validity of the opinions (Instituto Nacional de Ciencias Forenses de Guatemala, 2021).

This laboratory has three professionals from chemical, environmental, and forestry engineering, respectively. It was included among the new forensic services given the high incidence of contamination of aquifers and also of soil suffered by certain areas of the country due to poor waste management.

Environmental Analysis

AÑO	Total Cases Admitted
2021	7
2022	27
2023	28
2024	37

Source: INACIF statistical tables 2021 to 2024.

9.2.3 Laboratory of Anthropology and Archaeology

The Laboratory of Forensic Anthropology and Archaeology of INACIF has been active since shortly after its founding in 2006 and is part of its technical structure as a specialized unit for the identification of human remains and the investigation of complex cases that require anthropological and archaeological techniques. This laboratory was consolidated in the 2010s as a fundamental element of the Guatemalan forensic system not only for cases associated with the internal armed conflict but also to deal with acts of common violence in the country ("Laboratorio de Antropología Forense, Uno de Los Pilares Del INACIF," 2025).

This area has been operating since December 2007 in INACIF because it is an essential service in criminal investigation. However, given the need to implement new technologies that allow the analysis of pre-Columbian archaeological pieces, among others, it has been strengthened and modernised recently, for example, in 2023 its main headquarters was renovated (Instituto Nacional de Ciencias Foreses de Guatemala, 2023).

9.2.4 Ballistics Laboratory

It is one of the largest laboratories with a total of 61 people, of which 39 are expert analysts and the rest are technical and administrative personnel. The experts are mostly from the areas of engineering and others with forensic studies.

This laboratory is made up of two areas: one is identification ballistics, which is responsible for carrying out analyses of firearms in order to establish their operation, generation of indubitable ballistic fingerprints, and identification of alphanumeric characters recorded on their structure in order to be individualized; When this data that is stamped has been erased for criminal purposes, the experts carry out analyses that allow the recovery of the same. The identification ballistics area will also be in charge of analyzing casings recovered at crime scenes, as well as projectiles recovered in autopsy processes in order to identify caliber and in case of having weapons suspected of having detonated or fired them to carry out the respective microscopic comparisons.

The other area is computer ballistics where there is the integrated ballistic information system (IBIS), whose database has allowed to have valuable information on the different weapons that are used at crime scenes.

The Ballistics Laboratory of INACIF Guatemala has received significant support from the United States Agency for International Development (USAID) through the Justice and Transparency Project. This support has made it possible to:

- *Acquisition and upgrade of specialized software:* Mainly for the IBIS (Brasstrax, Bullettrax and Matchpoint), which has strengthened the technical capabilities for the analysis of casings and projectiles.
- *Forensic equipment:* Updating and acquisition of ballistic instruments and tools to strengthen the quality of the expert reports carried out in the laboratory.
- *Accreditation under international standards:* USAID's technical and financial support made it possible to meet the requirements of ISO accreditation and ensure the maintenance, reaccreditation, and expansion of nationally and internationally endorsed methods.
- *Training and professionalization:* The assistance included training of personnel in new technologies, ensuring the effective use of the systems and the assurance of quality in the processes.

Types of USAID Intervention

Type of Support	**Actions Carried Out**
Equipment and Software	IBIS upgrade, acquisition of hardware and software
Technical Assistance and Accreditation	Documentation, closure of corrective actions, compliance with ISO standards
Training and Fees	Training, payment of evaluators and international professionals
Accreditation Maintenance	Payment for regulatory services and reaccreditation

Impact on INACIF and the Justice System

- Improvement in traceability and ballistic linkage in criminal investigations.
- Increased international recognition and confidence in expert results.

- Strengthening of institutional capacity for effective criminal prosecution and compliance with international quality standards (Memoria de Labores, 2022).

9.2.5 Forensic Entomology Laboratory

The Forensic Entomology Laboratory of the National Institute of Forensic Sciences (INACIF) of Guatemala was inaugurated on July 13, 2021. This laboratory allows the incorporation of entomological evidence as a new source of evidence in judicial processes, especially to determine times related to deaths, such as the post-mortem interval and mobility of corpses, supporting medico-legal and criminal investigations (Memoria de Labores, 2022). It has biology professionals.

The strengthening of INACIF's Forensic Entomology Laboratory in Guatemala has been part of a strategy since its creation in 2021 to improve scientific and technical capacity in criminal investigation, especially in cases of crimes against life. This strengthening includes:

- The hiring and training of specialized personnel, including professionals in biology who were trained, for example, in Medellín, Colombia, to acquire a broad and specialized vision in forensic entomology.
- Provision of necessary infrastructure and equipment, such as stereoscopes, microscopes, breeding cages, and incubators with a controlled environment to study immature forms of insects relevant to criminal cases.
- Implementation of modern analytical methodologies and approved protocols under quality management systems, with the future vision of accrediting procedures in accordance with international standards, such as ISO 17025:2017.
- Technical support for the taxonomic identification of entomological evidence recovered at crime scenes or exhumations, which contributes to establishing post-mortem intervals and determining body movement.
- The official incorporation of this insect-based evidence into the Guatemalan judicial process, providing reliable scientific information to clarify medical-legal and criminal cases.
- Coordination with institutions such as the Public Prosecutor's Office, the National Civil Police, and the Judiciary for joint work to ensure an effective and timely system in forensic investigations.

This approach is a historic milestone for INACIF, seeking to position Guatemala as a forensic benchmark in the region and continue promoting advanced scientific research in criminalistics (Instituto Nacional de Ciencias Forenses de Guatemala, n.d.-c).

Forensic Entomology

AÑO	Total cases admitted
2022	35
2023	48
2024	38

Source: INACIF statistical tables 2022–2024.

9.2.6 Documentoscopy Laboratory

The INACIF Document Laboratory in Guatemala began operating in 2007, one year after the institute began its operations in 2006–2007. This laboratory was created in order to support justice through scientific and internationally recognized techniques for the analysis of documents, including authenticity, falsehood, trademark matching, signatures, and data recovery in public and private documents.

The laboratory carries out document and graphotechnical studies that allow, among other analyses, to verify authenticity, detect alterations such as erasures or cross-outs, compare signatures to identify authors, and compare brands or printed stamps. It has modern technological equipment that helps to carry out these analyses (Instituto Nacional de Ciencias Forenses de Guatemala, n.d.-b).

This area is made up of a total of 18 expert analysts who are in charge of carrying out forensic analysis of documents whose origin is doubtful.

The Document Laboratory of INACIF Guatemala has incorporated a strengthening process that includes formal accreditation under the international standard ISO/IEC 17025:2017, which guarantees the standardization and technical competence of its analytical procedures. This accreditation focuses on specific services, such as the comparison of signatures and handwriting to establish graphonomic correspondences, which ensures the reliability and validity of the results issued for the Guatemalan justice system (Instituto Nacional de Ciencias Forenses de Guatemala, n.d.-b).

Documentoscopy Laboratory

AÑO	Total Cases Admitted
2017	2580
2018	2780
2019	3217
2020	1917
2021	3095

AÑO	Total Cases Admitted
2022	3613
2023	3671
2024	3544

Source: INACIF statistical tables 2017–2024.

9.2.7 Physical Chemistry Laboratory

The Physical Chemistry Laboratory of INACIF Guatemala has five professional pharmaceutical chemical experts, as well as chemical engineers. This laboratory is responsible for carrying out a variety of chemical analyses on different indications found at crime scenes in order to establish their chemical composition, cutting patterns, etc. It also carries out a search for gunpowder in clothing in order to establish firing distances and analysis of primer residues in hands through scanning electrotechnical microscopy. In addition, the laboratory provides services in areas such as herbicide analysis, alcohol analysis in suspicious samples using gas chromatography and mass spectrometry, and accelerant analysis in fire-related samples (Instituto Nacional de Ciencias Forenses de Guatemala, n.d.-d).

The laboratory is accredited under the international standard ISO/IEC 17025, initially the 2005 version, for specific methods such as the analysis of primer residues using scanning electron microscopy. This accreditation certifies technical competence, the validity of its methods and results, and compliance with an internationally recognized quality management system.

The laboratory is currently in the process of transitioning to update this accreditation to the most recent version of the standard, ISO/IEC 17025:2017, which incorporates additional requirements on impartiality, confidentiality, staff qualifications, and risk management. This upgrade further strengthens the laboratory's operational capacity and ensures that its results are accepted with confidence in the Guatemalan judicial system.

Accreditation provides important benefits, such as technically demonstrating competence to generate valid results, promoting continuous improvement, managing preventive risk management, and establishing standardized activities for staff (Instituto Nacional de Ciencias Forenses de Guatemala, n.d.-e, n.d.-f, n.d.-d).

9.2.8 Vehicle Identification Laboratory

INACIF's Vehicle Laboratory in Guatemala specializes in the determination of alterations in vehicles, including the identification and verification of serial numbers, chassis, and engine. Its main function is to establish whether a vehicle has been modified or adulterated, which contributes to the individualization of vehicles and the clarification of criminal cases related to altered vehicles or linked to organized crime. The experts mostly belong to the mechanical engineering area who have also received training to perform trajectory analysis of Shot. This expertise is not carried out by ballistics since most cases related to firearm attacks are in vehicles, so for strategic purposes this area was located in this laboratory.

Among other activities they carry out this to establish whether the vehicles have been subject to color changes, as well as modifications in their structure for the illicit transport of drugs, weapons, or other illicit objects.

The services currently provided by the Vehicle Laboratory have methodologies accredited under the International Quality Standard ISO/IEC 17025:2017 (Instituto Nacional de Ciencias Forenses de Guatemala, 2023e).

9.2.9 Computer Forensic Laboratory

INACIF's Computer Forensics Laboratory in Guatemala specializes in the acquisition, preservation, extraction, analysis, and interpretation of digital evidence related to crimes committed using electronic devices or information and communication technologies (ICTs).

Made up of seven expert analysts from the areas of computer engineering, this laboratory is responsible for extracting and analyzing electronic devices whose structure or operation has data storage systems. Among the services it currently offers is the examination of SIM cards, which is developed according to a methodology accredited under the International Quality Standard ISO/IEC 17025:2017.

To carry out these tasks, the lab uses specialized software and hardware tools, such as EnCase, FTK (Forensic Toolkit), Magnet AXIOM, forensic imaging devices (e.g. Tableau Forensic Imager), and secure servers for storing digital evidence (Instituto Nacional de Ciencias Forenses de Guatemala, 2023a).

9.2.10 Linguistics Laboratory

This service is little requested; however, it provides great contributions, especially to investigations where indications related to discrimination, abuse through foul language, and others are obtained. It works only with one professional expert and they carry out an average of 10 expert reports per month.

9.2.11 Controlled Substances Laboratory

Its objective is to analyze evidence that is seized from drug trafficking. The analysis procedures are established to identify the substances and in cases where it is feasible, quantify illicit drugs, the most common being cocaine, marijuana, heroin, and *Papaver somniferum* (poppy). The professional pharmaceutical chemical experts of this laboratory are also trained to perform analyses of chemical substances and precursors that are illicitly used for the clandestine production of drugs.

9.2.12 Toxicology Laboratory

It has 22 professionals in the area of pharmaceutical chemistry who are trained to perform analyses to establish the presence of ethanol, volatile substances, pesticide drugs, and other substances in biological fluids consisting of samples of blood, urine, gastric contents, tissue fragments, vitreous humor, and other indications taken in necropsy processes. Blood and urine tests are also carried out on living people who are victims of a crime or in judicial proceedings to establish drug use.

9.2.13 Lophoscopy Laboratory

The Lophoscopy Laboratory of INACIF Guatemala is a laboratory of great forensic interest. It is mainly responsible for analyzing evidence that contains fingerprints, palm, or plantar prints, either obtained by ink, live scanning, digital images, or latent prints found on different types of surfaces and objects related to criminal investigations. Its function is to support the individual identification of people involved in criminal or suspicious acts, as well as in cases of traffic and mass disasters (Instituto Nacional de Ciencias Forenses de Guatemala, 2023b).

It is made up of 12 expert analysts. It has a database that allows searches and identification of people suspected of committing a crime through fingerprints.

This laboratory is also of special support in the processes of necroidentification of deceased people who enter the different forensic thanatology services and who are under investigation.

To carry out these comparison analyses, there is interconnection to the criminal and civil databases through the AFIS system.

This laboratory uses scientific methodologies accredited under the ISO/IEC 17025:2017 standard, which guarantees standardization and technical competence in its analytical procedures. Joint work with other institutions in the justice sector (Public Prosecutor's Office, Judicial Branch, National Civil Police) is essential for their results to be timely and reliable within the Guatemalan judicial system (Instituto Nacional de Ciencias Forenses de Guatemala, 2023b).

9.2.14 Serology and Genetics Laboratory

The two areas that make it up are specialized in the analysis of evidence from crime scenes, as well as clinical evaluations of living victims of a crime and evidence collected during the autopsy processes. The main objective is to establish the presence of blood, semen, sperm, saliva, and hair elements, and if these are of human origin. With these results and depending on the investigation process, the evidence goes through genetic analysis in order to isolate genetic profiles useful for correlating scene, victim, and suspect.

The Serology and Genetics Laboratory of the INACIF has been part of the national forensic system since the first years of operation of INACIF, consolidating itself as a strategic area in genetic and serological analysis for criminal, civil, and humanitarian investigations. It maintains an active role in the administration of the Genetic Data Bank for forensic use, in compliance with Decree 22-2017 of the Congress of the Republic and its regulations, an aspect that has consolidated the importance and modernization of this laboratory in the last decade (Instituto Nacional de Ciencias Forenses de Guatemala, 2023c, 2023d).

9.3 Support from International Cooperation

The laboratory has received important contributions from international organizations that have been key to its strengthening and modernization:

- Advanced Equipment Donations: Received Hamilton Microlab Nimbus automated robots, donated through the "Mechanisms for Human Identification" project, promoted by the Center for Human Identification at the University of North Texas (USA) and Gordon Thomas Honeywell (USA). This equipment allows the automation of critical processes in genetic analysis, reducing the risk of contamination and optimizing analysis times.
- Training and Technology Transfer: International collaboration has made it possible to train laboratory personnel in new methodologies and in the use of donated automated equipment, contributing to maintaining international standards and the scientific validity of the procedures.
- Projects for the Search and Identification of Missing Persons: In coordination with the Ministry of Foreign Affairs (MINEX) and international organizations, the laboratory participates in campaigns and projects aimed at the collection and genetic analysis of DNA samples for the identification of missing persons, using internationally recognized protocols and methodologies (Instituto Nacional de Ciencias Forenses de Guatemala, 2023c; *MINEX e INACIF Implementan Iniciativa Humanitaria Para Identificación de Guatemaltecos Desaparecidos En El Extranjero*, 2023).

9.3.1 Accreditation Process

INACIF's Serology and Genetics Laboratory is certified under the ISO/IEC 17025:2017 International Standard, which guarantees:

- Validity, reliability, and standardization of its analytical processes, including extraction, quantification, amplification, and typing of DNA in both filiation and criminalistics cases.
- Official recognition by national and international organizations (Guatemalan Accreditation Office, ILAC, IAAC) that endorse the technical competence of the laboratory.
- The accreditation covers analysis of DNA fragments in filiation and criminalistics, ensuring that the results issued are judicially and scientifically sustainable (Instituto Nacional de Ciencias Forenses de Guatemala, 2023c).

- *Continuous updating and improvement:* The laboratory maintains its quality management system with the commitment to adapt to new regulatory requirements and expand accredited methods, collaborating closely with other institutions in the justice sector and international organizations.

Forensic Genetics

AÑO	Total cases admitted
2017	4843
2018	8673
2019	10393
2020	6351
2021	10739
2022	13078
2023	12001
2024	12207

Source: INACIF statistical tables 2017–2024.

This laboratory plays an important role in the necroidentification process, being part of the lines of evidence that are used to identify corpses; especially in complex cases where due to the state of the corpse it is no longer feasible to identify by fingerprints and there are few lines of evidence that support a scientific identification.

Since 2014, the laboratory has had a CODIS database that was donated by the FBI and operates independently. It currently has more than 50,000 profiles entered.

In summary, the INACIF has made significant progress in strengthening its crime laboratories. Between October 2022 and May 2023, the accreditation of six new laboratories was obtained (October 19, 2022) and the second cycle of institutional accreditation for 10 additional laboratories began, a process that culminated in their reaccreditation on May 17, 2023 (Primer Informe Anual de Gestión, n.d.).

As part of the organizational structure of INACIF, from its inception it had the vision of having an office in charge of documenting all procedures, forms, etc. that officially become part of the documents that any service must have to carry out its activities.

In the organizational structure of the institution, the quality management and accreditation section was created, being in its beginnings, a dependency directly dependent on the general management.

During the first five years of INACIF's operation, all work procedures, forms, etc. are implemented.

However, despite having a specific section in charge of documentation since its inception, due to the fact that there was a lot of work ahead to build the institution, it was only possible to implement work protocols with the clear objective of accrediting the analytical processes.

Different situations, especially lack of a budget allocation according to the needs of the institute, after carrying out various procedures and international cooperation, the institute finally in 2014 agreed to support the project to accredit procedures under ISO standards. The program started with laboratories whose impact had greater impact on the courts of justice.

In 2014, USAID provided INACIF with support to start the accreditation program and from this account the work teams were formed to implement all the necessary documentation to accredit the chosen laboratories.

To begin with the accreditation project, as mentioned above, four laboratories with the greatest impact at the level of the justice system were chosen, both for the number of applications, and for the incidence in debates.

The laboratories chosen for being framed in the above were Genetics, Ballistics, Toxicology, and Physicochemistry.

In 2015, the project was closed and the dream of accrediting forensic services ended.

Again in 2016 the projects were resumed, always with international cooperation through USAID and after the hard work of all the collaborators who accepted the challenge; finally on March 6, 2019, the procedures for the analysis of ethanol and volatile substances, analysis of residues of primer in hands, analysis of ballistic fingerprints through the IBIS computer system, and the procedures of genetic analysis to establish paternity received their respective certificates of accreditation under the ISO 17025-2005 standard.

As guarantors of quality systems, in October 2022, the serology, vehicle identification, controlled substances, computer forensics, lophoscopy, and document collection laboratories were accredited, including both the new accreditation of laboratories and the reaccreditation of previously been accredited laboratories, under the ISO 17025-2017 standard.

To date, after different external audits, the accreditation has been maintained and the quality system is increasingly robust.

Currently, INACIF has a solid quality system and is committed, however, to face different challenges such as lack of budget and a few personnel in charge of the quality improvement office, comprising only three people in charge.

During 2024, a total of 288 documents were included in the quality system, among which we can mention:

- Manuals
- Procedures
- Instructional
- Forms

The approval process includes the preparation or updating of the document, its evaluation by peers and the corresponding leaderships, a technical review by the Quality Management and Accreditation unit, and, finally, formal approval by the General Directorate (Instituto Nacional de Ciencias Forenses de Guatemala, 2024).

9.3.2 The Role of International Cooperation in the Strengthening and Accreditation of INACIF's Crime Laboratories

Between 2012 and 2024, international cooperation has been a strategic pillar for the development, modernization, and accreditation of the INACIF crime laboratories. External support, both financial and technical, has made it possible to promote technological updating, the training of human resources, the establishment of quality procedures, and the obtaining of international accreditations that endorse the technical competence of the institution.

Key Areas of Support

1. Technical Strengthening and Modernization
    - *Provision of equipment:* International institutions and projects have equipped laboratories with modern instruments and advanced systems, essential for ballistic, genetic, chemical, and toxicological analysis.
    - *Infrastructure update:* External financing has allowed the expansion and modernization of facilities, facilitating compliance with international standards (Instituto Nacional de Ciencias Forenses de Guatemala, n.d.-e; Lopez Orantes, 2017).
    - *Implementation of forensic technology:* Initiatives supported by the EU and USAID, among others, have made possible the integration of systems such as IBIS for ballistics and genetic analysis platforms (Instituto Nacional de Ciencias Forenses de Guatemala, n.d.-e; Lopez Orantes, 2017).
2. Staff Training and Professionalization
    - *International training:* Training programs have been coordinated with universities and laboratories of recognized prestige, such as the University of Granada (Spain), the Institute of Forensic Sciences of Puerto Rico, and expert offices in Colombia.
    - *Specialized training:* The cooperation has facilitated postgraduate courses, diplomas, technical workshops, and direct advice on quality management, expert procedures, and new analytical methodologies.
3. Accreditation Assistance
    - *Guide in the implementation of quality management systems:* Multilateral organizations have advised INACIF to adopt and implement the ISO/IEC 17025 standard, the international quality standard for testing laboratories.
    - *Financing of audit and certification processes:* Cooperation has covered the costs of external audits, which are essential to obtain and maintain accreditation

by organizations such as the Guatemalan Accreditation Office (OGA) and international agreements such as ILAC and IAAC.

- *Regulatory knowledge transfer:* Guidelines and good practices have been received from accredited laboratories in Europe, North America, and South America, accelerating the process of validation and standardization of methods.

4. Project-Specific Support and Capacity Building
   - *Development of databases and information systems:* Projects such as the strengthening of the Genetic Data Bank have had capital and assistance for its expansion and continuous operation.
   - *Support for research and pilot projects:* International funds have made it possible to carry out studies, pilot tests and validation of critical processes for forensic work.

Highlights

- *Laboratory accreditation:* Ballistics, Genetics, Toxicological, and Physicochemical have achieved certification under ISO/IEC 17025-2017, demonstrating technically valid methods and competent personnel.
- *Regional recognition:* INACIF is recognized as a benchmark in Central America for its level of specialization, quality, and results, in part thanks to the international support received.
- *Improvement in judicial reliability:* The validity of the expert reports and scientific analyses generated by INACIF increased, derived from the rigor in the procedures and the institutional and technical support provided by the cooperation.

Concrete Examples of Cooperation (2012–2024)

Year	Organization/Project	Area of Support	Achievements/ Destinations
2012–2017	SEJUST (European Union)	Modern equipment, technical training, studies, infrastructure	Scientific consolidation and regional expansion
2015–2023	USAID (United States)	Modernization, IBIS implementation, auditing, training	Accreditation of key laboratories
Various	University of Granada, ICF-PR, Colombia	Academic commitment, postgraduate studies, workshops, DNA support	Professionalization and consolidation of methods

International cooperation has been decisive for INACIF to achieve quality standards, technological modernization, and regulatory compliance between 2012 and 2024. Thanks to the integration of resources, techniques, and knowledge provided by multilateral organizations and international partners, INACIF's crime laboratories today enjoy regional recognition, have highly trained personnel, and have accreditations that guarantee the expert validity of their results and opinions.

The institutional mission is:

> "To be a benchmark institution at the national and international level, for its competent human resources, technological capacity, good forensic practices, quality and transparency in institutional management and respect for human dignity"

Through international certification, we are sure that we have achieved this; and today, INACIF is positioned as an international benchmark laboratory.

9.3.3 Challenges for INACIF to Maintain the Accreditation of Its Laboratories

Since its founding in 2006, Guatemala's National Institute of Forensic Sciences (INACIF) has faced significant financial challenges in maintaining accreditation for its laboratories. Throughout its history, the institution has had considerable financial support from international cooperation. However, this dependence has created a structural challenge in ensuring the financial sustainability of projects and programes that were initially funded externally but now need to be supported and maintained with their own resources.

Main Financial Challenges

- *Budget insufficiency:* Of the more than Q500 million that INACIF requests annually, they only receive about half (Barreno, 2022). This limits the ability to invest in equipment, supplies, and technological modernization.
- *High maintenance and renovation costs:* Laboratory equipment requires constant renewal due to technological obsolescence and wear and tear, which implies considerable expenses in spare parts, licences, and system upgrades (Barreno, 2022).
- *Accreditation expenses:* The maintenance of accreditation under international standards, such as ISO/IEC 17025, involves payments to certifying bodies, external audits and continuous personnel training, which represents a recurring and high cost compared to the budget obtained.
- *Strengthening of administrative processes:* The continuous optimization of administrative processes represents a key opportunity to improve financial and operational management, thus facilitating the timely acquisition of inputs, reagents, and software licenses essential for the efficient development of expert tasks.

- *Lack of sustainable investment:* The shortage of funds prevents a robust strategy of training and technical training, key to maintaining accreditation standards, and facing external evaluation visits.

Recommendations for Overcoming Challenges

- *Efficient financial management:* Improve internal processes and budget planning to maximize available resources.
- *Income diversification:* Explore charging for specialized services to external entities and alliances with national academic or private institutions for self-financed projects.
- *Planning by accreditation cycles:* Prepare financial projections and five-year reserve funds, considering the peaks of expenditures on renovation and audits.
- *Process modernization and digitalization:* Invest in technology that optimizes resources, reduces operating costs, and improves process traceability.
- *Influence the legal framework:* Promote public policies that ensure progressive increases in the budget allocated to forensic sciences.

9.4 Conclusion

INACIF's 10-year experience shows that achieving internationally recognized accreditation is the start of a strong commitment to quality, modernization, and credibility rather than the end of a process. Sustained international cooperation has played a significant role in the remarkable progress made from the consolidation of specialized laboratories to the successful implementation of ISO/IEC 17025:2017 standards. Crucial pillars in this transition have included technical support, the provision of cutting-edge equipment, infrastructure modernization, specialized training, and reimbursement of accreditation expenses.

But upholding these standards is a structural problem that goes beyond technical ability; it calls for consistent institutional, financial, and strategic backing. Strict recurring audits, continuous employee training, method updates, and the replacement of advanced equipment are all necessary for laboratory accreditation, despite their high operating costs. There is a chance that quality standards and, by extension, judicial reliability will regress in the absence of mechanisms to guarantee the sustainability of these investments.

Therefore, international cooperation is an important long-term partner in preserving these accomplishments as well as an initial catalyst. In the 21st century, forensic science is complex and requires a level of technical and methodological rigor that many nations, particularly in developing contexts, cannot sustain without external partnerships. This is because scientific validity, the integrity of the chain of custody, and impartiality are all crucial. In addition to financial resources, cooperation makes it easier to integrate into transnational forensic expertise networks, transfer state-of-the-art techniques, and expose people to similar experiences. When combined, these components support the institution and the legal system overall.

Additionally, forensic science needs to function within standardized frameworks of quality and recognition in a globalized criminal landscape where organized crime, cybercrime, and environmental crimes are increasingly transnational. Cross-border cooperation in criminal investigations and prosecutions is made possible by international accreditation, which guarantees that Guatemala's forensic findings are recognized and trusted in other jurisdictions. This reciprocity solidifies Guatemala's standing as a trustworthy partner in international justice initiatives and upholds the rule of law.

But depending entirely on foreign assistance is risky. To sustain momentum, Guatemala needs to integrate quality management into INACIF's core operational culture, institutionalize continuous professional development, and ensure a budget that accurately reflects the true costs of accreditation. Strategic planning must anticipate accreditation cycles, equipment replacement requirements, and new forensic disciplines that will require infrastructure and new skills.

In this sense, the way forward needs to be balanced: national commitment guarantees stability, a sense of ownership, and resilience to political or economic ups and downs, while international cooperation continues to offer innovation, training, and external validation. Guatemala can only guarantee that currently accredited laboratories not only keep their accreditation but also adapt to new legal and scientific challenges by taking this two-pronged approach.

In the end, preserving accreditation is a reaffirmation of the institutional values of objectivity, openness, and scientific rigor rather than a technical exercise. Alongside national will, international cooperation ensures that these values endure, establishing the progress made as a lasting foundation for justice in Guatemala rather than a short-term solution.

References

Barreno, C. (2022, June 11). A qué retos y desafíos se enfrentará quien dirija por los próximos cinco años el Instituto Nacional de Ciencias Forenses? *Prensa Libre*.

Instituto Nacional de Ciencias Forenses de Guatemala. (2021, November 16) Inauguración Laboratorio Forense de Análisis Ambiental.

Instituto Nacional de Ciencias Forenses de Guatemala. (2023a) Laboratorio de Informática Forense. https://www.inacif.gob.gt/docs/guias_tablas_otros/guias_tablas_otros/2023_Informatica_Forense.pdf (accessed August 15, 2024).

Instituto Nacional de Ciencias Forenses de Guatemala. (2023b) Laboratorio de Lofoscopía. https://www.inacif.gob.gt/docs/guias_tablas_otros/guias_tablas_otros/2023_Informatica_Forense.pdf (accessed August 15, 2024).

Instituto Nacional de Ciencias Forenses de Guatemala. (2023c). Laboratorio de Serología y Genética ÁREA DE GENÉTICA. https://www.inacif.gob.gt/docs/guias_tablas_otros/guias_tablas_otros/2023_Genetica.pdf (accessed August 15, 2024).

Instituto Nacional de Ciencias Forenses de Guatemala. (2023d). Laboratorio de Serología y Genética ÁREA DE SEROLOGÍA. https://www.inacif.gob.gt/docs/guias_tablas_otros/guias_tablas_otros/2023_Serologia.pdf (accessed August 15, 2024).

Instituto Nacional de Ciencias Forenses de Guatemala. (2023e). Laboratorio de Vehículos. https://www.inacif.gob.gt/docs/guias_tablas_otros/guias_tablas_otros/2023_Identificacion_de_Vehiculos.pdf (accessed August 15, 2024).

Instituto Nacional de Ciencias Forenses de Guatemala. (2024) Memoria de Labores.

Instituto Nacional de Ciencias Forenses de Guatemala (n.d.-a) Laboratorio de Acústica Forense. Retrieved July 24, 2025, from https://www.inacif.gob.gt/docs/guias_tablas_otros/guias_tablas_otros/2023_Acustica_Forense.pdf (accessed August 15, 2024).

Instituto Nacional de Ciencias Forenses de Guatemala. (n.d.-b) Laboratorio de Documentoscopía. Retrieved July 24, 2025, from https://www.inacif.gob.gt/docs/guias_tablas_otros/guias_tablas_otros/2023_Documentoscopia.pdf (accessed August 15, 2024).

Instituto Nacional de Ciencias Forenses de Guatemala. (n.d.-c) Laboratorio de Entomología Forense. Retrieved July 24, 2025, from https://www.inacif.gob.gt/docs/guias_tablas_otros/guias_tablas_otros/2023_Entomologia.pdf (accessed May 9, 2025).

Instituto Nacional de Ciencias Forenses de Guatemala. (n.d.-d) Laboratorio de Fisicoquímica. Retrieved July 25, 2025, from https://www.inacif.gob.gt/docs/guias_tablas_otros/guias_tablas_otros/2023_Fisicoquimica.pdf (accessed May 9, 2025).

Instituto Nacional de Ciencias Forenses de Guatemala. (n.d.-e) Laboratorios de Criminalísticas del INACIF reciben acreditación de calidad internacional.

Instituto Nacional de Ciencias Forenses de Guatemala. (n.d.-f) Transición hacia la norma ISO 17025:2017.

Instituto Nacional de Ciencias Foreses de Guatemala. (2023, April 11). Inauguran remozamiento en el laboratorio de Antropología Forense.

Laboratorio de Antropología Forense, uno de los pilares del INACIF. (2025) *Revista Científica Diálogo Forense*, 47–49.

Lopez Orantes, A. R. (2017) Evaluación del impacto del programa de la Unión Europea en apoyo a la seguridad y justicia SEJUST 2013-2015 en el fortalecimiento del Instituto Nacional de Ciencias Forenses INACIF [*Univerisdad de San Carlos de Guatemala*]. http://biblioteca.usac.edu.gt/tesis/28/28_0988.pdf (accessed July 13, 2025).

Memoria de Labores. (2022). Instituto Nacional de Ciencias Forenses de Guatemala (2022) Memoria de Labores. (accessed July 13, 2025).

(2023, July 11) *MINEX e INACIF implementan iniciativa humanitaria para identificación de guatemaltecos desaparecidos en el extranjero. Ministerio de Relaciones Exteriores de Guatemala.*

Primer Informe Anual de Gestión. (n.d.) Retrieved July 25, 2025, from https://www.inacif.gob.gt/docs/guias_tablas_otros/informe_anual_primer.pdf (accessed July 13, 2025).

CHAPTER 10

Latin America in Forensic Action: Quality Standards Alone Do Not Provide an Infallible Quality Assurance

Roberto C. Parra[1,*], Gian Carlo Iannacone[2], Allan G. Alvarez-Godoy[3], Daniel Castellanos[4], Ruth Garcia-Marroquin[5], and Jorge L. Vasquez-Guerrero[2]

[1] *The Specialized Forensic Team of the United Nations Joint Human Rights Office (UNJHRO) in the Democratic Republic of the Congo*

[2] *Institute of Legal Medicine and Forensic Sciences of Peru, Lima, Peru*

[3] *International Forensic Consultant, The Hague, Netherlands*

[4] *University of Antioquia, Medellin, Colombia*

[5] *Forensic Science Laboratories, INACIF-Guatemala, Guatemala City, Guatemala*

10.1 Introduction

As has been extensively discussed in other chapters, the standardization of processes and the use of quality management systems are now the most important topics in forensic science (Wilson-Wilde, 2018; Ballantyne and Wilson-Wilde, 2020). The use of standards like ISO/IEC 17025 for testing laboratories and ISO/IEC 17020 for inspection bodies has been pushed as a necessary way to make sure that technical reliability, procedural traceability, operational transparency, and institutional credibility are all in place. In this context, accreditation has been characterized not merely as a mechanism to enhance the technical competencies of forensic services but also as a crucial prerequisite for their legitimacy in the eyes of the judicial systems and the public (Wilson-Wilde, 2018).

This model has been well-received in Latin America, and in some countries, it has made significant progress. Forensic institutions have begun to align their practices with international standards, put in place quality assurance measures, and made progress in formalizing procedures that aim to improve the chain of custody, analytical reproducibility, and technical independence. The process has not been the same for all countries, though. This is because of historical, political,

*The views expressed herein are those authors and do not necessarily reflect the views of the United Nations.

Forensic Science and Quality Management: Addressing the Era of Standardization in Challenging Environments, First Edition. Edited by Roberto C. Parra and Allan G. Alvarez-Godoy.

budgetary, and cultural factors that affect each country's ability to adopt, adapt, and maintain these standards over time. The increasing concern regarding the standardization of technical and methodological procedures is a principal factor.

The aim of this chapter is to provide a critical and contextual analysis of the current role of quality standards in the consolidation, or at least the ongoing advancement, of forensic science in Latin America. It specifically looks at the danger of treating accreditation as an end in itself, separate from the institutional conditions that make good, ethical, and scientifically sound forensic practice possible. In many instances, obtaining certification may foster a semblance of quality that, in the absence of a significant structural and cultural transformation among technical and professional personnel, risks devolving into a mere symbol rather than a reliable assurance. This phenomenon, which we might call the "mirage of accreditation" and quality, needs to be taken seriously and carefully. This is not to undermine the technical formalization efforts that some countries in the region have made but to find its true place in a bigger and more complicated forensic ecosystem.

There are different examples in the region that show this tension. Countries like Colombia, Panama, Chile, Guatemala, and Brazil have made a lot of progress in setting up quality systems. They now have more integrated forensic structures, formalized processes, and institutional policies that focus on technical assurance. Nonetheless, even in these instances, difficulties remain concerning territorial equity, budgetary sustainability, and the collaboration between technical entities and legal professionals. Conversely, there are situations where, despite the presence of national regulations or Institutes of Legal Medicine and Forensic Science, as seen in Peru, institutional fragmentation, inadequate forensic governance, or insufficient political will impede the establishment of quality standards beyond regulatory discussions.

In this case, accreditation cannot be seen as a separate thing or a single goal. Instead, it needs a complete institutional plan that takes into account real-world situations, local technical skills, staff training, resource availability, and the ability of scientific criteria to stand on their own without outside influences. Forensic quality is not just based on documents and audits; it is also based on ethical, responsible, and long-lasting practices that meet both international standards and local needs. But for now, this is still a "forensic delusion" in Latin America.

So, this chapter starts with two ideas. It acknowledges the significance of international standards as essential tools for enhancing forensic science. Conversely, it contends that its efficacy is intrinsically connected to the presence of institutional conditions that facilitate its authentic implementation, internalization in quotidian practice, and sustainability beyond political or economic cycles. In this context, we suggest a critical evaluation of the trajectories undertaken by various Latin American nations, pinpointing advancements, effective practices, enduring challenges, and insights gained. We do not aim to examine the specifics but to pinpoint generalizable elements that characterize the phenomenon.

Finally, we draw inspiration from the conceptual framework of the Sydney Declaration (SD) (Roux et al., 2022; Willis, 2022), a new tool that aims to add to traditional quality frameworks by focusing on core ideas such as scientific integrity, institutional resilience, and contextual relevance (also discussed in Chapter 1 of this volume). This approach expands the view of forensic quality beyond official regulatory standards and includes moral and operational aspects that are necessary for working in difficult situations. We want to add a more nuanced and realistic discussion about the problems the region faces with forensic quality by showing that standards are necessary but not enough on their own. We can only move forward toward forensic science that is truly reliable, accessible, and serves justice if we work together on rules, professional practice, and institutional commitment.

10.1.1 The Mirage of Forensic Quality in Latin America

Popularly, as in professional belief, often say that accreditation means quality, but in many cases it has become an empty symbol: a formal recognition that doesn't always mean that everyday forensic practices have gotten better. This "mirage of quality" is most obvious when forensic systems try to meet the standards set by accreditation bodies without questioning the scientific validity of the methods used or thinking about whether the procedures are right for the situations they are used in. In Queensland, Australia, for example, accreditation can happen alongside questionable methods if auditors just make sure that "what is said is done is done" without carefully checking the scientific basis of the method.

A lot of forensic systems in Latin America try to follow ISO standards without first building the scientific, ethical, and institutional foundations that would make that adaptation long-lasting and useful. So, more effort is put into making documents, making sure that standards are followed, and passing audits than into thinking critically about the methods and how they apply. It's time for an inspection! Let's make sure everything is in order. We need to pass it this year to keep our accreditation! What really makes something good is not how scientifically sound it is, but how well it follows the rules. This creates a dangerous false sense of validity, which is a forensic delusion.

Also, accreditation tends to create a centralized and rigid model, which makes it harder to use in places or countries where things work differently. But this limit can also be a chance. ISO standards don't directly check the validity of methods; instead, they check how well the management system follows the rules. This allows for flexibility, which means that other systems can come up with scientifically sound, though unusual, methods as long as they are well-documented and make sense on their own. This broader interpretation would allow for the accreditation of forensic models designed for adverse contexts, supported by contextualized quality standards, without sacrificing scientific rigor.

Another important thing to remember is that working in the field is different from working in the lab. The first one works best when things are changing, and there is uncertainty, risk, and logistical problems. The second one is better for audits that are structured and in controlled environments. Using the same quality logic in both cases can be wrong in terms of knowledge and not helpful at all. Fieldwork requires adaptability, professional judgment, and goal-oriented methodologies rather than those centered on form. Quality should be thought of as a balance between strict methods and flexible operations, not as a single model that everyone has to follow.

The real challenge is not to refuse accreditation, but to change what it means and why it is there. It's about getting back its useful side, not just for the sake of it, and adding it to a bigger picture of forensic practice that values honesty, relevance, and openness over just following the rules. This means building a scientific culture that values real-world evidence, ongoing professional development, and the capacity of institutions to learn, adapt, and be held responsible. If not, there is a chance that a decorative quality model will keep going, which protects institutions but not the truth or the victims.

10.2 International Standards: Foundations and Limitations in their Forensic Applicability

In the last few decades, quality assurance in forensic science has become very important. This is because there is a growing need for forensic evidence to be clear, traceable, and technically reliable. The use of international standards, especially ISO/IEC 17025 for testing laboratories and ISO/IEC 17020 for inspection bodies, has been pushed as a key part of this change. These standards, created for metrology and industrial testing, have been gradually adopted in forensic practice with the hope that using them will help reduce mistakes, strengthen institutions, and make the technical side of things more legitimate in the eyes of the courts and the public.

However, as Neuteboom et al. (2023) caution in their critical review, this integration has encountered tensions, limitations, and inquiries. The authors conducted an international survey encompassing six regional networks of forensic laboratories, including participants from Latin America via the Ibero-American Academy of Criminalistics and Forensic Studies (AICEF). They pinpointed structural elements of the accreditation model that necessitate reevaluation to ensure that quality management aligns with the requirements and intricacies of forensic practice.

One of the main problems is what the authors call the questioning of the "fitness for purpose" of the standards that are currently in use. In other words, do these standards do a good enough job of covering the full range of issues that arise in the forensic process? The study's answer is complicated, but it points to a clear truth: the ISO/IEC 17025 standard has done a good job of formalizing laboratory analytical procedures, but it doesn't cover other important parts of forensic practice, especially those that happen outside the lab, like on-scene investigation, coming up with interpretive hypotheses, or making conclusions when there is uncertainty. These dimensions are precisely the most critical in institutional environments such as those in Latin America, where traceability and contextualization are essential to guarantee justice.

10.2.1 A Standard Outside Its Original Context

The ISO/IEC 17025 standard was designed for testing and calibration laboratories in controlled industrial or scientific settings. Its focus is on the technical validation of procedures, document management, and measurement traceability. Its application to the forensic field was, at the time, a pragmatic decision, given the absence of discipline-specific standards. However, as Neuteboom et al. (2023) point out, there is a disconnect between the standard's prescriptive approach and the inherently uncertain, interpretive, and multidisciplinary nature of forensic science.

In Latin America, this disconnect is accentuated by operational realities that do not always allow these standards to be implemented under ideal conditions. Peru is a clear example of this problem; its own mobile infrastructure does not guarantee an appropriate physical location, as it must be rented on numerous occasions. How to organize quality systems when the path is uncertain and adequate budgets are required to maintain them, as well as a vision for development and political will, which is currently nonexistent or even precarious. Laboratories with staff shortages, institutions with frequent management turnover, chronic budget constraints, and a lack of digital infrastructure make the uniform application of complex standards difficult. In many cases, attempts to implement ISO end up being formal exercises, oriented more toward the production of documentary evidence for audits than toward the substantive improvement of forensic practice.

Furthermore, the pressure to achieve accreditation can generate unintended adverse effects, such as over-documentation, increased technical bureaucracy, and the prioritization of form over substance. This phenomenon has been described as one of the main obstacles to continuous improvement: quality is measured by adherence to written procedures, rather than by the scientific or interpretive quality of the results (Neuteboom et al., 2023). In Latin American contexts, where forensic science is often practiced under adverse conditions, this situation can lead to a troubling paradox: institutions that meet the formal standard continue to face systematic errors, a lack of technical independence, or deficient, even extreme, expert interpretations.

10.2.2 The Risk of Operational Fragmentation

Another important finding from the survey is that the current quality model doesn't fully include the forensic process as a whole. More than half of the people who answered the survey did not think that crime scene investigation (CSI) was an important part of a forensic scientist's job. This is concerning because the crime scene is where the whole analytical process starts, and how it is handled directly affects how valid the results are. This fragmentation is especially clear in Latin America. For example, in Colombia and Chile, crime scenes are only handled by trained police or other criminal investigation groups. Laboratories, on the other hand, work under different rules and don't have many ways to get feedback or work together to evaluate cases.

Quality assurance systems are less effective because the different parts of the forensic process don't work together. For instance, if evidence collection is not traceable or if decisions about which samples to send for analysis are made without clear technical criteria, the validity of laboratory results is compromised, even if they have been generated under an accredited system. The study indicates that a comprehensive quality model must encompass the entire forensic continuum: from the crime scene, through the laboratory, to interpretation and presentation in court. This systemic approach is essential for nations where forensic evidence may represent the sole objective component in intricate judicial scenarios.

10.2.3 The Internal Logic of the Accreditation Drive

One of the most interesting things about Neuteboom et al.'s (2023) work is that it shows that most accreditation processes have come from within forensic institutions themselves, not from outside demands from the justice system or the public. This brings up an important question: who is the laboratory accredited for? In Latin America, forensic science is still new to politics, and judges and other legal officials don't always know the technical details of expertise. They need accreditation because they hear about it or read about it in the news. Instead of being a requirement of the criminal justice system, accreditation is more often a way for peers to recognize each other or a requirement for joining international networks and legitimizing certain competitions between "scientific" power groups.

This discovery has significant ramifications for the formulation of public policy. If standards are not linked to the ultimate beneficiaries of the service (prosecutors, judges, victims), they may devolve into a self-referential practice, serving merely to illustrate institutional order while remaining detached from the tangible effects on the administration of justice. The survey also shows that external evaluation tools, like user satisfaction surveys or reviews by judges, are not often used to help things get better all the time. As a result, quality is often measured internally in these technical fields, without taking into account the actual needs of the situation.

10.2.4 Costs, Documentation, and Sustainability

Respondents also said that the costs of the accreditation process were one of the biggest problems. This is especially important in countries where forensic budgets rely on discretionary funds, international donations, or tight fiscal budgets.

In Latin America, several attempts to get accreditation have failed or been put on hold because they couldn't find enough money, staff, or political changes.

Similarly, a propensity for superfluous documentation accumulation was noted in reaction to inadequately assessed nonconformities. This practice doesn't improve quality; instead, it can put too much stress on already small technical teams, making it harder for them to focus on important scientific tasks. A defensive mindset can take over instead of a culture of improvement. This mindset is based on avoiding audit observations without really thinking about how well the processes that were put in place are working.

10.2.5 Toward a Contextual and Integrated Vision of Quality

In light of these constraints, the study advocates for a transition to a more contextual, systemic, and outcome-focused perspective on forensic quality assurance. In this regard, the framework suggested by the SD (examined in Chapter 1) becomes pertinent. It acknowledges that quality is not merely the application of a standard, but an institutional construct that must consider scientific integrity, resilience to adverse conditions, and contextual relevance.

This method works best in Latin America, where many forensic institutions work in places where there is structural violence, limited resources, and a lack of coordination between institutions. Adapting quality standards to these settings does not entail lowering expectations; instead, it acknowledges that the pursuit of technical excellence must be grounded in actual operational conditions rather than unmodified imported normative ideals. Neuteboom et al. (2023) assert that quality systems must transition toward more open and dynamic frameworks that emphasize the fundamental objectives of forensic science: advancing truth and facilitating access to justice.

10.3 Accreditation and Forensic Practice: Diverse Trajectories in Latin America

The evolution of forensic systems in Latin America has been heterogeneous (see Table 10.1), determined by historical, political, regulatory, and budgetary factors that vary significantly among countries (see also Chapters 7–9). Some states have been able to set up technical and scientific institutions that are working toward accreditation and putting together integrated quality policies. Other states, on the other hand, are still in the process of putting these policies into place or have structural problems that make it hard to start long-term accreditation processes. This section looks at five examples that show how different trajectories can be: Colombia, Chile, Brazil, Guatemala, and Peru. Chapter 9 examines the situation in Panama in greater depth.

Table 10.1 Forensic QMS Evolution of the most prominent forensic systems in Latin America.

Country	Evolution of the forensic QMS (estimated)	Highlights
Brasil	Advance	High density 9001; tradition 17025 in the Federal Police; proficiency testing and extended LIMS Strengths: Scale, investment, and leadership in the region related to the culture of quality; general presence of 17025 and multi-center validations. Typical gaps: Challenges of greater process standardization across states, which will impact the integration of 21043. Signs of maturity: Presence of audits and maintenance of the QMS focused on performance.
Colombia	Advance	Notable 17025 coverage; process culture; indicators and regular proficiency testing. Strengths: Risk management, proficiency testing, metrological traceability; coordination between agencies within the administration of justice; and a solid chain of custody. Typical gaps: Quality standards established for crime scenes across all regions; uniform modernization regarding LIMS use. Signs of maturity: Quality management system performance indicators and trend analysis implemented.
México	Upper intermediate	Extensive accreditations (EMA) and 9001 governance; presence of state heterogeneity Strengths: Scale and experience; validations and attitude testing; strengthening of chain of custody and LIMS across multiple entities. Typical gaps: Disparities across states; maintenance of 17025 scope in complex disciplines; staff turnover impacting competency. Signs of maturity: Consolidated practices in DNA and toxicology; advanced risk management and periodic audits.
Chile	Upper intermediate	Formal ISO adoption (NCh); SML/Police with 17025; consolidating 17020/LIMS

Table 10.1 (Continued)

Country	Evolution of the forensic QMS (estimated)	Highlights
		Strengths: Tradition of formal adoption of ISO standards; consistent metrological traceability and document control; stable internal audit culture. Gaps: LIMS interoperability between stakeholders (SML, police, prosecutor's offices); expansion of 17025 scope to all disciplines. Signs of maturity: Systematic use of proficiency tests and interlaboratory testing, risk management and improvement in annual reports; integration with growing digital chain of custody.
Argentina	Intermediate	Centers of Excellence; Federal Variability in 17025 Coverage and Maintenance Strengths: High technical capacity in DNA, fingerprints, and document examination; academic environments promote robust validation. Typical Gaps: Interjurisdictional Heterogeneity; Uneven 17025 Coverage; Uneven Crime Scene Standardization (17020). Signs of Maturity: Best practices in core disciplines; Need to close gaps in ancillary disciplines.
Perú	Low intermediate	Quality management system implemented in institutions related to the administration of justice with ISO 9001; forensic application still limited; potential under consolidation. Strengths: Institutional presence of ISO 9001 in organizations in the justice and prosecution sectors. Culture of continuous improvement in public management. Typical gaps: Low 17025 accreditation in forensic laboratories. Regional fragmentation and limited traceability. Limited use of assay tests, analytical validations, and LIMS. Signs of maturity: Low, although still dispersed and under development.
Panamá	Upper intermediate	Formal ISO, further information in Chapter 7. Signs of maturity: Systematic use of proficiency tests.

10.3.1 Colombia: Institutional Articulation and Technical Maturity

Colombia is one of the most advanced examples of institutional consolidation in forensics in the region, and it is even an example for other countries to follow. The National Institute of Legal Medicine and Forensic Sciences (INMLCF) was established at the start of the last century and is now an agency of the Attorney General's Office. It is the main agency for forensic investigations in the country. Its national, decentralized, and hierarchically integrated structure has helped standardize procedures, make human resources more professional, and slowly adopt quality management systems based on ISO standards.

The INMLCF has received important accreditations in important fields like forensic genetics, chemistry, ballistics, and human identification. Its laboratories are certified under the ISO/IEC 17025 standard. This process has been able to continue because there is clear political will and forensic science is seen as an important part of the judicial system and human rights policy, especially in the context of the internal armed conflict. Working with the Accusatory Criminal System and the Special Jurisdiction for Peace has made the institute more important to the government and strengthened its culture of quality.

But even in this fairly stable situation, there are still problems that may not be obvious from the outside. But if we look more closely at its inner workings, where the systems need to be more flexible to support the impressive equipment that the ISOs need, we would find a lot of surprises. The realities of Bogota, Medellín, or Cali do not differ from those of Pasto, Montería, or Villavicencio, which is a city very close to the core of the Institute. The INMLCF's technical and scientific mandate and the judicial system's operational needs can sometimes conflict, which can limit technical autonomy. The long-term success of processes for continuous improvement depends on the stability of institutions and budgets. The Colombian model has also been criticized for putting too much focus on the lab and not enough on fully integrating crime scene work into the quality system.

10.3.2 Chile: Expert Modernization and Systemic Approach

Chile has developed a technically sound and legally consolidated forensic model, based on two main institutions: the Legal Medical Service (SML), under the Ministry of Justice and Human Rights, and the Criminalistics Laboratory of the Carabineros de Chile (LABOCAR), under the Ministry of the Interior. This institutional duality, far from generating fragmentation, has been accompanied by strategic planning and the progressive adoption of quality systems in line with international standards.

The SML has implemented institutional policies aimed at quality assurance, with accreditation processes in areas such as genetics, toxicology, and forensic pathology. These initiatives have been supported by a clear regulatory framework and a growing institutional awareness of the importance of forensic traceability and transparency. Chile has also incorporated external evaluations, systematic audits, and ongoing training processes as part of its quality model.

What is noteworthy in the Chilean case is its systemic approach, which seeks to integrate forensic production with the needs of the administration of justice, while maintaining an independent technical and scientific profile. This balance has allowed Chile to position itself as a regional benchmark in forensic institutions, although it still faces challenges in the homogeneous territorial expansion of its standards and in the consolidation of a scientific culture that prioritizes applied forensic research.

10.3.3 Brazil: Technical Leadership in Tension with Structural Inequality

Brazil is a complicated and mixed case. The country has some of the most advanced forensic laboratories in the area, with state units that have gotten ISO certification in areas like molecular biology, forensic chemistry, and ballistics. For instance, the Federal Police has laboratories that are known around the world for their high quality. This high level of technical skill, on the other hand, exists alongside a huge gap in the availability of resources, technical skills, and access to forensic services among the different states.

The Brazilian forensic system is very decentralized. Each state has its own forensic structure, which is overseen by the Ministry of Public Security in that state. This has led to the development of many quality models, some of which are very professionalized and accredited, while others still don't have standardized processes or clear outside oversight. In some instances, accreditation endeavors have been upheld by local initiatives that are not aligned with national policies.

So, Brazil's biggest problem is getting its quality standards to work together at the federal level. This will make sure that the technical achievements of some laboratories don't become islands of excellence that are cut off from the rest of the judicial system. Even though things are getting better, the lack of a national forensic quality policy with clear goals and a separate budget limits the impact of accreditation as a way to change institutions.

10.3.4 Guatemala: Technical Advances and Sustained Institutional Will

Guatemala has been one of the Central American countries that has shown the most institutional consistency in its efforts to improve the quality of forensic work. The National Institute of Forensic Sciences (INACIF) was set up in 2007 and has been putting quality assurance policies into place in different areas over time. The main goal is to help the justice system and meet international standards. They have received ISO accreditation, which means they follow standard procedures, technical protocols, performance evaluations, and do regular internal audits.

INACIF has always been clear about its commitment to making forensic practice more professional by encouraging ongoing training, building capacity, and improving infrastructure. Guatemala has chosen technical centralization of the forensic system, which has made it easier to consistently put quality policies into action. Furthermore, direct engagement with the judicial system has facilitated the alignment of forensic methodologies with the evidentiary requirements of criminal proceedings.

However, challenges persist. International technical cooperation is a big part of INACIF's financial stability. If this issue can't be fixed through the public budget, it could affect the future of its improvement projects. Also, the best practices will only work if the judicial system can correctly understand and use forensic evidence in court.

10.3.5 Peru: Structural Fragmentation and Quality Stagnation

The long-running case in Peru shows how the formal existence of forensic institutions can cause problems when there aren't any long-term public policies in place to make sure they are doing their jobs well. The Institute of Legal Medicine and Forensic Sciences (IMLCF) is connected to the Public Prosecutor's Office, but it has not been able to become a governing body or a model for how the forensic system works at the national level. Its way of doing things has been around for a long time in Latin America, but it wasn't officially recognized as an institute until the early 1980s. Even though the country has internal rules, a national hierarchy, and a system of regions that seems to be well-organized, like Colombia's, and even though there are some efforts to improve things, the country still doesn't have any processes that meet ISO standards or a national medium- or long-term forensic quality management strategy, like Chile, Colombia, Panama, and Guatemala do. There is also a worrying trend: the rise of several ad hoc forensic units within supranational prosecutor's offices. These units work alongside the IMLCF and are a type of atomized forensic system that is only used for certain types of investigations. This situation has led to a formal system of broken forensic practices, with no technical oversight or institutional integration, even though they all belong to the Public Prosecutor's Office. There has been no scientific policy vision or performance evaluation mechanisms to go along with the choices that led to this model. Actually, they have only made the IMLCF weaker.

The conversation about quality has been added to strategic documents and guidelines that are well-meaning but lack proper follow-up, which has not led to long-term action, separate budgets, or major changes in institutions. Technological progress has been overlooked, including the potential to enhance its infrastructure. In this regard, the Peruvian case exemplifies a scenario of structural stagnation, wherein accreditation has not been emphasized as a technical imperative or as an institutional obligation. This reality underscores the significance of political will, the absence of vision, and, most importantly, the enhancement of a culture of quality grounded in analytical reflection as a crucial component for advancing towards resilient and dependable forensic systems.

10.4 Myths and Realities of Quality Discourse: Between the Normative Symbol and Effective Transformation

In the last few decades, the idea of quality has become the most important part of the global reform and professionalization of forensic services. People have said that following international standards like ISO/IEC 17025 is the same as being reliable, legitimate, and scientifically rigorous. In many situations, especially in Latin America, this conversation has become more symbolic than practical. It has become a way to make things seem more legitimate without actually changing how forensic work is done.

This phenomenon, characterized as normative fetishism or the illusion of quality, prompts inquiries regarding the actual function of standards in enhancing forensic systems and the potential peril that documentary compliance may supplant scientific integrity and operational efficacy. This part looks at the main myths that come up when people talk about quality in forensic science, what they mean in practice, and what needs to be done to keep standards from becoming meaningless and not related to the real problems that forensic institutions in the area face.

10.4.1 Myth 1: Accreditation as an Automatic Guarantee of Quality

A common myth is that if a lab is accredited by ISO standards, it means that there is a reliable, open, and ethical forensic system in place. This premise, while intuitively appealing, lacks empirical support. Accreditation verifies adherence to a set of documented and validated procedures; however, it does not directly evaluate factors such as scientific autonomy, the validity of expert interpretation, or the contextual significance of the reports generated.

In some Latin American countries, the quest for accreditation has been driven more by political or strategic imperatives – such as enhancing the institutional reputation, fulfilling international cooperation mandates, or integrating into technical networks – or by the observation of external circumstances, under the assumption that these efforts yield quality, rather than by a sincere commitment to improving practice. In these instances, accreditation processes may evolve into objectives in their own right, emphasizing the development of manuals, policies, and records, while neglecting a critical evaluation of the suitability of these procedures for the local operational context. So, there is a chance of building a "facade of quality" that hides deeper problems with the structure, such as not having enough resources, having too many institutions, not having enough training, and not having a scientific culture.

10.4.2 Myth 2: The Standard Is Universally Applicable Without Adaptation

Another common myth is that international standards can be used in any setting without needing to be changed or put into context. This reasoning, partially derived from industrial paradigms, overlooks the distinctive characteristics of forensic science, whose methodologies are not solely technical but also interpretative, contingent, and intricately connected to specific judicial, cultural, and institutional frameworks.

Many forensic laboratories and services in Latin America work in bad conditions. For example, they don't have enough specialized technical staff, the authorities change too often, they are under pressure to get results right away, they don't invest enough in applied research, and there isn't enough coordination between the people who work in the justice system. In these circumstances, the strict adherence to normative standards may be counterproductive, leading to operational tensions, staff frustration, and a disconnect between established procedures and the actual requirements of the criminal justice system. Neuteboom et al. (2023) propose that standards be assessed according to their suitability for purpose, specifically their capacity to adapt to the intended objective. If a standard does not encompass the entire forensic process, including the on-scene investigation, the interpretation of results, and the generation of contextualized expert knowledge, its practical utility is constrained. The challenge is not to dismiss standards, but to comprehend them as instruments that require appropriation, adaptation, and critical integration.

10.4.3 Myth 3: More Documentation Equals More Control

In a lot of situations, the talk about quality has made a direct link between the amount of documents and the level of control. This reasoning suggests that an increase in written procedures, records, forms, and audits enhances traceability, thereby improving the system's quality. This perspective neglects the examination of the actual utilization of this documentation, its comprehension by technical personnel, and its significance to the fundamental aims of forensic science.

Many laboratories in Latin America, like those in Peru and Guatemala, have said that the process of getting accredited has caused "document overload." In some cases, policies and procedures are made because the standard says they have to be, but they don't have anything to do with how the technical team works every day. This makes people unhappy, unmotivated, and uninterested in the purpose of forensic work. Instead of encouraging a culture of quality, a culture of formalistic compliance is created, where passing audits is more important than improving scientific skills.

Quality management experts say that a good documentation system isn't one that has the most paperwork (real or virtual). Instead, it's one that turns quality principles into useful tools for everyday work. To keep documentation from becoming an end in itself, it is important to simplify it intelligently, review it regularly, involve people in the design of procedures, and keep training people.

10.4.4 Myth 4: Technical Quality Guarantees Scientific Integrity

A fourth myth is the idea that technical controls like methodological validations, proficiency testing, and equipment traceability always make forensic results scientifically sound. These components are essential, yet insufficient to ensure that expert conclusions are founded on rigorous, critical, and contextualized scientific reasoning.

In forensic fields where interpretation is paramount, including forensic anthropology, fact reconstruction, pattern analysis, and probabilistic inference, quality hinges on both the technical integrity of hypothesis formulation and the practitioner's cognitive proficiency, logical reasoning, and capacity to convey uncertainty. Neuteboom et al. (2023) caution that these dimensions are frequently overlooked in contemporary accreditation frameworks, resulting in essential components of forensic practice being excluded from the quality system.

Moreover, scientific integrity entails the autonomy of experts to express independent opinions, even when such opinions are at odds with institutional or political expectations. A quality system that doesn't take into account the moral and epistemological aspects of forensic work could end up validating results that are technically correct but not scientifically sound or fair.

10.4.5 Conditions for Overcoming Quality Fetishism

To get rid of normative fetishism in forensic science, we need to move away from just following the rules and toward creating an institutional culture that values quality. This change means realizing that standards are useful tools, but their usefulness depends on how they are understood, used, and applied in each situation.

The first condition is the contextual appropriation of standards. This does not mean making technical principles less important; it means adjusting how they are used to fit each country's legal, institutional, and operational needs. It entails creating pragmatic, forward-thinking, and inclusive roadmaps that enhance technical autonomy without enforcing frameworks that are incongruous with local contexts.

Second, it's very important to support quality systems that put people first. It is the teams that put the manuals into action that make quality happen.

Including technical staff in the creation of procedures, knowledge management, and processes for ongoing improvement builds trust, motivation, and a sense of shared responsibility.

A third requirement is the evaluation of cognitive and interpretive skills, which are lacking in many accreditation programs. Forensic quality encompasses not only precise measurement but also the capacity to reason, articulate uncertainty, and provide well-founded opinions. Adding these dimensions makes the forensic process more scientifically sound.

Finally, we need a systemic approach that considers the crime scene, the laboratory, and interpretation as a technical-scientific continuum. Colombia is a clear example of this, but essentially due to its disconnect between the various forensic components that drive the evidentiary system. There is an ISO-certified Institute of Legal Medicine and Forensic Sciences, recognized worldwide as an example of good quality practices, but its procedures are limited and even disconnected from the external reality of its own traceable organization, from those other Colombian state systems responsible for evidence collection at crime scenes. This approach highlights anomalies, and its communicable improvement would ensure that quality is not just a set of separate elements but a clear institutional policy based on impartiality, scientific accuracy, and real-world utility. This is the only way to prevent standardization from becoming an empty symbol and, instead, to give it real value.

10.4.6 Toward a Meaningful Culture of Quality

The challenge is not to dismiss standardization but to reframe it. It is essential to perceive quality not as a fixed, certified, and attained objective but as a dynamic, interactive, and contextual process. A meaningful culture of quality is built on principles, not just rules, and on what people can do, not just what they can control from the outside.

This means bringing together institutions that value scientific integrity more than just following the rules, that encourage critical thinking, that respect technical independence, and that understand that there are many different ways to do forensic science. It also means rethinking how professionals are trained, making interpretive skills, probabilistic thinking, and ethical sensitivity necessary parts of being good at forensics.

Latin America is in a good position to take the lead in this change. The area has seen violence, impunity, and weak institutions that have put traditional management models to the test. These challenges ought not to be perceived as impediments, but rather as catalysts for contextual innovation. From this point of view, forensic quality should be measured not only by how well it follows the rules, but also by how much it helps people get to the truth, get justice, and keep their dignity.

10.5 Elements for Contextual and Comprehensive Quality: From the Sydney Declaration to Its Applicability in Latin America

Quality in forensic science should not be limited to compliance with international standards; it should encompass the ability of forensic systems to respond contextually, scientifically, and ethically to the social and judicial demands they encounter. The SD on forensic science has provided a conceptual framework that enables a reevaluation of quality from its epistemological foundations, particularly at a time when conventional quality assurance methods, which concentrate solely on laboratory accreditation, exhibit considerable shortcomings. Recent proposals for the African context (Olckers and Ben Khelil, 2024; Smith and Horne, 2024) suggest that the critical adoption of SD constitutes a strategic opportunity for Latin America, serving not only as a technical framework but also as a philosophical foundation for the comprehensive transformation of forensic systems in challenging environments.

10.5.1 Shifting the Focus: From Tools to Fundamentals

One of the most important things the SD does is ask us to rethink what makes forensic science good, moving the focus from tools to the basics. This conceptual reformulation facilitates a departure from the dominant paradigm that equates quality solely with the presence of modern equipment, accredited laboratories, or standardized procedural manuals. The SD, on the other hand, says that quality should be based on the scientific method's guiding principles: logical coherence, reasoned traceability, empirical validation, and an awareness of the context in which one works.

In the African context, authors like Olckers and Ben Khelil (2024) contend that this methodology enables nations lacking advanced industrial frameworks to establish dependable, legitimate, and effective forensic systems. This change in focus lets forensic science be based on how clear the process is, how clear the inference is, and how committed to the truth it is, instead of copying external models that don't work. This proposal does not downplay the need for standards; instead, it puts it in a bigger epistemological hierarchy where the instrument itself is not the most important thing, but how and why it is used.

This reasoning is particularly pertinent in Latin America, where forensic institutions frequently navigate a precarious balance between selective technological advancement and enduring structural deficiencies. It is common to find well-equipped laboratories that don't have technical governance, or highly trained professionals who have to work under institutional pressures that limit their ability to interpret data freely. In this situation, a system that puts tools first can make it seem like the quality is good, but it doesn't deal with the most important parts of the forensic process, which are scientific judgment, critical inference, and methodological honesty.

Putting the Latin American forensic debate back on its foundations opens up new possibilities. It entails the education of professionals who comprehend the limitations and applications of their instruments, who engage in evidence-based reasoning, and who perceive forensic practice as a scientific endeavor rather than a mere administrative duty. This change in how we think about things is necessary if we want to create a forensic science that is useful, long-lasting, and legitimate, even in difficult institutional settings.

10.5.2 Overcoming the Illusion of Accreditation as the Ultimate Goal

One of the most persistent challenges in the debate on forensic quality in Latin America is the growing belief, especially among legal authorities (judges and prosecutors) and administrators of forensic systems, that ISO standards, especially ISO/IEC 17025, are the best and most reliable way to ensure quality. This perspective, though comprehensible from a normative and administrative governance standpoint, is inadequate and may misrepresent reality when quality is regarded as a scientific, ethical, and contextualized practice. Accreditation is a useful way to improve traceability, standardize procedures, and make comparisons between countries. Nevertheless, it is neither an end in itself nor should it be, as extensively evidenced in the scholarly literature (Weyerman and Roux, 2021; Roux et al., 2021, 2022; Neuteboom et al., 2023; Ross and Neuteboom, 2020a,b; Neuteboom and Ross, 2024; Smith and Horne, 2024; Willis, 2010, 2022 among numerous others).

Smith and Horne (2024) conducted analyses based on African experiences, revealing that even accredited laboratories have committed significant errors or generated subpar reports when their personnel operated under institutional pressure, lacked adequate training, or were devoid of ethical oversight. So, true quality isn't just about following the rules; it also needs a mix of critical thinking, scientific culture, interpretive skills, and technical independence. In short, it means making the forensic system stronger by creating a culture of quality at all levels—technical, administrative, reflective, and interpretive. It also means making sure that reports are clear, logical, and, above all, written in plain language that doesn't use technical jargon. In many Latin American countries, the quest for accreditation has been driven more by the need to improve the image of institutions, work together with other countries, or meet financial needs than by a deep understanding of its goals and limits. This has made people more anxious about getting accredited to improve processes.

This phenomenon can result in normative forensic fetishism: an excessive valuation of the standard as a symbol of modernization, which undermines the substantive assessment of the knowledge generated. Forensic laboratories or units in this situation put writing manuals, making sure that documents are in order, and getting ready for outside audits ahead of more important things like thinking about their methods, adapting to the situation, and peer review.

To get past this false idea, we need to change how we think about accreditation: it is a useful tool, but not one that can stand on its own. The effectiveness of this will depend on the institutional environment it is in, the governance that supports it, and how advanced the technical team is in their field. In Latin America, this redefinition is necessary to avert the degradation of quality into a mere administrative task and to foster a forensic science focused on truth, relevance, and social responsibility.

10.5.3 Building Systems Centered on Human Potential and Knowledge

A contextual and comprehensive approach to quality must focus on the individuals who utilize scientific knowledge. The SD stresses how important it is to use logical reasoning, do research in context, and be aware of your own limits as an expert. Training professionals in Africa to think critically, weigh options, and understand the uncertainty continuum through logical reflection (SD Principles 3 and 5) is more important than giving laboratories the newest technology. Technology is a useful addition that makes the expert's logic and the way they think and see things more rigorous, but it never takes the place of those things. Chapter 2 looks at how artificial intelligence works and what it needs to work well. Its main job is to help with reasoning and bringing ideas together. Latin America needs a major overhaul of its forensic programs' curricula, adding epistemology, inferential logic, scientific communication, and forensic ethics. This training must be continuous, accessible, and regionally coordinated, fostering a critical mass of experts equipped to endorse scientifically valid and socially responsible practices.

The SD's recognition that forensic systems are not sustained solely by regulatory frameworks or advanced technologies, but by the expert knowledge of the people who comprise them, is one of its most innovative aspects. This idea is supported by the work of Smith and Horne (2024) and Olckers and Ben Khelil (2024). In this framework, quality transcends mere written procedures or calibrated instruments; it fundamentally resides in the cognitive, interpretive, and ethical competencies of technical and scientific personnel. This statement, while appearing straightforward, carries significant structural ramifications, particularly in regions like Latin America, where the education, professional acknowledgment, and institutional advancement of forensic personnel remain markedly inequitable. This is why ongoing certification and strict training programs need to be much more useful. In Africa and Latin America, the absence of consistent investment in human capacity has resulted in an excessive dependence on external models, an uncritical adoption of standards, and a forensic practice that frequently emphasizes formal compliance over analytical reasoning. In this way, the documents that were looked at call for a radical change in how things are done: moving from systems that are based on norms to systems that are based on knowledge and people. This means, among other things, valuing local knowledge, setting up institutional rewards for ongoing training, and making sure that there are stable career paths that keep scientific talent.

In Latin America, forensic experts frequently encounter unstable working conditions, restricted technical autonomy, and institutional fragmentation that hinders the formation of robust epistemic communities. To build people-centered systems in this situation, we need more than just technical training. We need to create a scientific culture that encourages curiosity, critical thinking, and a dedication to the truth. It also means making sure that employees have good working conditions, places to talk about technical issues, and institutional structures that value professional independence as a key part of quality.

Lastly, forensic science that is based on people and knowledge is not only better, but it also lasts longer. African experiences show that professionals who are trained in scientific reasoning and making decisions when things are uncertain can keep quality standards even in weak institutions, as long as they have support from the institution, technical freedom, and social recognition.

10.5.4 Ensure Systemic Approach and Operational Coherence

It is not possible to understand or guarantee forensic quality in a piecemeal way. The Sydney Declaration, along with contributions from Smith and Horne (2024) and Olckers and Ben Khelil (2024), emphasizes the necessity of a systemic approach, wherein forensic science is perceived as a continuous and interdependent process extending from the crime scene to the presentation of the expert report in court. This approach is particularly pertinent to Latin America, where quality is frequently regarded as a characteristic solely of the laboratory, overlooking the upstream and downstream connections that significantly impact the validity of scientific outcomes.

Forensic practice in many countries in the region has big problems: crime scenes that aren't well-preserved, evidence that isn't collected properly, no standard protocols, state forensic agencies that aren't working together, and no chains of custody that work across borders. Technology or partial accreditation won't fix these problems. Instead, we need to use a logic of operational coherence, where each step is linked by common principles of accountability, traceability, and validation.

The African experience shows that even in places where resources are scarce, a systemic approach can improve quality by putting clear workflows, clear lines of responsibility, and technical trust-based collaboration between institutions at the top of the list. Latin America can benefit from this integrative model by moving toward the consolidation of forensic networks that articulate police, prosecutors, laboratories, forensic scientists, criminalists, and judges under common protocols, but with room for contextual adaptation.

To ensure operational coherence, we also need to make information systems that can work together, make it easier to track documents outside of the lab, and make sure that the different people in the system can give each other useful feedback. Additionally, it necessitates an institutional dedication to collaborative training and the formulation of quality indicators that evaluate not only technical precision but also the judicial applicability and societal significance of forensic science.

If there isn't a systemic approach, forensic quality could become disorganized and weak, which is already happening in some parts of Latin America. A disjointed scientific practice is unlikely to endure in contentious litigation contexts, where technical precision, argumentative validity, and institutional legitimacy are essential.

10.5.5 Promote a Scientific Culture Instead of an Administrative Culture

One of the most persistent problems in Latin American forensic systems is the establishment of an administrative culture that undermines a genuinely scientific culture. In numerous institutional contexts, quality management has been bureaucratized to such an extent that documentation, form signatures, and audit preparation have become ends in themselves, supplanting critical thinking, methodological reflection, and technical innovation. The SD, along with the thoughts of Olckers and Ben Khelil (2024) and Smith and Horne (2024), suggests that this trend should be reversed: forensic practice should return to its scientific roots and become an investigative, interpretive field dedicated to finding the truth.

In places like Latin America where there aren't enough people to do the work and the courts are busy, it's understandable that productivity indicators, response times, and report standardization are more important. But when these things take the place of critical analysis, empirical validation, or a balanced reading of the results, the scientific integrity of the expert process is at risk. As demonstrated, an overly bureaucratic culture can yield "good" indicators while compromising sound scientific decision-making (Neuteboom and Ross, 2024).

Encouraging a scientific culture means encouraging values like reasonable doubt, being open to peer review, talking about methods, and knowing the limits of what we know. It also means knowing that not all evidence can be measured or automated and that forensic interpretation needs a full understanding of the case that goes beyond what can be measured. This necessitates institutional settings that safeguard technical autonomy, permit time for contemplation, and promote the collaborative development of scientific criteria tailored to the context.

It is not easy or quick to change from an administrative culture to a scientific culture. To change what quality means, we need technical leadership, political will, and institutional will. This is the only way to create a Latin American forensic science that can stand on its own, not because it has a lot of reports but because the knowledge it produces is solid, relevant, and legitimate.

10.5.6 Toward a Contextualized Normative Architecture

One of the biggest problems that forensic systems in Latin America face is that there aren't clear, well-thought-out rules that fit the needs of the region. In numerous nations, forensic regulations are disjointed, incomplete, or adopted from foreign jurisdictions without appropriate modification processes. In light of this situation, the SD and comparative analyses in Africa (Olckers and Ben Khelil, 2024; Smith and Horne, 2024) advocate for the development of a contextualized regulatory architecture, which entails a regulatory framework that acknowledges the universal principles of forensic science while adapting them to operate within complex, unequal, and legally diverse contexts. The Ibero-American Network of Legal Medicine and Forensic Science Institutions (https://redforenseiberoamericana.org/) can be very helpful in this effort. Instead of copying regulatory models from countries with stable infrastructure, unified governance, and significant investment in science, Latin America requires regulations that address its unique challenges: institutional fragmentation, the politicization of evidence, the coexistence of forensic actors with varying oversight frameworks, and, in certain instances, overlapping functions among prosecutors' offices, police, and medical services. This situation calls for a flexible but strict architecture that balances scientific standards with human rights principles, technical independence, and long-term viability.

The successful establishment of national forensic authorities in certain African nations, including Zambia, which possess regulatory, supervisory, and inter-institutional coordination functions, serves as a significant precedent (Smith and Horne, 2024). A similar idea could work in Latin America if national forensic councils were set up. These councils would be hybrid regulatory bodies with input from technical, judicial, and academic experts. Their job would be to set minimum standards, make sure they are followed, and make sure that all parties are on the same page. Also, a contextual regulatory framework needs to include scalable regulatory tools, such as step-by-step technical manuals, flexible implementation paths, and functional minimum standards that don't leave out institutions because they don't have enough money. In other words, standards that make things more technically advanced without making it impossible for new systems to meet them. This proposal would let local laboratories, universities, and community forensic networks all work together under one quality framework, which would promote fairness, cooperation, and progress.

To put it simply, a contextualized regulatory framework does not mean less strictness; it means more relevant regulation. It is about making rules that fit with what people can do in their area, will last over time, and will help forensic science become more independent, trustworthy, and dedicated to justice and human rights.

10.5.7 Applicability and Projection of the Sydney Declaration in Latin America

The SD is a once-in-a-lifetime chance to change the way forensic systems work in Latin America from a strategic, scientific, and moral point of view. In the region, it should not be limited to a symbolic or merely declarative adoption; instead, it should serve as an operational framework that transcends the constraints of traditional approaches centered solely on accreditation, formal compliance, and the technification of processes. The SD provides a strong basis for rethinking forensic quality in Latin America, just as it has begun to do in Africa, where its principles have started to shape the design of new, more suitable, and long-lasting forensic structures.

One of the most important things about SD for Latin America is that it focuses on how different forensic contexts are. The statement makes it clear that quality can't be defined by unique models or standardized recipes, and that it has to be sensitive to the institutional, economic, and cultural realities of each environment. This methodological flexibility is essential for a region characterized by the coexistence of technologically advanced forensic systems, as seen in Brazil, Colombia, or Chile, alongside others severely constrained by institutional fragmentation, a lack of technical autonomy, or the absence of clear normative frameworks, such as in Peru, Ecuador, Bolivia, Paraguay, and Honduras. In this regard, the SD facilitates the development of distinct yet complementary pathways for forensic enhancement, honoring national specificities while upholding universal scientific principles.

The SD also has a forward-looking view of regional cooperation, which it sees as more than just sharing technical knowledge; it sees it as a way to build forensic knowledge together. Olckers and Ben Khelil (2024) say that regional alliances can be very important for putting the SD principles into practice in Africa. They can help create learning networks, validate each other's practices, and come up with adaptive standards. In Latin America, this means that spaces like Mercosur, the Andean Community, CELAC, or the Ibero-American Network of Institutions of Legal Medicine and Forensic Sciences can work together to push for common forensic goals in the region, strengthen regional protocol banks, encourage joint training, and make it easier for countries with different levels of institutional development to get technical help.

To use the SD effectively in Latin America, it is important to create political will and institutional commitment. The ISO frames are often adopted because of outside pressures, like international cooperation, conditional financing, or pressure from the courts. The SD, on the other hand, requires a commitment to scientific integrity and social responsibility from within the organization. For this, decision-makers must understand that the quality of forensic work cannot rely solely on technical initiatives or short-term projects; it necessitates a structural investment in scientific governance, institutional infrastructure, and technical autonomy. The judicial and public ministries, as well as the legislative bodies and control agencies, must all agree on this.

The SD's proposal to make scientific training and continuing education two of the main parts of forensic quality is another important part of it. Peru is a clear example of this; its forensic scientists do not routinely publish their work in any journal with these international characteristics. This is due to several clear reasons that would hinder scientific research, such as a lack of research culture, administrative blockages or rigorous investigation procedures, research budgets, the excessive number of cases that must be managed in a short period of time, leaving little time for investigation, among many others. In Latin America, where there are big gaps in training and forensic models based on random empirical experience are still very important, SD suggests a cultural shift: training experts not just as people who follow procedures, but as scientists who can think critically, make arguments, recognize uncertainties, and adapt to new situations. The influence of SD in this domain can be manifested in the establishment of minimum regional curricula, the enhancement of forensic academic networks, and the creation of centers of excellence that facilitate the ongoing professionalization of the field.

Also, SD is a way for forensic science to be accepted as legitimate in Latin America. In a continent where people don't trust the courts very much and where mistakes made by forensic scientists can have serious effects on the protection of rights, using strict, ethical, and scientific quality standards can help restore trust. This process needs ways to hold people accountable, make forensic results clear, let the public see technical information, and connect forensic science with public opinion, especially when it comes to violence, disappearances, or human rights violations. Colombia is a very important example to follow. The INMLCF has a big social media presence, an informative website, and a document called Forensis that comes out every year and helps people make decisions about public policy. It is very important for countries in the region to follow and use these best practice methods.

The SD is a proposal for a slow, structural, and deeply moral change in forensic science, which Colombia has been working toward for a long time without saying so. In Latin America, its usefulness and effect will depend on how its ideas are used in public policy, professional training, regional cooperation, and institutional governance. The SD can be the foundation of a new Latin American forensic model that is critical, contextual, scientific, and very human if people really believe in it.

10.5.8 Final Reflection: A New Look at Latin American Forensic Quality

Forensic science in Latin America cannot remain confined to the complacency of standardized procedures or the fixation on adhering to seals and audits that, while essential, have frequently been regarded as unequivocal truths. Forensic quality cannot be reduced to a technical exercise or a management objective in a region where structural violence, forced disappearances, extrajudicial executions, organized crime, and institutional mistrust persist like open wounds. It must be unequivocally positioned at the forefront of the struggle against impunity.

According to Willis (2022) forensic science, despite its crucial role in justice systems, has not yet reached full professional maturity. The field still lacks a unified knowledge base, consistent entry requirements, and effective self-regulation. Historically, areas such as fingerprint analysis, ballistics, DNA, toxicology, and digital forensics have evolved independently, creating separate cultures with limited knowledge sharing. This fragmentation weakens training and research, especially in the Global South, where forensic work is indispensable for addressing violence, institutional fragility, and resource scarcity. Large-scale, efficiency-focused organizational models can manage routine tasks, but they restrict the expert judgment needed for complex case assessments, particularly in challenging environments where evidence is degraded, resources are scarce, and pressure is considerable. Weak barriers to entry and the absence of a coherent ethical framework further undermine consistency and public trust. We agree with Willis (2022) that the Sydney Declaration provides a fundamental basis for unifying principles, strengthening training and supporting meaningful self-regulation, especially in contexts with demanding forensic realities.

The SD asks us to rethink how we think about quality. Not as a goal that can only be reached through certified laboratories or manuals that are in line with international standards, but as a practice that is epistemologically sound, ethically guided, and socially relevant. This statement doesn't say that the tools aren't useful; it just reminds us that their value comes from how, why, and for whom they are used. In this situation, it is important to get rid of the "normative fetishes" that have taken over how we think about quality. The institutional anxiety to achieve accreditation, while comprehensible, has produced a perilous distortion: conflating form with substance, procedure with knowledge, and seal with truth. This illusion has led to a forensic culture that cares more about not failing an audit than about correctly interpreting important evidence for a victim, their family, or the community.

But there is a chance. Latin America can and must develop a distinct form of forensic science: one that is not constrained by formalism, but rather serves as a partner to justice and humanitarian efforts; not limited to laboratory settings, but dedicated to a global and holistic understanding of what it means to practice forensic science in the pursuit of a society that demands accountability and truth in the battle against impunity. A discipline that recognizes that quality is assessed not solely by technical accuracy, but also by the capacity to convert scientific truth into social truth, particularly in instances where silence has facilitated violence. The SD can be the starting point for this change. Its strength comes not only from its principles but also from the fact that it can remind us that forensic science can be a powerful tool against impunity when used with honesty and integrity. And that real quality is what lets the truth come out, even in the worst situations.

References

Ballantyne, K.N. and Wilson Wilde, L. (2020) Assessing the reliability and validity of forensic science – An industry perspective. *Australian Journal of Forensic Sciences*, **52**(3), 275–281. https://doi.org/10.1080/00450618.2019.1704058.

Neuteboom, W. and Ross, A. (2024) Shall the twain ever meet? *Australian Journal of Forensic Sciences*. https://doi.org/10.1080/00450618.2024.2363823.

Neuteboom, W., Ross, A., Bugeja, L., Willis, S., Roux, C., and Lothridge, K. (2023) Quality management in forensic science: A closer inspection. *Forensic Science International*, 111779. https://doi.org/10.1016/j.forsciint.2023.111779.

Olckers, A. and Ben Khelil, M. (2024) *The Sydney Declaration – An unique opportunity for Africa*. *Forensic Science International*, **357**, 111969. https://doi.org/10.1016/j.forsciint.2024.111969.

Ross, A. and Neuteboom, W. (2020a) ISO-accreditation – Is that all there is for forensic science? *Australian Journal of Forensic Sciences*. https://doi.org/10.1080/00450618.2020.1819414.

Ross, A. and Neuteboom, W. (2020b) Implementation of quality management from a historical perspective: The forensic science odyssey. *Australian Journal of Forensic Sciences*. https://doi.org/10.1080/00450618.2019.1704058.

Roux, C., Bucht, R., Crispino, F., de Forest, P., Lennard, C., Margot, P., *et al.* (2022) The Sydney Declaration – Revisiting the essence of forensic science through its fundamental principles. *Forensic Science International*, **332**, 111182. https://doi.org/10.1016/j.forsciint.2022.111182.

Roux, C., Willis, S., and Weyermann, C. (2021) Shifting forensic science focus from means to purpose: A path forward for the discipline? *Science & Justice*, **61**, 678–686. https://doi.org/10.1016/j.scijus.2021.08.005.

Smith, J.H. and Horne, J.S. (2024) Quality management system in forensic science: An African perspective. *Forensic Science International: Synergy*, **8**, 100476. https://doi.org/10.1016/j.fsisyn.2024.100476.

Weyermann, C. and Roux, C. (2021) A different perspective on the forensic science crisis. *Forensic Science International*, **323**, 110779. doi: 10.1016/j.forsciint.2021.110779.

Willis, S. (2010) Power, process, people: A critical look at ISO accreditation and what it means for the forensic science community. *National Institute of Forensic Science*.

Willis, S. (2022) The professionalisation of forensic science. *WIREs Forensic Science*, **5**(1), e1478. *Advance online publication*. https://doi.org/10.1002/wfs2.1478.

Wilson-Wilde, L. (2018) The international development of forensic science standards – A review. *Forensic Science International*, **288**(1), 9. https://doi.org/10.1016/j.forsciint.2018.04.009.

CHAPTER 11

The Sydney Declaration as an Operational Approach to Challenging Forensic Environments

Roberto C. Parra[1,*] and Claude Roux[2]

[1] *The Specialized Forensic Team of the United Nations Joint Human Rights Office (UNJHRO) in the Democratic Republic of the Congo*

[2] *Centre for Forensic Science, University of Technology Sydney, Sydney, Australia*

11.1 Introduction

Forensic science faces significant challenges globally, yet its role in advancing justice and societal resilience remains crucial, particularly in the Global South amid complex social, legal, and humanitarian conditions. There is growing global pressure for international standards that aim to improve traceability, transparency, and confidence in results (the era of standardization). Simultaneously, forensic science must maintain its purpose, especially in places where resources are scarce, and institutions are weak. This broader aim requires the field to rely on its foundations. This book delves into this complex terrain, exploring how quality management can be understood not only as a system of standards and audits but as a broader framework. The so-called challenging environments, which define the core of this book, require perspectives that differ substantially from those developed in stable contexts. First and foremost, they demand a genuine understanding of the social, institutional, and humanitarian complexity that characterizes these settings. These are not merely scenarios marked by limited resources or weak structures, but spaces with substantial needs, where forensic science is increasingly required as a tool to support justice processes and the safeguarding of rights.

In such contexts, forensic practice can only be effective if it is built upon the most fundamental principles of the discipline, as emphasized in the Sydney

*The views expressed herein are those authors and do not necessarily reflect the views of the United Nations.

Forensic Science and Quality Management: Addressing the Era of Standardization in Challenging Environments, First Edition. Edited by Roberto C. Parra and Allan G. Alvarez-Godoy.

Declaration: grounding work in scientific foundations, rigorous interpretation of traces, solid inferential reasoning, and a reflective understanding of the purpose of forensic science (Roux et al., 2022; Willis 2022). This means recognizing that standardization alone cannot address the magnitude of the challenges; rather, it is essential to integrate epistemological principles, methodological rigor, and contextual sensitivity so that forensic science can fulfill its role in challenging environments (see also Chapter 1).

11.2 Reflections Throughout the Volume

The 10 chapters in this volume explore scenarios that attempt to answer a key question: how can we ensure high quality in forensic science in difficult situations involving structural problems, limited resources, and institutional pressures? The answer outlined here recognizes that quality cannot be limited to technical parameters or administrative certifications alone; rather, it must be perceived as a scientific, rigorous, and socially determined effort to promote justice and combat impunity. The contextual view of the episodes of social reality in which forensic science operates must be fully visible, beyond sole technical arguments.

The opening chapter establishes the theoretical foundation that will guide the entire volume. It shows how the idea of quality emerged in medieval guilds, was consolidated in the industrial logic of standardization, and then transferred to forensic science. However, it is observed that industrial logic, based on repetition and uniformity, is inadequate in a field that addresses distinct and unrepeatable traces and has an important interpretive dimension. In this context, two complementary dimensions can be identified. The first, inspired by the Sydney Declaration, reaffirms the epistemological core of the field: central role of the trace, unambiguous interpretation, open communication, and the duty to acknowledge uncertainty. The second, represented by international standards such as ISO/IEC 17025 and ISO 21043, seeks to ensure traceability, comparability, and global recognition. The chapter concludes that both dimensions are mutually essential: the first ensures validity even in contexts of extreme precariousness and the second reinforces legitimacy when institutional conditions allow.

The Book examines the current challenges of forensic practice in difficult environments within this framework. The analysis of artificial intelligence in Chapter 2 is an excellent example. It recognizes that it can handle a large amount of information and make processes more efficient, but it also recognizes that there are risks such as inaccurate algorithms, repetitive biases, and the possibility of replacing expert judgment. The conclusion is clear: AI can only be an ally if it is framed within the principles of the Sydney Declaration. Technology can never replace the ethical responsibility of forensic practitioners or their critical capacity, especially in situations where institutions are weak.

Chapter 3 uses the Minnesota Protocol as an example to demonstrate the importance of adaptable universal frameworks. This tool not only establishes technical standards for investigating deaths that may have been unlawful but also offers advice on how to protect human rights in times of crisis. Its flexible application illustrates that forensic quality takes on full meaning when it becomes a resource for combating impunity, even where institutions are weak or resources are scarce.

In Chapter 4, the problem of deaths in custody in Burkina Faso starkly reveals the structural limitations of prison systems and the difficulties of working in environments marked by precariousness and a lack of safeguards. An inescapable principle is reaffirmed: in any complex environment, every death in custody must be considered suspicious and addressed as part of the fight against impunity.

Chapter 5 shifts the focus to humanitarian action. The International Committee of the Red Cross demonstrates that quality management is not limited to accredited laboratories; it can also work in places where conflict and violence are present. Governance, ongoing training, and international collaboration are identified as fundamental pillars supporting quality in situations where formal accreditation is unattainable, but dedication to justice and human dignity is essential.

Chapter 6 is even more dramatic because it addresses sexual violence in armed conflict. It redefines forensic quality in this context: it is not enough to ensure that reports are technically correct; it is also important to protect victims and prevent them from becoming victims again. In these situations, rigorous documentation becomes a humanitarian act and an important weapon in the fight against impunity. This demonstrates that quality in difficult situations cannot be separated from ethical and social sensitivity.

The implicit second part of this book discusses how forensic science is practiced in Latin America from a quality assurance perspective. Chapter 7 examines Panama as an example of how accreditation processes can help institutions modernize. However, it also demonstrates that accreditation can only have a limited effect without a strong scientific culture and long-term resources. In Chapter 8, Peru faces a different problem: institutional fragmentation and territorial inequalities hinder the full implementation of international standards. In this context, the Sydney Declaration is highlighted as a good way to maintain good practices, especially in rural and marginalized areas. In Chapter 9, Guatemala shows how international cooperation has driven the advancement of laboratory accreditation. However, the greatest challenge remains building a lasting culture of quality that does not depend solely on external aid.

Chapter 10 concludes with a look at Latin America. This chapter warns against the "quality mirage," the false idea that accreditation means high quality. It clarifies the idea that more procedures imply more control or that good technical quality is sufficient to guarantee scientific integrity. The main challenge, it is argued, is creating systems that utilize international standards relevant to the field, enhance people's capabilities, and can survive in the region's difficult conditions.

The 10 chapters teach us a clear lesson: it is not enough to simply consult and operationalize procedural accreditation manuals to determine the usefulness and quality of the contribution of forensic science. It is an active, dynamic, and reflective practice that requires solid scientific and epistemological support, the ability to adapt to adverse situations, and a commitment to combating impunity. The Sydney Declaration offers us a way of thinking that works in any situation, and international standards legitimize it when necessary. Forensic science must adapt to evolving contexts by integrating these approaches.

11.3 Conclusion

This volume affirms that uniformity of processes (standardization) and reflection on fundamental principles (Sydney declaration) should not be considered contradictory forces, but rather synergistic dimensions that improve and strengthen forensic practice even in challenging environments. Internationally standardized frameworks offer consistency, transparency, and institutional credibility; conversely, thoughtful engagement with scientific and argumentative foundations ensures relevance and adaptability to diverse contexts. In this constructive convergence, quality management transcends mere administrative oversight and establishes itself as a dynamic instrument for integrating effective practices with significant social and humanitarian impact.

From this perspective, the book underscores the importance of the Sydney Declaration as a guiding framework and educational awareness-raising tool. It allows for the alignment of international harmonization with academic and professional values by providing an adaptable and foundational strategy. This achieves a balance between global frameworks and local needs. The book proposes a forensic management model that, beyond formal accreditation, serves as a tool for continuous improvement, collaboration, and institutional strengthening in contexts characterized by structural constraints and growing demands.

Ultimately, this volume represents only the opening of a broader and absolutely necessary debate. It invites forensic scientists and other actors committed to combating impunity to look beyond the dominant perspectives shaped in the Global North and to recognize that multiple and diverse realities demand greater attention and differentiated responses. The era of standardization, when applied to challenging environments, cannot rely on uniform solutions; instead, it requires approaches grounded in explicit scientific principles, contextual reasoning, and operational adaptability. Only by acknowledging this diversity of realities and articulating the fundamental purposes of the discipline can meaningful progress be achieved. The conclusions of Chapter 1 reflect this system of dimensions, which may serve as a source of guidance for future approaches.

References

Roux, C., Bucht, R., Crispino, F., de Forest, P., Lennard, C., Margot, P., *et al.* (2022) The Sydney Declaration – Revisiting the essence of forensic science through its fundamental principles. *Forensic Science International,* **332**, Article 111182. https://doi.org/10.1016/j.forsciint.2022.111182.

Willis, S. (2022) The professionalisation of forensic science. *WIREs Forensic Science,* **5**(1), e1478. Advance online publication. https://doi.org/10.1002/wfs2.1478.

Index

Forensic Science and Quality Management: Addressing the Era of Standardization in Challenging Environments, First Edition. Edited by Roberto C. Parra and Allan G. Alvarez-Godoy.

Printed and bound by CPI Group (UK) Ltd, Croydon, CR0 4YY

16/08/2026

14942674-0006